I0470968

MCQs

In

RADIOLOGY

NAGENDRA KUMAR SINHA

MBBS,MD (Radiodiagnosis)

First edition. 2013

ISBN-13:978-1492826538

ISBN-10:1492826537

All rights reserved

No part of this publication may be reproduced or transmitted in any form or any means ,electronic, mechanical ,photocopy ,recording ,translated ,or any information storage and retrieval system, without permission in writing from this author/publisher

TO

MY WIFE ---RINA

AND

MY SON----RAJAT AND ANMOL

FOR THEIR SACRIFICE

PREFACE

MCQs are standard format to assess the conceptual and factual knowledge . This book is an humble effort to provide enough MCQs (more than 20000) for SELF-ASSESSMENT and ,thereby to improve the chance of top ranking in the entrance exams.

Questions in this book cover all aspects of radiology including radiophysics and radioprotection which is heart of radiology . All the formulated questions has been picked up from common standard textbooks (Harrison,Nelson,Swartz,Dutta,Grainger,Sutton,Chapman ,Rumack,Christenson etc).

The questions have been arranged chapter-wise and answers are given at the end of each chapter with explanations. I will advise to read textbooks to augment and stenghthen the asked concepts and facts .However, the answers provided may be used independently as HIGH YIELDING POINTS for rapid review at the time of exam.,thus serving the dual purpose of self assessment and speedy review at time of exams.

Some of the questions has been repeated and asked in different ways to emphasize the importance of the topics.

This book is useful for those appearing for FRCR exams and clinicians to refresh the facts and concepts

Any suggestions to improve the book are welcome .

I wish all the best for all the examinee.

NAGENDRA KUMAR SINHA

ACKNOWLEDGEMENTS

First of all,I thank ALMIGHTY GOD for giving me inspiration to undertake this project and giving me strength to complete it.

I am grateful to all my teachers ,especially Dr N K Gogoi ,Dr R K Gogoi,Dr Khound,Dr P K Deowra,and Dr Bhouiyan who chided me for my ignorance and who prodded me for excellence .

I am extremely happy to aknowledge constant blessing of my parents Sri Dwarika Prasad and Smt Kaushalya Devi.

I am indebted to my bother Er S K P Sinha who taught me "Never to Quit"

It is my priviledge to acknowledge constant support of my wife Rina Sinha without whom the book couldnot have seen the light of the day.

No words can compensate the sacrifice made by my sons Rajat and Anmol, my most precious possession and mission of my life.

I am especially thankful to DR Akshay Dharmah,who instilled idea of writing such book in my mind.

I feel highly indebted to my resident Dr Prashant who shared the load of my work and gave valuable inputs .

I am grateful to my colleagues and seniors for their support,cooperation and suggestions,to name a few :Dr Amarjeet Singh,Dr M L Jaipal,Dr Naveen Niraj, Dr Surendra ,Dr Pawan Pandey,Dr Mukesh Verma,Dr Vidya,Dr Jyotsana,Dr Surendra Singh,Dr Suman Bharati,Dr Dhruv Pathak,Dr Anil

Shahni,Dr D K Jha,Dr Mukesh Prasad,Dr Mukesh Singh,Dr lokesh,Dr ansari,Dr sharaf,Dr yogesh,Dr K K Sinha,Dr Purvey,Dr Permanand, Dr Dr B P Sharma,Dr Sharaf

Last but not the least , I am thankful to all members of Facebook fraternity and different Facebook plateforms (Radiology golden points and MCQs,FRCR group etc) who responded and appreciated to my questions posted during manuscripts preparation.

At last I am grateful to CreateSpace.com who provided me plateform to launch the book .

CONTENTS

RADIOPHYSICS

1.Who discovered x ray

a.Wilhelm Conrad Roentgen

b.Madame Curie

c.Bloch and Felix

d.Coulomb

2.X ray was discovered in

a.8th Nov. 1895

b. a.8th Nov. 1896

c.8th Nov. 1897

d.8th Nov. 1898

3.Wave length of diagnostic x ray is

a.1 to 0.1 A

b. 1 to 10 A

c.10 to 50 A

d.50 to 100 A

4.SI unit of absorbed dose of radiation

a.rad

b.gray

c.curie

d.roentgen

5. SI unit of magnetic flux denslty

a.Tesla

b.weber

c.curie

d.roentgen

6.All are true regarding x ray tube

a.tube filled with helium gas

b.cathode and anode made of tungsten

c.rotating anode used to withstand generated heat

d.pyrex glass used as encasing

7.Elecron cloud produced at cathode filament by thermionic emission is known as

a.thomson effect

b.edison effect

c.jule effect

d.crompton effect

8.Tungsten is used as filament and target material due to all except

a.low atomic no.(34)—so more efficient producer of x rays

b.high melting point(3370) —so withstand high generated heat

c.little tendency to vaporize – so long life expectancy of filament

d.can be drawn into thin wire that is quite strong

9.Limit to anode angle in x ray tube is due to

a.heel effect

b.edison effect

c.jule effect

d.crompton effect

10.Purpose of use of rotating anode is

a.to produce more x ray

b. to withstand high generated heat

c.to produce air for cooling

d.to focus produced x ray

11.Rotating anode is primarily made up of

a.cupper

b.tungsten

c.silver

d.ceramics

12.All are true regarding x ray production except

a.interaction with nucleus of the target produce general radiation

b.interaction with electrons in the the inner shell of the target produce characteristic radiation

c.atomic number of target determine the quality of radiation

d.molybdenum target used in breast radiography

13.general radiations produced by interaction of target nucleus is known as

a.general radiation(bremsstrahlung)

b.characteristic radiation

c.both

d.none

14.Ways of x ray interaction with matter are all except

a.coherent scattering

b.photoelectric effect

c.Compton effect

d.Edison effect

15.Which x ray interaction produce radiographic image of excellent quality

a.pair production

b.photoelectric effect

c.Compton effect

d.photodisintegration

16.Scatter radiation encountered in diagnostic radiology comes from which interaction

a.pair production

b.photoelectric effect

c.Compton effect

d.photodisintegration

17.Purpose of filter is

a.reduce patients radiation dose

b.to enhance x ray production

c.to protect anode from heat

d.to protect x ray tube from voltage fluctuation

18.All material may be used as filter except

a.molebdynum

b.cupper

c.aluminium

d.tungsten

19.Purpose of using beryllium window is

a.reduce patients radiation dose

b.to produce unfiltered x ray beam

c.to protect anode from heat

d.to protect x ray tube from voltage fluctuation

20.Which material is used as filter in breast mammography

a.molebdynum

b.cupper

c.aluminium

d.tungsten

21.Which material is used as filter

a.beryllium

b.zinc

c.aluminum

d.tungsten

22.The reduction in the intensity of an x ray beam as it traverses matter is known as

a.filtration

b.attenuation

c.scattering

d.none

23.Factors affecting attenuation

a.energy of x ray

b.density of matter

c.atomic number and electrons/gram of matter

d.all

24.Half value layer in radiography refers to

a.absorber thickness

b.absorber atomic number

c.absorber density

d.absorber volume

25.All can be used as K-edge filter except

a.aluminum

b.holmium

c.molybdenum

d.gadolinium

26.Barium and iodine is used as contrast agent because of

a.k edge

b.availability

c.cheapness

d.low toxicity

27.All are true regarding filters except

a.sheets of metal

b.placed in path of x ray beam near the x ray tube housing

c.absorb high energy radiation

d.reduce patient'exposure to useless radiation

28.Recommended thickness of aluminum filter for diagnostic radiography

a.2.5mm

b.3.5mm

c.4.5mm

d.5.5mm

29.Devices attached to opening in the x ray tube housing to regulate size and shape of an x ray beam is

a.filter

b.target

c.filament

d.beam restrictors

30.All are beam restrictors except

a.filter

b.aperture diaphragms

c.cones and cylinders

d.collimators

31.Which regulate size and shape of x ray beam

a.collimators

b.filter

c.target

d.grid

32.The radiographic device consisting of a series of lead foil strips seprated by x ray transparent spacers is known as

a.collimators

b filter

c.grid

d.target

33.The most effective of removing scatter radiation from large radiographic field is

a.collimators

b filter

c.target

d.grid

34.Bucky factor is related to

a.collimators

b filter

c.grid

d.target

35.All are located near/in x ray tube except

a.filament

b.target

c.collimatror

d.grid

36.All are true regarding intensifying screen except

a.located in pair x ray cassette

b.calcium tungstate serves as phosphor

c.decrease x ray dose to patients

d.requires higher exposure (more mAs)

37.Light sensitive material in emulsion of x ray film is made up of

a.gelatin

b.silver iodobromide

c.polyester

d.cellulose nitrate

38.Developing solutions used in radiography contain all except

a.developing agents

b.an acid

c. preservative(sodium sulfite)

d.restrainers or antifogants(potassium bromide)

39. Developing agents used in radiography is all except

a.hydroquinone

b.phenindone

c.metol

d.potassium bromide

40. Which is used as fixer in radiography

a.sodium or ammonium thiosulphate

b.hydroquinone

c.phenindone

d.sodium sulfite

41.What controls image contrast

a.exposure (mAs)

b.kVp

c.voltage of current source

d.all

42.What controls film density

a.exposure (mAs)

b.kVp

c.voltage of current source

d.all

43.The speed of film –screen system is defined as the ------ of the exposure in roentgens to produce a density of 1.o above base plus fog density

a.proportional

b reciprocal

c. both depending on multiple factors

d.lograthmic

44.Ortho x ray film is sensitive to

a.green

b.red

c.both

d.none

45.Pan x ray film is sensitive to

a.all light colors

b.only red color

c.only blue colors

d.only violet colors

46.Darkroom safelight for ortho film is

a.amber

b.red

c.green

d.blue

47.The amount of blackening of an x ray film is expressed by the term

a.contrast

b.photographic density

c.speed of film

d.film gamma

48.Which is used as input phosphor in image intensifier in radiology

a.cesium iodide

b.calcium tungstate

c.zinc-cadmium sulfide

d.titanium oxide

49.Which is used as output phosphor in image intensifier in radiology

a.cesium iodide

b.calcium tungstate

c.zinc-cadmium sulfide

d.titanium oxide

50.Term used for difference in density between areas in the radiograph is

a.contrast

b.photographic density

c.speed of film

d.film gamma

51.Effect of fog and scatter on film is

a.to reduce radiographic contrast

b.to reduce radiographic density

c.to increase radiographic clarity

d.all

52.Radiographic contrast depend on

a.subject contrast

b.film contrast

c.scatter radiation plus fog

d.all

53.The production of a visible image utilizing the charged surface of a photocnductor (amorphous selenium) is known as

a.xeroradiography

c.fluoroscopy

c.tomogaraphy

d.stereoscopy

54.Who discovered Computerised axial transverse scanning in 1972

a.G.N.Hounsfield

b.Oldendorf

c.Chester F. Carlson

d.Kuhl and Edwards

55.All are true regarding different generation of CT scan except

a.1ˢᵗ generation (translate – rotate ,one detector)

b.2ⁿᵈ generation(translate – rotate,multiple detector)

c.3ʳᵈ generation(rotate-fixed)

d.4ᵀʰ generation(rotate-fixed)

56.All are true regarding 3ʳᵈ and 4ᵗʰ generation CT scan except

a.both x ray tube and detectors rotate around the patient(rotate-rotate) in 3ʳᵈ generation

b. x ray collimated into a fan beam (use of 'fan beam' geometry) in 3ʳᵈ generation and 4ᵗʰ generation

c.a ring of detectors around the patient which does not move in 4ᵗʰ generation

d.the x ray tube rotates in a circle outside the detectors ring a in 4ᵗʰ generation

57.Back projection,iterative methos ,and analytical methods used in CT are meant for

a.image acquisition

b.image reconstruction

c.image display

d.image retrieval

58.CT number refers to

a.relationship between the linear absorption coefficient of a pixel and fat linear attenuation coefficient

b.relationship between the linear absorption coefficient of a pixel and water linear attenuation coefficient

c.relationship between the linear absorption coefficient of a pixel and protein linear attenuation coefficient

d.relationship between the linear absorption coefficient of a pixel and fat and water linear attenuation coefficient

59.CT number is calculated by formula

a.magnification constant(pixel linear attenuation constant+water linear attenuation constant)/ water linear attenuation constant

b.magnification constant(pixel linear attenuation constant x water linear attenuation constant)/ water linear attenuation constant

c.magnification constant(pixel linear attenuation constant— water linear attenuation constant)/ water linear attenuation

d.magnification constant(pixel linear attenuation constant— fat linear attenuation constant)/ fat linear attenuation constant

60.Contraidications of MR imaging are(H)

a.internal defibrillatory device

b.bone growth stimulators

c.spinal cord stimulators

d.all

61. Contraidications of MR imaging are(H)

a.elecronic infusion devices

b.ocular metallic foreign body

c.tattooed eyeliner

d.all

62.Contraidications of MR imaging are(H)

a.McGee stapedectomy piston prostheses

b.Swan Ganz catheter

c.magnetic dental implants

d.all

63.All are true regarding MR angiography except(H)

a.vascular map rather than anatomical map

b.fast flowing blood returns no signal(flow void) on routine T1or T2 sin echo image

c.most frequently used technique is Time-of- flight

d.higher patial resolution than conventional film-based angiography

64.CT can display objects with density difference of

a.0.5% or less

b.1.0% or less

c.1.5% or less

d.2.0% or less

65.For film –screen radiography,a density difference of --% is required for contrast resolution

a.1.0%

b.10%

c.15%

d.20%

66.Utrasound ,by definition , has a frequency of grater than

a.10,000 Hz

b.20,000 Hz

c.30,000 Hz

d.40,000 Hz

67.A device used to convert electrical energy into ultrasound and reflected ultrasonic enery into electrical signal is known as

a.transducer

b.transformer

c.gradient

d.radiofrequency coil

68.The principle of piezo-electricity is used in
a.Digital radiography
b.CT
c.USG
d.MRI

69.The most important component of transducer is
a.piezoelectric crystal
b.radiofrequency coil
c.gradients
d.none

70.Curie temperature is related to
a.trasnsducer of USG
b.transformer of x ray machine
c.heat generated in body by MRI
d.heat produced in x ray tube

71. Concept of acoustic impedence is related to
a.MRI
b.CT
c.USG
d.PET

72.Doppler effet refers to
a.change in perceived frequency of sound emitted by a moving structures
b.change in perceived intensity of sound emitted by a moving structures
c.change in perceived velocity of sound emitted by a moving structures
d.change in perceived frequency of sound emitted by a stationary structures

73.Doppler USG is primarily used for
a.study of blood vessel
b.study of liver
c.study of spleen
d.study of pancreas

74.Unit of biological effectiveness of radiation
a.roentgen
b.rad and gray
c.rem and sievert
d.none

75.SI unit of absorbed dose of radiation
a.rad
b.rem
c.gray
d.sievert

76.SI unit of absorbed dose equivalent
a.rad
b.rem
c.gray
d.sievert

77.All are true regarding stochastic effect of radiation except

a.probability of occurrence increases with increasing absorbed dose

b.severity of the effect depend on the magnitude of the absorbed dose

c.no dose threshold

d.an all-or- none phenomenon

78.The stochastic effect of radiation is

a.cancers

b.genetic effects

c.both

d.none

79.The first imaging technique of MRI is attributable to

a.Hounsefield

b.Lauterbur

c.Felich and bloch

d.none

80.Gyromagnetic ratio and larmor frequency are related to physics of

a.USG

b.CT

c.MRI

d.PET

81.MRI make use of all except

a.magnet

b.radiofrequency coil

c.gradient coils

d.transducer

82.Gas which is used in MRI for cooling is

a.helium

b.nitrogen

c.oxygen

d.hydrogen

83.The temperature at which entire magnetic system must be maintained is

a.about 4 degree Kelvin

b.about 8 degree kelvin

c.about 12 degree kelvin

d.about 16 degree Kelvin

84.The superconducting material used in magnet of MRI is

a.NbTi

b.SbTi

c.CdTi

d.AlTi

85.Magnetic resonance imaging is based on

a.precession of proton

b.precession of electron

c.precession of neutron

d.precession of positron

86.Larmor frequency of ^1H is

a.29.16MHz/T

b.40.05MHz/T

c.42.58MHz/T

d.17.24MHz/T

87.All are true regarding MRI except

a.T1 weighted image uses a short TE and sort TR

b.T2 weighted image uses a long TE and long TR

c.Spin density images use short TR and long TR

d.T1weighted image use long TR and short TR

88.Which weighted image is used for display of anatomy

a.T1W

b.T2W

c.Spin density image

d.all

89. Which weighted image is most commonly used when looking for tumour

a.T1W

b.T2W

c.Spin density image

d.all

90.Which molecule in body provide the best MRI signal

a.hydrogen

b.nitogen

c.carbon

d.oxygen

91.MRI make use of

a.microwave

b.radiowave

c.infrared

d.all

92.Earth 's magnetic field is about

a.100 microT

a.50 microT

a.1000 microT

a.500 microT

93.Usual range magnetic field used in MRI machine is

a.0.15 to 3 T

a.0.5 to 1 T

a.1 to 1.5T

a.1 to 2.5T

94.Which tissue has relatively smallest T1 recovery time

a.water

b.compact bone

c.CSF

d.fat

95.Which tissue has reltively longest T2 decay

a.water

b.gray matter

c.white matter

d.fat

96. Which tissue has relatively smallest T1 recovery time and smallest T2 decay

a.water

b.compact bone

c.CSF

d.fat

97.Which tissue has reltively

longest T2 decay and longest T1 recovery

a.water

b.gray matter

c.white matter

d.fat

98.All are correct regarding signal on MRI

a.fat appears dark on T1W and bright on T2W

b.water and CSF appear dark on T2W

c.water and CSF appear brighter than fat on T2W

d.CSF and fat appear bright on proton density

99. All are true regarding signal of brain tissue except

a.gray matter appear brighter than white matter on proton density weighted image

b.gray matter appear brighter than white matter on T2W weighted image

c.white matter appear brighter than gray matter on T1W weighted image

d.gray matter appear brighter than whitematter on T1 weighted image

100.Which is used for slice selection and thickness

a.superconducting coil

b.radiofrequency coil

c.gradients

d.none

101.Tip angle concept is useful in

a.USG

b.MRI

c.CT

d.PET

102.In GRE sequence of MRI ,all moving blood appears

a.bright

b.dark

c.signal void

d.none

103.TOF and phase contrast are methods of angiography in

a.catheter angiography

b.CT angiography

c.MR angiography

d.none

104.Which contrast is used in perfusion study in MRI

a.iodine

b.barium

c.gadolinium

d.none

105.Claustrophobia is a specific side effect of

a.CT

b.MRI

c.USG

d.x ray

106.K-edge of barium is

a.20 keV

b.50 keV

c.37 keV

d.88 keV

107.The device used to measure radiation dose is

a.dosimeter

b.ammeter

c.polarimeter

d.photometer

108.Critical molecules for radiation damage

a.proteins like enzymes

b.nucleic acid principally DNA

c.both

d.none

109.Threshold dose of radiation for cataracts

a.1 gray

b.2 gray

c.3 gray

d.5 gray

110.Typical absorbed dose in PA view of chest

a.0.15mGy

b 0.50mGy

c.0.75mGy

d.1.0mGy

111. The MRI technique used to null signal from fluids is(GRAINGER)

a.FLAIR

b.STIR

c.GRE

d.Spin-echo

112.The MRI technique used to null signal from fat is(GRAINGER)

a.FLAIR

b.STIR

c.GRE

d.Spin-echo

113.ALARA stands for(GRAINGER)

a. as low as reasonably achievable

b. as least as reasonably achievable

c. as low as rationably achievable

d. as least as reasonably achievable

114.Typical dose in CT head scan

a.1mSv

b.2mSv

c.3mSv

d.4mSv

115.ALARP in radioprotection stands for

a.as least as reasonably practicable

b.as low as rationally practicable

c.as light as reasonably practicable

d.as low as reasonably permissible

116.Annual dose limit for public

a.1 mSv

b.2 mSV

c.3 mSV

d.4mSV

117.Annual dose limit for employees

a.10 mSv

b.20 mSV

c.30 mSV

d.40mSV

118.Annual dose limit for employees for abdomen of women of reproductive capacity(in any consecutive 3-month period)

a.10 mSv

b.13 mSV

c.20 mSV

d.25mSV

119. Annual dose limit for fetus of pregnant employee

a.1mSv

b.2 mSV

c.3 mSV

d.4mSV

120.Target material for mammography x ray tube

a.molybdenum

b.rhodium

c.both a and b

d.tungsten

121.All are true regarding digital radiography

a.computed radiography use barium fluorohalide doped with europium as photostimulable phosphor

b.Cesium iodide(indirect) and amorphous selenium(direct) are used as detectors in digital radiography

c.both

d.none

122.All are true regarding approximate range of CT numbers except

a.bone 500 to 1500

b.grey matter 35 to 45

c.lung   -300 to -800

d.fat   60 to 150

123.All are true regarding helical CT scan except

a.use of slip ring technology

b. continuous rotation of gantry

c.continuous acquisition of data

d.longer scan time

124.Correctly matched half-lives are all except

a.Technetium-99m---6hrs

b.iodine 123----------- 13hrs

c.iodine 131----------- 8days

d.iodine ---------- 60hrs

125.Gamma rays are emitted by

a.^{99m}Tc

b.^{123}I

c.both

d.none

126.All are correct use of Technetium linked molecule except

a.methylene diphosphonate for bone imaging

b.HMPAO for cerebral imaging

c.DMSA and MAG3 for renal studies

d.HIDA for cardiac finction

127. All are correct use of Technetium linked molecule except

a.HSA macroaggregates for lug perfusion study

b.DTPA aerosol for lung ventilation studies

c.HIDA for biliary study

d.sestamibi or tetrofosmin for cerebral imaging

128.Which radionuclide is used in PET

a.beta emitter

b.gamma emitter

c.alpha emitter

d.positron emitter

129.positron emitter is

a.^{18}F

b.^{99m}Tc

c.^{123}I

d.none

130. True regarding transducer of ultrasound is

a.made up of piezo-electric material

b.loses piezo-electricity below Curie temperature

c.should be autoclaved for sterilization

d.generally should be immerged in water for cleaning

131.The Fresnel region and the Fraunhofer region is related to

a.USG

b.MRI

c.PET

d.SPECT

132.Coupling gel is used in ultrasound to

a. increase speed of ultrasound

b. to remove air bubbles between transducer and patient surface c.to remove patients discomfort

d.for easy movement of transducer

133.Contrast agent used in ultrasound imaging is

a.iodine

b.gadolinium

c.omnipaue

d.low solubility gas encapsulated in a lipid shell

134.Effective dose for CT head is(GRAINGER)

a.50 chest x ray

b.100 chest x ray

c.150 chest x ray

d.175 chest xray

135.Imaging of blood flow by ultrasound is based on

a.edison effect

b.doppler effect

c.crompton effect

d.heel effect

136.PACS refers to

a.patient archiving and communication system

b a.picture archiving and commputation system

c.picture archiving and communication system

d.patient archiving and commputation system

137.Iodinated nonionic monomer contrast is

a.coray

b.omnipaque

c.hexabrix

c.visipaque

138.Iodinated nonionic dimer contrast is

a.coray

b.omnipaque

c.hexabrix

c.visipaque

139.In radiation therapy ,major mode of interaction of photons with tissues (dutta)

a.Compton scattering

b.photoelectric effect

c.pair-production

d.all

140.Acoustic shadowing on USG is noted in

a.stone

b.cyst

c.solid tumor

d.all

141.Acoustic enhancement on USG is noted in

a.stone

b.cyst

c.solid tumor

d.all

142.All are true regarding radiations except (H)

a.radiation exposure may be natural (50%) or man-made(50%)

b.Radon gas account for majority of(37%) natural radiation exposure

c.CT account for 50% of man-made radiation exposure

d.CT is responsible for 5% of all radiation exposure

143.All imaging uses radiation except (H)

a.x ray

b. CT

c.PET

d.USG

144.Unit of radiation absorbed dose is(H)

a.curie(common unit) and Becquerel(new unit)

b.rem (common unit)and Sievert(new unit)

c.roentgen

d.rad(common unit) and gray(new unit)

145. Unit of equivalent dose and effective dose for biologic response to radiation is(H)

a.curie and Becquerel

a.curie(common unit) and Becquerel(new unit)

b.rem (common unit)and Sievert(new unit)

c.roentgen

d.rad(common unit) and gray(new unit)

146. Unit of radiation exposure (H)

a.curie(common unit) and Becquerel(new unit)

b.rem (common unit)and Sievert(new unit)

c.roentgen

d.rad(common unit) and gray(new unit)

147. Unit of radioactivity (H)

a.curie(common unit) and Becquerel(new unit)

b.rem (common unit)and Sievert(new unit)

c.roentgen

d.rad(common unit) and gray(new unit)

148.1 gray= ?rad(H)

a.1 rad

b.10 rad

c.100 rad

d.1000 rad

149.1 Sievert =?rem(H)

a.1 rem

b.10 rem

c.100 rem

d.1000 rem

150.All are true regarding stochastic effect of radiation except(H)

a.occur at any dose

b.no threshold

c.prabability increases with increasing dose

d.of less concern than deterministic effect

151.Correct matching for deterministic effect and its threshold are all except(H)

a.temporary epilation --200 rad

b.permanant epilation—700 rad

c.acute cataract--200 rad

d.trasient erythema—50 rad

152.All are true regarding radiation(H)

a.effect primarily from effect on DNA

b.children 10 more sensitive than adult

c.boys more sensitive than girls

d.dose generally used in diagnostic radiology <0.1gray

153.Hematopoietic syndrome results from acute whole-body radiation doses above(H)

a.200 rad

b.150 rad

c.100 rad

d 50 rad

154.Gastrointestinal syndrome results from acute whole-body radiation doses above(H)

a.200 rad

b.600 rad

c.800 rad

d 400 rad

155.drugs used in case of internal contamination with cesium and thallium(H)

a.prussian blue

b.potassium iodide

c.oral phosphate

d.ammonium chloride

156.MRI is a technique based on magnetic properties of(H)

a.oxygen nuclei

b.hydrogen nuclei

c.carbon nuclei

d.nitrogen nuclei

157 .Disadvantages of CT (SW)

a.significant radiation

b.cannot be used during pregnancy

c.contast allergy

d.all

158.All are true regarding Doppler USG (SW)

a.detect presence of blood vessel

b.determine direction of blood flow

c.determine velocity of blood flow

d.all

159.All are true regarding MRI except(SW)

a.magnetic field align the hydrogen atoms in the body

b.magnetic waves alter the alignment of magnetization

c.different tissues absorb and release radiowaves energy at similar rates

d.most tissues can be differentiated by differences in their characteristic T1 and T1 relaxation times

160.All are true regarding MRI except

a.T1 is a measure of how quickly a tissue can become magnetized

b.T2 measures how quickly a tissue lose its magnetization

c.breath- holding imaging technique incerases motion artefact

d.Gadopentenate dimeglumine is an MRI contrast agent

161.All are MRI contrast agent except(SW)

a.Gadopentenate dimeglumine

b.ferumoxides

c.iminodiacetic acid derivative –radionuclides

d.omnipaque

162.Metabolic molecule used in PET imaging(SW)

a.fluorodeoxyglucose

b.Gadopentenate dimeglumine

c.ferumoxides

d.iminodiacetic acid derivatives

163.Advantages of USG are all except(SW)

a.noninvasive

b.painless

c.no radiation

d.easy to examine obese patient

164.All hepato-biliary specific agent are taken up by reticulo-endothelial system except(GRAINGER)

a.Ferrumoxides

b.SHU-555A

c.AMI-227

d.Mn-DPDP

165.All are hepato-specific paramagnetic agents except(GRAINGER)

a.Mn-DPDP

b.Gd-BOPTA

c.Gd-EOB-DTPA

d.Ferrumoxides

166.All are true regarding digital radiography are all except(H)

a.No possibility of postprocessing

b.immediate availability of images

c.electronic storages

d.facility of transfer

167.Advantages of CT scan over routine chest radiography are all except(H)

a.distintion between densities

b.characterization of tissue densities

c. accurate size assessment of lesions

d.less radiation exposure.

168.Effects of helical CT technology are all except(H)

a.faster scan (single breath holding maneuver)

b.improved contrast enhancement

c.thinner collimation

d.more motion artefact

169. True regarding helical CT technology(H)

a.allows collection of continuous data over large areas

b.reconstruction of data to produce sagittal/coronal planes

c.vertual bronchoscopy possible

d thicker collimation

170. All are true regarding multidetector CT(MCDT)except(H)

a.additional detector along scanning axis (z-axis)

a.especially beneficial for children,the elderly and critically ill patients

c.less radiation as compared to single detector CT

d.improved imaging of pulmonary vasculatures

171. True regarding MDCT (H)

a.enhanced resolution

b.increased image reconstruction ability

c.shorter breath holds

d.All

172. All are true regarding MRI(H)

a.avoided in unstable and /or ventilated patients

b.pacemaker and aneurysm clip precludes use of MRI

c.the use of nonionising electromagnetic radiation

d.contast always needed to distinguish vascular from non vascular structures

173. Intravascular contrast agent used for MR angiography is(H)

a.gadolinium

b.gastrograffin

c.iodinated contrast

d.barium

174. FDG is used in(H)

a.MDCT

b.MRA

c.PET SCAN

d. ventilation perfusion scan

175.^{18}F-FDG emit (SW)

a.alpha particle

b.beta particle

c.gamma rays

d.positron

176.Which MR sequence is sensitive to the microscopic motion of water(H)

a.Diffusion MR

b.Perfusion MR

c.MR spectroscopy

d.functional MR

177.All are true regarding alpha radiation except

a.negatively charged particles

b.contains two protons and two neutons

c.limited penetrating power(cannot penetrate skin)

d.small risk with external exposure

178.All are true regarding beta radiation except

a.consists of electrons

b.few cm of penetration

c.platic layers and clothing stop most of beta radiation

d.released by radioactive iodine

179.All are true regarding Gamma rays and x-rays except

a.no charge

b.no mass

c. just energy

d.different biologic effect

180.The principle type of radiation that cause total body exposure

a.x-rays and gamma rays

b.alpha particles

c.beta particles

d.none

181.Penetrating radiations are

a.x-rays

b.gamma rays

c.both

d.none

182.The unit used to measure

energy deposited in living
matter
a. gray
b.rem
c.sievert
d.roentgen
183.All are true regarding
neutrons except
a.heavy particle
b.charged
c often emitted during nuclear
detonation
d.has wide energy range
184.True regarding radiation
a.Alpha particles donot
penetrate beyond skin
b.Beta particles can cause
significant cutaneous burns
and scarring
c.gamma radiation cause local
damage as well as whole body
radiation
d.all
185.all emit beta and gamma
radiation except
a.cobalt 60
b.iodine 131
c.technetium
d.polonium
186.P-32 emit only
a.alpha particles
b.beta particles
c.gamma rays

d.neutrons
187.Radiologic half life of
technetium is
a.6hrs
b.16hrs
c.12hs
d.2hrs
188 .Correct matching for
biological half life are all
except
a.iodine 123—33hrs
b.molybdenum—66.7days
c.iodine 131—8.1days
d.phosphorus 32---14.3days
189.Without medical
support,$LD_{50/30}$(a dose that
causes a 50% mortality at 30
days) for whole-body
exposure is
a. approx.1 gray
b. approx.4 gray
c. approx.8 gray
d. approx.10 gray
190 .All are true regarding
acute radition syndrome(ARS)
a.ARS is mild with exposure to
<5gray
b.whole body exposure with
doses >9-10 gray is almost
always fatal
c.neurovascular syndrome
predominate with whole body
exposure>20gray

d.Haemopoietic syndrome predominate with whole body exposure to 6-10 gray

191.Which boold cell show most rapid declin eafter radiation exposure

a.lymphocyte

b.platelets

c.neutrophil

d.erythrocyte

192.The least vulnerable blood element to radiation exposure

a.lymphocyte

b.platelets

c.neutrophil

d.erythrocyte

193.All are true regarding lymphocyte in radition exposure

a.Absolute lymphocyte count is a sensitive marker for radiation damage

b.Absolute lymphocyte count correlate with exposure but not prognosis

c.Lymphocyte chromosomal analysis detect radiation exposure as low as .03-.06gray

d.dicentric chromosome and ring forms aberration noted in lymphocyte after radiation exposure

194.Relative contraindications of MRI are(H)

a.pacemakers

b.internal defibrillator

c.cerebral aneurysm clip

d.all

195.incidence of severe anaphylactoid reactions due to contrast is(H)

a.0.1% to 0.2%

b.0.3% to 0.4%

c.0.5%to 0.6%

d.0.7%to 0.9%

196.True about contrast induced nephropathy are all except(H)

a.increase in creatine>0.5mg/dl within 48-72 hrs of contrast administration

b.occurs in 20% of patients

c. DM and CHF are risk factors

d.intrvascular volume expansion limits the risk

197.A modern CT scanner is capable of obtaining slice thickness as thin as(H)

a.0.5mm-1mm

b.2mm-2.5mm

c.3mm-3.5mm

d.4mm-4.5mm

198.Radition exposure for routine brain CT study is(H)

a.2-5mSv

b.6-7mSv

c.8-10mSv

d.11-12mSv

199.Contrast nephropathy is defined by a rise of serum creatinine of at least ------- mg/dl within 48hrs of contrast administration(H)

a.1mg/dl

b.2mg/dl

c.3mg/dl

d.4mg/dl

200.Risk factors for contrast nephropathy include all except(H)

a.age>80yrs

b.serum ceatinine exceeding 2mg/dl

c.solitary kidey

d.diabetes insipidus

201.Risk factors for contrast nephropathy include all except(H)

a.diabetes mellitus

b.paraprotenemia

c.overhydration

d.high dose of contrast

202.All are true regarding contrast nephropathy except(H)

a.usually need dialysis

b.serum creatinine level return to baseline within 1-2 weeks

c.risk of nephropathy increases with estimated GFR<60ml/min/1.73m^2

d.hydration,bicarbonate,acetyl cysteine reduce contrast nephropathy

203.Exact estimated GFR below which iodinated contrast should not be given(according to American college of Radiology) (H)

a.45ml/min/1.73m^2

a.50ml/min/1.73m^2

a.55ml/min/1.73m^2

a.60ml/min/1.73m^2

204. In what % of cases severe allergic reactions is noted with nonionic iodinated contrast(H)

a.0.04%,six fold lower than with ionic media

b. 0.08%,eight fold lower than with ionic media

c.0.10%,eight fod lower than with ionic media

d.0.12%,six fod lower than with ionic media

205.All are true regarding contrast except(H)

a.noninic contrast is preffered

b.glucocortcoids used as premedication in patients with prior contrast allergy

c.patents with allergic reaction to iodinated contrast usually react to gadolinium based MR contrast

d.nonionic contrast relatively costly

206.MRI image is result of interaction of except(H)

a.hydrogen protons in biologic tissues

b.a static magnetic field (magnet)

c.radiofrequency waves of specific frequency

d.earth's magnetic field

207.All are true about MRI except(H)

a.coils produce radiofrequency

b.magnetic gradients help in spatial localization

c.field strength of magnet is not directly related to signal-to- noise ratio

d.3T-8T magnets available

208.All are true regarding MRI imaging except(H)

a.Rf pulses transiently excites energy states of hydrogen protons

b.hydrogen protons release Rf energy (echo) during relaxation

c.Echo is detected by gradients

d.Fourier analysis is used to form image

209.All are true regarding MR angiography except(H)

a.Phase contrast MRA takes longer time than TOF

b.Phase contrast MRA reveal velocity and direction of blood flow

c.Phase contrast MRA provide excellent suppression of high signal- intensity backround structures

d.Selective venous and arterial MRA images cannot be obtained with Phase contrast MRA

210.All are true regarding T1-weighted image except(H)

a.use of relatively short TR and TE

b.fat and subacute hemorrhage has reatively short T1 relaxation time

c.fat and subacute hemorrhage produce relatively higher signal intensity

d.water gives bright signal

211.All are true about gadolinium except(H)
a.heavy metal element
b.paramagnetic substance
c.used as MR contrast agent
d.increase T1 and T2 relaxation time of nearby water protons

212.A ll are true about Gd DTPA contrast except(H)
a.chelated to DTPA which allows safe renal excretion
b.dose is approx. 0.2mg/kg body weight
c.does not generally cross BBB
d.produce low signal on T1 and high signal on T2

213.All are true regarding Gadolinium contrast except(H)
a.enhance lesions lacking BBB
b.cause renal failure
c.avoided in <6moths of age
d.nephrogenic systemic fibrosis in patients with renal insufficiency

214.Contraindications of MR imaging are all except(H)
a.cardiac pacemaker or permanent pacemakers leads
b.intracranial aneurysm clip
c.chochlear prostheses
d.ferromagnetic IVC filters,coils,stents (six weeks after implantation)

215.Maximum radiation exposure is noted in
a.bone scan
b.CT
c.MRI
d.chest x ray

216.Which show maximum ionization potential
a.helium ion
b.y-ray
c.electron
d.proton

217.Systemic radionuclides are all except
a.Samarium 153
b.Strontium 89
c.phosphorus 32
d.iridium 192

218.Radiocontrast is contraindicated in all except
a.hypovolemia
b.chronic renal insufficiency
c.metformin treatment
d.obesity

219.Photoelectric effect refers to interaction between
a.low energy incident photon and the outer shell electron
b. low energy incident photon and the inner shell electron

c.high energy incident photon and the outer shell electron

d.high energy incident photon and the inner shell electron

220.Crompton effect refers to interaction between

a.low energy incident photon and the outer shell electron

b. low energy incident photon and the inner shell electron

c.high energy incident photon and the outer shell electron

d.high energy incident photon and the inner shell electron

221.Wall of CT scanner room is coated with

a.iron

b.lead

c.glass

d.tungsten

222.The difference between light and x ray is

a.type of wave

b.speed

c.energy

d.mass

223.the most Ionizing radiation is

a.Alpha

b.Beta

c.x rays

d.Yamma rays

224.Background radiation refers to

a.radiation in the background of nuclear reactors

b. .radiation present constantly from natural resources

c.radiation in the background of radiological investiations

d.radiation from nuclear fallout

285.Amount of radition delivered to an organ in the radiation field is known as

a.exposure dose

b.effective dose

c.equivalent dose

d.absorbed dose

286.True regarding stochastic effect

a.severity dose dependent

b.probability dose dependent

c.has threshold

d.erythema and cataract are examples

287.True statement regarding contrast agent is

a.osmolar contrast agents may be ionic or non ionic

b.Gadolinium cross BBB

c.iohexol is a high contrast media

d.ionic monomers have three iodine atoms /two particles in solution

289.Dose of radiation during whole body exposure that leads to hematological syndrome is

a.2Gy

b.10Gy

c.100Gy

d.200Gy

290.All are true regarding magic angle phenomenon in MRI imaging except(G)

a.artefactual increased signal from tendons on short TE imaging sequence

b.angle of alignment of tendon to static magnetic field is apprex.55 degree

c.magic angle effect is not seen in ligament ,cartilage or menisci`

d.magic angle effect is not persistent on long TE sequence

291.Black synovium on MRI is noted in all except(G)

a.pigmented villonodular synovitis

b.amyloid deposition

c.hemophiliac arthropathy

d.rheomatoid arthritis

292.Appearance of water/edema in mri imaging(G)

a.dark on T1W

b.bright on T2W

C.both

d.none

293.Which MR sequence is sensitive to the microscopic motion of water(H)

a.Diffusion MR

b.Perfusion MR

c.MR spectroscopy

d.functional MR

294.What is the most sensitive technique for detecting acute ischemic stroke (H)

a.perfusion MR

b.diffusion MR

c.MR spectroscopy

d.functional MR

RADIOPHYSICS (ANSWERS)

1.a---Wilhelm Conrad Roentgen discovered x ray

2.a---X ray was discovered in 8th Nov. 1895

3.a---Wave length of diagnostic x ray is1 to 0.1 A

4.b---SI unit of absorbed dose of radiation is gray

5. a---SI unit of magnetic flux density Tesla

6.a---Regarding x ray tube: .tube is vacuumated ,cathode and anode made of tungsten,rotating anode used to withstand generated heat,pyrex glass used as encasing

7.b---Elecron cloud produced at cathode filament by thermionic emission is known as edison effect

8.a---Tungsten is used as filament and target material due to high atomic no.(74)—so more efficient producer of x rays,high melting point(3370) –so withstand high generated heat,little tendency to vaporize –so long life expectancy of filament,can be drawn into thin wire that is quite strong

9.a---Limit to anode angle in x ray tube is due to heel effect

10.b---Purpose of use of rotating anode is to withstand high generated heat

11.b---Rotating anode is primarily made up of tungsten

12.c---Regarding x ray production: interaction with nucleus of the target produce general radiation,interaction with electrons in the the inner shell of the target produce characteristic radiation,the quality of radiation produced depend almost entirely on the x ray tube potential(kVp),molybdenum target used in breast radiography

13.a----general radiations produced by interaction of target nucleus is known as general radiation(bremsstrahlung)

14.d---Ways of x ray interaction with matter are coherent scattering,photoelectric effect,Compton effect

15.b---Which x ray interaction produce radiographic image of excellent quality photoelectric effect

16.c---Scatter radiation encountered in diagnostic radiology comes from which interaction Compton effect

17.a---Purpose of filter is reduce patients radiation dose

18.d---All material that may be used as filter molebdynum,cupper,aluminium

19.b---Purpose of using beryllium window is to produce unfiltered x ray beam

20.a---molybdenum is used as filter in breast mammography

21.c---Aluminium is used as filter

22.b---The reduction in the intensity of an x ray beam as it traverses matter is known as attenuation

23.d----Factors affecting attenuation energy of x ray,density of matter,atomic number and electrons/gram of matter

24.a---Half value layer in radiography refers to absorber thickness

25.a---Used as K-edge filter holmium ,molybdenum,gadolinium

26.a---Barium and iodine is used as contrast agent because of k edge

27.c---Regarding filters :sheets of metal,placed in path of x ray beam near the x ray tube housing,absorb low energy radiation,reduce patient'exposure to useless radiation

28.a---Recommended thickness of aluminum filter for diagnostic radiography 2.5mm

29.d---Devices attached to opening in the x ray tube housing to regulate size and shape of an x ray beam is beam restrictors

30.a---Beam restrictors: aperture diaphragms,cones and cylinders,collimators

31.a---Collimators regulate size and shape of x ray beam

32.c---The radiographic device consisting of a series of lead foil strips seprated by x ray transparent spacers is known as grid

33.d---The most effective of removing scatter radiation from large radiographic field is grid

34.c---Bucky factor is related to grid

35.d---Located near/in x ray tube:filament ,target,collimatror

36.d---Regarding intensifying screen located in pair x ray cassette,calcium tungstate serves as phosphor,decrease x ray dose to patients,requires lower exposure (less mAs)

37.b---Light sensitive material in emulsion of x ray film is made up of silver iodobromide

38.b---Developing solutions used in radiography contain developing agents,an alkali, preservative(sodium sulfite),restrainers or antifogants(potassium bromide)

39. d---Developing agents used in radiography are:hydroquinone,phenindone,metol

40. a---Used as fixer in radiography:sodium or ammonium thiosulphate

41.b---KVp controls image contrast

42.a—Exposure (mAs)controls film density

43.a---The speed of film –screen system is defined as the proportional of the exposure in roentgens to produce a density of 1.o above base plus fog density

44.a---Ortho x ray film is sensitive to green

45.a---Pan x ray film is sensitive to all light colors

46.b---Darkroom safelight for ortho film is red

47.b---The amount of blackening of an x ray film is expressed by the term photographic density

48.a---cesium iodide is used as input phosphor in image intensifier in radiology

49.c---zinc-cadmium is used as output phosphor in image intensifier in radiology

50.a---Term used for difference in density between areas in the radiograph is contrast

51.a---Effect of fog and scatter on film is .to reduce radiographic contrast

52.d---Radiographic contrast depend on subject contrast,film contrast,scatter radiation plus fog

53.a---The production of a visible image utilizing the charged surface of a photocnductor (amorphous selenium) is known as xeroradigraphy

54.a--- G.N.Hounsfield discovered Computerised axial transverse scanning in 1972

55.c---Regarding different generation of CT scan :1st generation (translate –rotate ,one detector),2nd generation(translate – rotate,multiple detector),3rd generation(rotate-rotate),4Th generation(rotate-fixed)

56.d---Regarding 3rd and 4th generation CT scan : both x ray tube and detectors rotate around the patient(rotate-rotate) in 3rd generation,x ray collimated into a fan beam (use of 'fan beam' geometry) in 3rd generation and 4th generation,a ring of detectors around the patient which does not move in 4th generation ,the x ray tube rotates in a circle inside the detectors ring a in 4th generation

57.b---Back projection,iterative methos ,and analytical methods used in CT are meant for image reconstruction

58.b---CT number refers to relationship between the linear absorption coefficient of a pixel and water linear attenuation coefficient

59.c---CT number is calculated by formula magnification constant(pixel linear attenuation constant—water linear attenuation constant)/ water linear attenuation

60.d---Contraidications of MR imaging are(H)internal defibrillatory device,bone growth stimulators,spinal cord stimulators

61. d---Contraidications of MR imaging are(H) elecronic infusion devices,ocular metallic foreign body,tattooed eyeliner

62.d---Contraidications of MR imaging are(H)McGee stapedectomy piston prostheses,Swan Ganz catheter,magnetic dental implants

63.d---True regarding MR angiography (H) vascular map rather than anatomical map,fast flowing blood returns no signal(flow void) on routine T1or T2 sin echo image,most frequently used technique is Time-of- flight,lower patial resolution than conventional film-based angiography

64.a---CT can display objects with density difference of 0.5% or less

65.b---For film-screen radiography,a density difference of 10% is required for contrast resolution

66.b---Utrasound ,by definition , has a frequency of greater than 20,000 Hz

67.a---A device used to convert electrical energy into ultrasound and reflected ultrasonic enery into electrical signal is known as transducer

68.c---The principle of piezo-electricity is used in USG

69.a---The most important component of transducer is piezoelectric crystal

70.a----Curie temperature is related to trasnsducer of USG

71. c---Concept of acoustic impedence is related to USG

72.a---Doppler effet refers to change in perceived frequency of sound emitted by a moving structures

73.a---Doppler USG is primarily used for study of blood vessel

74.c---Unit of biological effectiveness of radiation is rem and sievert

75.c---SI unit of absorbed dose of radiation gray

76.d---SI unit of absorbed dose equivalent sievert

77.b-- Regarding stochastic effect of radiation probability of occurrence increases with increasing absorbed dose,severity of the effect does not depend on the magnitude of the absorbed dose,no dose threshold,an all-or- none phenomenon

78.C---The stochastic effect of radiation is cancers and genetic effects

79.b---The first imaging technique of MRI is attributable to Lauterbur

80.c---Gyromagnetic ratio and larmor frequency are related to physics of MRI

81.d---MRI make use of magnet,radiofrequency coil,gradient coils

82.a---Gas which is used in MRI for cooling is helium

83.a---The temperature at which entire magnetic system must be maintained is about 4 degree Kelvin

84.a---The superconducting material used in magnet of MRI is NbTi

85.a---Magnetic resonance imaging is based on precession of proton

86.c---Larmor frequency of ^1H is 42.58MHz/T

87.d---Regarding MRI :T1 weighted image uses a short TE and sort TR,T2 weighted image uses a long TE and long TR,Spin density images use short TR and long TR

88.a----T1W weighted image is used for display of anatomyT1W

89.b----T2W weighted image is most commonly used when looking for tumour

90.a---Hydrogen molecule in body provide the best MRI signal

91.b---MRI make use of radiowave

92.a---Earth 's magnetic field is about 50 microT

93.a---Usual range magnetic field used in MRI machine is 0.15 to 3 T

94.d---Fat tissue has relatively smallest T1 recovery time

95.a---Water tissue has relatively longest T2 decay

96.d---fat has relatively smallest T1 recovery time and smallest T2 decay

97.a---water has reltively longest T2 decay and longest T1 recovery

98.c---Regarding signal on MRI :water and CSF appear brighter than fat on T2W

99. d---Regarding signal of brain tissue gray matter appear brighter than white matter on proton density weighted image,gray matter appear brighter than white matter on T2W weighted image,white matter appear brighter than gray matter on T1W weighted image

100.c---Gradients is used for slice selection and thickness

101.b---Tip angle concept is useful in MRI

102.a---In GRE sequence of MRI ,all moving blood appears bright

103.c---TOF and phase contrast are methods of angiography in MR angiography

104.c---Which contrast is used in perfusion study in MRI gadolinium

105.b---Claustrophobia is a specific side effect of MRI

106.a---K-edge of barium is 37 keV

107.a---The device used to measure radiation dose is dosimeter

108.c---Critical molecules for radiation damage proteins like enzymes ,nucleic acid principally DNA

109.d----Threshold dose of radiation for cataracts 5 gray

110.a---Typical absorbed dose in PA view of chest 0.15mGy

111.a--- The MRI technique used to null signal from fluids is(GRAINGER) FLAIR

112.b---The MRI technique used to null signal from fat is(GRAINGER) STIR

113.a---ALARA stands for(GRAINGER) as low as reasonably achievable

114.b---Typical a dose CT head scan .2mSv

115.a---ALARP in radioprotection stands for as least as reasonably practicable

116.a---Annual dose limit for public 1 mSv

117.a---Annual dose limit for employees 10 mSv

118.b---Annual dose limit for employees for abdomen of women of reproductive capacity(in any consecutive 3-month period) 13 mSV

119.a--- Annual dose limit for fetus of pregnant employee 1mSv

120.c---Target material for mammography x ray tube molybdenum,rhodium

121.c---Regarding digital radiography computed radiography use barium fluorohalide doped with europium as photostimulable phosphor,Cesium iodide(indirect) and amorphous selenium(direct) are used as detectors in digital radiography

122.d---Regarding approximate range of CT numbers :bone 500 to 1500,grey matter 35 to 45,lung   -300 to -800

123.d---Regarding helical CT scan use of slip ring technology, continuous rotation of gantry,continuous acquisition of data,shorter scan time

124.d---Matched half-lives are Technetium-99m---6hrs,iodine 123----------- 13hrs,iodine 131----------- 8days

125.c---Gamma rays are emitted by $^{99m}Tc, ^{123}I$

126.d--- Use of Technetium linked molecule :methylene diphosphonate for bone imaging,HMPAO for cerebral imaging,DMSA and MAG3 for renal studies,HIDA for hepatobiliary finction

127. d---Use of Technetium linked molecule HSA macroaggregates for lug perfusion study,DTPA aerosol for lung ventilation studies,HIDA for biliary study,sestamibi or tetrofosmin for cardiac imaging

128.d----radionuclide is used in PET positron emitter

129.a---positron emitter is ^{18}F

130.a--- Regarding transducer of ultrasound :made up of piezo-electric material,loses piezo-electricity above Curie temperature,should never be autoclaved for sterilization,generally should not be immerged in water unless waterproof

131.a---The Fresnel region and the Fraunhofer region is related to USG

132.b---Coupling gel is used in ultrasound to to remove air bubbles between transducer and patient surface

133.d---Contrast agent used in ultrasound imaging is low solubility gas encapsulated in a lipid shell

134.b---Effective dose for CT head is(GRAINGER)100 chest x ray

135.b---Imaging of blood flow by ultrasound is based on doppler effect

136.c---PACS refers to picture archiving and communication system

137.b---Iodinated nonionic monomer contrast is omnipaque

138.c---Iodinated nonionic dimer contrast is visipaque

139.a---In radiation therapy ,major mode of interaction of photons with tissues (dutta) Compton scattering

140.a---Acoustic shadowing on USG is noted in stone

141.b--Acoustic enhancement on USG is noted in cyst

142.d---Regarding radiations:(H)radiation exposure may be natural (50%) or man-made(50%),Radon gas account for majority of(37%) natural radiation exposure,CT account for 50% of man-made radiation exposure

143.d-- Imaging uses radiation (H) x ray, CT,PET

144.d---Unit of radiation absorbed dose is(H) rad(common unit) and gray(new unit)

145. b----Unit of equivalent dose and effective dose for biologic response to radiation is(H) rem (common unit)and Sievert(new unit)

146. c---Unit of radiation exposure (H)roentgen

147.a--- Unit of radioactivity (H) curie(common unit) and Becquerel(new unit)

148.c---1 gray= 100 rad(H)

149.c---1 Sievert = 100rem(H)

150.d---Regarding stochastic effect of radiation (H) occur at any dose,no threshold,prabability increases with increasing dose

151.d---Correct matching for deterministic effect and its threshold :(H) temporary epilation --200 rad,permanant epilation—700 rad,acute cataract--200 rad

152.c---Regarding radiation(H) effect primarily from effect on DNA,children 10 more sensitive than adult,girls more sensitive than boys,dose generally used in diagnostic radiology <0.1gray

153.a----Hematopoietic syndrome results from acute whole-body radiation doses above(H) 200 rad

154.c---Gastrointestinal syndrome results from acute whole-body radiation doses above(H) 800 rad

155.a---drugs used in case of internal contamination with cesium and thallium(H) prussian blue

156.b---MRI is a technique based on magnetic properties of(H) hydrogen nuclei

157 .d---Disadvantages of CT (SW) significant radiation,cannot be used during pregnancy,contast allergy

158.d--Regarding Doppler USG (SW) detect presence of blood vessel,determine direction of blood flow,determine velocity of blood flow

159.c---Regarding MRI :(SW)magnetic field align the hydrogen atoms in the body,magnetic waves alter the alignment of magnetization,different tissues absorb and release radiowaves energy at different rates,most tissues can be differentiated by differences in their characteristic T1 and T1 relaxation times

160.d---Regarding MRI: T1 is a measure of how quickly a tissue can become magnetized,T2 measures how quickly a tissue lose its magnetization,breath- holding imaging technique decreases motion artefact,Gadopentenate dimeglumine is an MRI contrast agent

161.d---MRI contrast agent are (SW) Gadopentenate dimeglumine ,ferumoxides,iminodiacetic acid derivative – radionuclides

162.a---Metabolic molecule used in PET imaging(SW) fluorodeoxyglucose

163.d---Advantages of USG are (SW) noninvasive,painless,no radiation,difficult to examine obese patient

164.d---All hepato-biliary specific agent are taken up by reticuloendothelial system except(GRAINGER) Ferrumoxides,SHU-555A,AMI-227

165.d---Hepato-specific paramagnetic agents (GRAINGER)Mn-DPDP,Gd-BOPTA,Gd-EOB-DTPA

166.a---Regarding digital radiography :(H)possibility of postprocessing ,immediate availability of images,electronic storages,facility of transfer

167.d---Advantages of CT scan over routine chest radiography are (H) distintion between densities,characterization of tissue densities,accurate size assessment of lesions

168.d---Effects of helical CT technology are (H) faster scan (single breath holding maneuver),improved contrast enhancement,thinner collimation,less motion artefact

169.d--- Regarding helical CT technology:(H)allows collection of continuous data over large areas,reconstruction of data to produce sagittal/coronal planes,vertual bronchoscopy possible,thinner collimation

170. c---Regarding multidetector CT(MCDT)(H)additional detector along scanning axis (z-axis),especially beneficial for children,the elderly and critically ill patients,more radiation as compared to single detector CT,improved imaging of pulmonary vasculatures

171. d---Regarding MDCT (H) enhanced resolution,increased image reconstruction ability,shorter breath holds

172. d---Regarding MRI:(H)avoided in unstable and /or ventilated patients,pacemaker and aneurysm clip precludes use of MRI,the use of nonionising electromagnetic radiation,contast not always needed to distinguish vascular from non vascular structures

173.a--- Intravascular contrast agent used for MR angiography is(H) gadolinium

174. c---FDG is used in(H) PET SCAN

175.d---^{18}F-FDG emit (SW)positron

176.a---Diffusion MR sequence is sensitive to the microscopic motion of water(H)

177.a---Regarding alpha radiation :positively charged particles, contains two protons and two neutons,limited penetrating power(cannot penetrate skin),small risk with external exposure

178.b---Regarding beta radiation consists of electrons,platic layers and clothing stop most of beta radiation,released by radioactive iodine

179.d---Regarding Gamma rays and x-rays :no charge,no mass, just energy

180.a---The principle type of radiation that cause total body exposure x-rays and gamma rays

181.c---Penetrating radiations are x-rays,gamma rays

182.a---The unit used to measure energy deposited in living matter: gray

183.b---regarding neutrons :heavy particle ,often emitted during nuclear detonation,has wide energy range

184.d---Regarding radiation :Alpha particles donot penetrate beyond skin,Beta particles can cause significant cutaneous burns and scarring,gamma radiation cause local damage as well as whole body radiation

185.d---Emmit beta and gamma radiation :cobalt 60,iodine 131,technetium

186.b---P-32 emit only beta particles

187.a---Radiologic half life of technetium is 6hrs

188 .a--Correct matching for biological half life are : iodine 123 —13hrs,molybdenum—66.7days,iodine 131— 8.1days,phosphorus 32---14.3days

189.b---Without medical support,$LD_{50/30}$(a dose that causes a 50% mortality at 30 days) for whole-body exposure is approx.4 gray

190 .a---Regarding acute radition syndrome(ARS):whole body exposure with doses >9-10 gray is almost always fatal,neurovascular syndrome predominate with whole body exposure>20gray,Haemopoietic syndrome predominate with whole body exposure to 6-10 gray

191.a---Which boold cell show most rapid declinE after radiation exposure lymphocyte

192.d---The least vulnerable blood element to radiation exposure erythrocyte

193.b---Regarding lymphocyte in radition exposureAbsolute lymphocyte count is a sensitive marker for radiation damage,Lymphocyte chromosomal analysis detect radiation exposure as low as .03-.06gray,dicentric chromosome and ring forms aberration noted in lymphocyte after radiation exposure

194.d---Relative contraindications of MRI are(H) pacemakers,internal defibrillator,cerebral aneurysm clip

195.a---incidence of severe anaphylactoid reactions due to contrast is(H) 0.1% to 0.2%

196.b---About contrast induced nephropathy :(H) increase in creatine>0.5mg/dl within 48-72 hrs of contrast administration,DM and CHF are risk factors,intrvascular volume expansion limits the risk

197.a---A modern CT scanner is capable of obtaining slice thickness as thin as(H) 0.5mm-1mm

198.a---Radition exposure for routine brain CT study is(H) 2-5mSv

199.a---Contrast nephropathy is defined by a rise of serum creatinine of at least 1mg/dl mg/dl within 48hrs of contrast administration(H)

200.d---Risk factors for contrast nephropathy include (H)age>80yrs,serum ceatinine exceeding 2mg/dl,solitary kidey

201.C---Risk factors for contrast nephropathy (H)diabetes mellitus,paraprotenemia,high dose of contrast

202.a---Regarding contrast nephropathy (H)serum creatinine level return to baseline within 1-2 weeks,risk of nephropathy increases with estimated GFR<60ml/min/1.73m^2,hydration,bicarbonate,acetylcysteine reduce contrast nephropathy

203.a---Exact estimated GFR below which iodinated contrast should not be given(according to American college of Radiology) (H) 45ml/min/1.73m^2

204. a---0.04% of cases(six fold lower than with ionic media) severe allergic reactions is noted with nonionic iodinated contrast(H)

205.c---Regarding contrast :(H) noninic contrast is preffered,glucocortcoids used as premedication in patients with prior contrast allergy,nonionic contrast relatively costly

206.c---MRI image is result of interaction of (H) hydrogen protons in biologic tissues,a static magnetic field (magnet),radiofrequency waves of specific frequency

207.c---True about MRI :(H) coils produce radiofrequency,magnetic gradients help in spatial localization,3T-8T magnets available

208.c--true regarding MRI imaging (H)Rf pulses transiently excites energy states of hydrogen protons,hydrogen protons release Rf energy (echo) during relaxation,Fourier analysis is used to form image

209.d--True regarding MR angiography (H) Phase contrast MRA takes longer time than TOF,Phase contrast MRA reveal velocity and direction of blood flow,Phase contrast MRA provide excellent suppression of high signal- intensity backround structures,Selective venous and arterial MRA images can be obtained with Phase contrast MRA

210.d---True regarding T1-weighted image :(H) use of relatively short TR and TE,fat and subacute hemorrhage has reatively short T1 relaxation time,fat and subacute hemorrhage produce relatively higher signal intensity ,water gives dark signal

211.d---True about gadolinium :(H) heavy metal element,paramagnetic substance,used as MR contrast agent

212.d---True about Gd DTPA contrast:(H) chelated to DTPA which allows safe renal excretion,dose is approx. 0.2mg/kg body weight,does not generally cross BBB,produce high signal on T1 and low signal on T2

213.b---True regarding Gadolinium contrast: (H)enhance lesions lacking BBB,avoided in <6moths of age,nephrogenic systemic fibrosis in patients with renal insufficiency

214.d---Contraindications of MR imaging are (H)cardiac pacemaker or permanent pacemakers leads,intracranial aneurysm clip,chochlear prostheses

215.a---Maximum radiation exposure is noted in bone scan

216.a---Helium ion shows maximum potential of ionization

217.d---Systemic radionuclides are Samarium 153,Strontium 89,phosphorus 32

218.d---Radiocontrast is contraindicated in hypovolemia,chronic renal insufficiency,metformin treatment

219.b--Photoelectric effect refers to interaction between low energy incident photon and the inner shell electron

220.c---Crompton effect refers to interaction between high energy incident photon and the outer shell electron

221.b---Wall of CT scanner room is coated with lead

222.c----The difference between light and x ray is energy

223.a---the most ionizing radiation is Alpha

224.b---Background radiation refers to radiation present constantly from natural resources

285.d----Amount of radition delivered to an organ in the radiation field is known as absorbed dose

286.a----True regarding stochastic effect severity dose dependent

287.d---True statement regarding contrast agent is ionic monomers have three iodine atoms /two particles in solution

289.a---Dose of radiation during whole body exposure that leads to hematological syndrome is 2Gy

290.c---Regarding magic angle phenomenon in MRI imaging :(G) artefactual increased signal from tendons on short TE imaging sequence,angle of alignment of tendon to static magnetic field is apprex.55 degree,magic angle effect is seen in ligament ,cartilage or menisci`,magic angle effect is not persistent on long TE sequence

291.d---Black synovium on MRI is noted in (G) pigmented villonodular synovitis,amyloid deposition,hemophiliac arthropathy

292.c---Appearance of water/edema in MRI imaging(G) dark on T1W,bright on T2W

293.a---Diffusion MR sequence is sensitive to the microscopic motion of water(H) Diffusion MR

294.a---Perfusion MR is the most sensitive technique for detecting acute ischemic stroke (H)

NERVOUS SYSTEM

1.Which MR sequence is sensitive to the microscopic motion of water(H)

a.Diffusion MR

b.Perfusion MR

c.MR spectroscopy

d.functional MR

2.What is the most sensitive technique for detecting acute ischemic stroke (H)

a.perfusion MR

b.diffusion MR

c.MR spectroscopy

d.functional MR

3.CT scan is pragmatic choice for initial evaluation of all except (H)

a.acute changes in mental status

b.suspected stroke/heamorrhage

c.intrcranial/spinal trauma

d.multiple sclerosis

4.What is pragmatic choice for initial evaluation of intracranial trauma/spinal trauma(H)

a.CT scan

b.MRI

c.X RAY

d.Nuclear scan

5.All are true regarding role of MRI and CT except (H)

a.In general,CT is more sensitive than MRI for lesions of CNS

b.MRI is more sensitive than CT for lesions of spinal cord,cranial nerves posterior fossa structures

c.CT is more sensitive than MRI for fine osseos detail

d.CT is indicated in iniatial evalution of conducting hearing loss

6.MRI with contrast is recommended technique for all except(H)

a.neoplasm(primary/metastatic)

b.infection /abscess

c.cranial neuropathy/menineal disease

d.acute trauma

7.MRI with coronal T2 imaging is recommended in(H)

a.partial complex/refractory seizure

b.subarachnoid hemorrhage

c.anerysm

d.acute trauma

8.Recommended technique for subacute /chronic hemorrhage is(H)

a.MRI

b.CT

c.nuclear scan

d.none

9.Recommended technique for acute parenchymal hemorrhage is(H)

a.CT

b.MRI

c.both

d.none

10.Recommended technique for subarachmoid hemorrhage are all except(H)

a.CT and CTA

b.lumbar puncture

c.Angiography

d.nuclear scan

11.Recommended technique for aneurysm is (H)

a.Angiography

b.CTA

c.MRA

d.none

12.Recommended technique for hemorrhagic infarction is (H)

a.CT

b.MRI

c.both

d.none

13.Recommended technique for vertebral /carotid dissection is (H)

a.MRI/MRA

b.CTA

c.both

d.none

14.CTA is recommended in (H)

a.subachnoid hemorrhage

b.vertebral basilar insufficiency

c.carotid stenosis

d.multiple sclerosis

15.MRI+gradient echo imaging is recommended in(H)

a.white matter disorder

b.demyelinating disease

c.shear injury/chronic hemorrhage

d.headache /migraine

16.MRI is recommended technique for (H)

a.vascular malformation

b.dementia,white matter diseases,

c.demyelinating disease

d.all

17.True regarding cysticerci in brain parenchyma

a.size 5-20mm in diameter

b.round

c.both

d.none

18.On CT scan bone appears as(H)

a.an area of high density due to greater x ray attenuation

b.an area of high density due to lesser x ray attenuation

c. an area of low density due to greater x ray attenuation

b.an area of low density due to lesser x ray attenuation

19.Advantages of MDCT are all except(H)

a.longer scan time

b.reduced patient and organ motion

c.CT perfusion study

d.CT angiography study

20. Role of iodinated contrast in CT scan are all except(H)

a.identify vascular structures

b.detect defect in blood-brain- barrier

c.pituitary gland,chroid plexux,dura normally enhance after contrast

d.High risk of allergic reactions

21.CT scan Is the primary study of choice in the evaluation of(H)

a.acute changes in mental status

b.focal neurologic finding

c.acute trauma to the brain and spine

d.subacute /chronic hemorrhage

22.CT is complimentary to MR in evaluation of(H)

a.the skull base

b. orbit

c.osseous structures of spine

d.all

23 True about CT cisternography is (H)

a.Indicated in CSF fistula

b.evaluate intracranial cisterns

c.intrathecal contrast injection

d.all

24.Cortical tuber,subependymal nodule and giant cell astrocytoma are features of

a.Von Hippel-lindau syndrome

b.tuberous sclerosis

c.Sturge –Weber syndrome

d.neurofibromatsis

25.'Tram track ' gyriform calcification is feature of

a.Von Hippel-lindau syndrome

b.tuberous sclerosis

c.Sturge –Weber syndrome

d.neurofibromatsis

26. Which is intraconal orbital mass lesion

a.optic nerve glioma/meningioma

b.rhabdomyosarcoma

c.orbital cellulitis

d.dermoid

27.Intradural spinal mass is (C)

a.meningioma

b.ependymoma

c.astrocytoma

d.prolapsed disc

28.Percentage of retinoblastoma showing calcification on CT(C)

a.over 90%

b.over 70%

c.over60%

d.over50%

29.Tram track sign is noted in which orbital lesion(C)

a.optic nerve glioma

b.optic nerve meningioma

c.retinoblastoma

d.toxocariasis

30.The most common type of cranial herniation is(H)

a. transtentorial herniation

b.uncal herniation

c.transfalcial herniation

d.forminal herniation

31.Kernohan-Waltman sign is seen in (H)

a. transtentorial herniation

b.uncal herniation

c.transfalcial herniation

d.forminal herniation

32.MRI abnormalities in mesial temporal lobes are seen in

a.paraneoplastic encephalitis

b.autoimmune encephalitis

c.HHV-6 encephalitis

d.multiple sclerosis

33.Meningeal involvement in tuberculos meningitis is pronounced at

a.convexity of brain

b.base of brain

c.both

d.none

34.In what % of cases of tuberculous meningitis has evidence of old pulmonary lesions or of milliary pattern

a.more than 50%

b.more than20%

c.more than 30%

d.more than 40%

35.Causes of ring enhancing lesion in brain in HIV infected patients are all except

a.toxoplasmosis

b.CNS lymphoma

c.TB/Fungal/bacterial abscess

d.acute infarction

36.All are neuro imaging finding suggestive of nerocysticercosis except

a.cystic lesions with or without enhancement

b.one or more nodular calcifactions

c.focal enhancing lesions

d.diffuse ceerebritis

37.Imaging modality of choice in patients with acute strokes(H)

a.contrast CT of head

b.noncontrast CT of head

c.contrast MRIof head

d.noncontrast MRI of head

38.All are true about T2-weighted signal except(H)

A use of longer TE and TR

b.Csf and edema produce high signal

c. more sensitive to demyelination,infarction and chronic hemorrhage

d.Csf has short T1 and T2 relaxation time

39 correct matching of signal produced (H)

	CSF	FAT	EDEMA
a.T1W	low	high	low
b.T2W	low	low	low
c.FLAIR	low	medium	low
d. Flair	high	medium	low

40.Correct matching of signal on T1W images(H)

a.fat --- high signal

b.subscute hemorrhage –low signal

c.CSF---high signal

d.brain—high signal

41.Correct matching of signal on T2W images are all exept(H)

a.CSF–high signal

b.fat—low signal

c.brain—high signal

d.edema –low signal

42. Correct matching of signal on FLAIR images are all exept(H)

a.CSF –low signal

b.fat—medium signal

c.brain—high signal

d.edema –high signal

43.All are true about MRI sequence except(H)

a.In FLAIR, csf signal is suppressed

b.FLAIR is more sensitive to edema or water containing lesions than standard spin echo c.susceptibility weighted imaging is indicated in lesions with microhemorrhages

d.Gradient echo imaging is less sensitive to magnetic susceptibility generated by blood,calcium and air

44.The most common intramedullary tumour of cord in children(SW)

a.ependymoma

b.astrocytoma

c.haemangioblastoma

d.teratomas

45.Insular ribbon sign is a finding of

a.Posteror cerebral artery infarction

b.anterior cerebral artery infarction

c.Middle cerebral artery infarction

b.anterior cerebellar artery infarction

46.Empty delta sign is a feature of

a. cerebral arterial infarction

b.acute venous infarction

c.both

d.none

47.Multiple arteriovenous malformations are noted in

a.Osler-Weber-Rendu syndrome

b.Wyburn-Mason syndrome

c.both

d.none

48.MRI of brain showing a central pop-corn core of high T1W with surrounding rim of hemosiderin(very lowT2W signal) is suggestive of

a.venous haemangioma

b.arteriovenous malformation

c.cavernous angioma

d.none

49.Rasmussen 's encephalitis is characterized by

a.atrophy localized to one cerebral hemisphere

b.atrophy involving both cerebral hemisphere

c.atrophy of basal ganglia

d.atrophy of bilateral perisylvian area

50.All are hyperdense leions of brain on CT except

a.meningioma

b.lymphoma

c.colloid cyst

d.glioma

51.C-shaped calcification in brain is due to

a.dural calcification

b.pineal gland calcification

c.habenular commissure calcification

d.parasellar ligament calcification

52.Sharply defined CSF-containing structures that surround small arteries as they penetrate the brain is known as

a.virchow-Robin space

b.ambient space

c.both

d.none

53.The standard technique for extracranial vascular MRA(H)

a.TOF

b.phase –contrast MRA

c.contrast –enhanced MRA

d.none

54. The most common primary CNS neoplasm(SW)

a.oligodendroglioma

b.astrocytoma

c.epedymoma

d.choroid plexus papilloma

55.Gray matter contain -- %more water than white matter(H)

a.10-15%

b.5-10%

c.15-25%

d.none

56 Echoplanar MR imaging is basis of all except(H)

a.diffusion imaging and tractography

b.perfusion imaging

c.functional imaging

d.MR angiography(TOF and phase contrast)

57.All are true regarding Diffusion weighted imaging(H)

a.assess microscopic motion of water

b.restricted motion of water appear as low signal

c.infarcted tissue reduces water motion within cells and interstitial tissue

d.sensitive to infarction,encephalitis,abscess

58.The most sensitive technique for detection of acute cerebral infarction of <7days(H)

a.diffusion weighted imaging

b.CT

c.MRA

d.Nuclear scan

59.Typical finding of infarction on perfusion imaging is(H)

a.delay in mean transit time

b.reduction in cerebral blood volume

c.reduction in cerebral blood flow

d.all

60.Imaging that assess the microscopic motion of water along white matter tracts (H)

a.diffusion tensor imaging

b.diffusion weighted imaging

c.perfusion imaging

d.functional imaging

61.EPI technique that localizes regions of activity in brain following task activation(H)

a.diffusion tensor imaging

b.diffusion weighted imaging

c.perfusion imaging

d.functional imaging

62.All are true regarding magnetic nerve neurography except(H)

a.indicated in rediculopathy with normal conventional MR study of spine

b.suspected peripheral nerve entrapement

c.peripheral nerve trauma

d.T1weighted image

63.PET finding in Alzheimer's diseases(H)

a.a lower activity of FDG in the parietal lobes

b.a higher activity of FDG in parietal lobes

c. a lower activity of FDG in the temporal lobes

d.a higher activity of FDG in temporal lobes

64.Present indications of conventional plan-film myelography are(H)

a.suspected meningeal or arachnoid cyst

b.localisation of spinal dural arteriovenous

c. localisation of spinal CSF fistula

d.All

65.Myelography should be prformed with caution in all except(H)

a. elevated intracranial pressure

b.evidence of spinal block

c.history of allergic reactions to intrathecal contrast

d.spinal csf fistula

66 The most commonly used route for angiography (H)

a.femoral route

b.axillary route

c.antecubital route

d.none

67.The most feared complication of cerebral angiography(H)

a.stroke

b.reversible brainstem dysfunction

c.acute short term memory loss

d.none

68.Prior to aortic artery aneurysm,spinal angiography is done to identify(H)

a.the artery of Adamkiewicz

b.the artery of labbe

c.the artery of Trolard

d.the artery of Rolan

69.Correct matching of interventional therapy(H)

a.carebral aneurysm—detachable coils

b.arteriovenous malformation—particulate or liquid adhesive emboisation

c.carotid-cavernous fistula—balloon occlusion

d.infarction---coils

70.The most common syndrome associated with focal seizure with dyscognitive features(H)

a.medial temporal lobe sclerosis

b.Lennox-Gastaut syndrome

c.juvenile myoclonic seizure

d. absence seizure

71.High resolution MRI finding of medial temporal lobe sclerosis are all except(H)

a.small hippocampus

b.small temporal lobe

c.enlarged temporal horn

d. increased signal on T1 weighted image

72.All are true about imaging in seizures except(H)

a.almost all patients with new-onset seizure should have brain imaging

b.CT is superior to MRI for detection of lesions associated with epilepsy

c.Hippocampal sclerosis is associated with medial temporal lobe sclerosis

d.PET and SPECT is used to evaluate some of patients with medical refractory seizures

73.Eligibility criteria for use of IV rtPA are all except(H)

a.<3 hr time window

b. hemmorrhage or edemaof >1/3 of MCA territory on CT

c.age = >18yrs

d.clinical diagnosis of stroke

74. Drop metastases is noted (SW)

a.oligodendroglioma

b.astrocytoma

c.epedymoma

d.choroid plexus papilloma

75.Puff of smoke appearance on conventional x ray angiography is noted in(H)

a.moyamoya disease

b.CADASIL

c.giant cell arteritis

d.mitochondrial disorder

76.Notch-3 mutation is noted in(H)

a.CADASIL

b.CARASIL

c.HERNS

d.CERNS

77.Role MRI in strokes are all except(H)

a.reliably document infarction in posterior fossa and cortical surface

b.DWI is more sensitive for early brain infarction than standard MRI sequences

c.Brain regions showing poor perfusion but no abnormality on diffusion are equivalent measure of ischemic penumbra

d.MR angiography is poorly sensitive for stenosis of extracranial internal crotd arteries and of large intracranial cessels

78.The Gold standard for identifying and quantifying atherosclerotic stenoses of cerebral arteries is(H)

a.conventional x ray cerebral angiography

b. CT angiography

c.MR angiography

d.Doppler

79. Conventional x- ray cerebral angiography is gold standard for identifying and characterizing(H)

a.aneurysm

b.vasospasm

c.intraliminal thrombi

d.all

80. Conventional x- ray cerebral angiography is gold standard for identifying and characterizing(H)

a.fibromuscular dysplasia

b.arteriovenous fistula

c.vasculitis

d.all

81.Investigation that can quantify cerebral blood flow (H)

a.xenon-CT

b.PET

c.both.

d.none

82.The most common type of intracranial hemorrhage (H)
a.ICH
b.EDH
c.SDH
d.sub-arachnoid hemorrhage

83.probably the most common cause of lobar hemorrhage in the elderly(H)
a.hypertention
b.cerebral amyloid angiopathy
c.trauma
d.cocaine

84.All are neuroimaging feature suggestive of dementia exept(H)
a.Alzheimer's disease---hippocampal atrophy and posterior dominant cortical atrophy
b.FTD—frontal,insular and or temporal atrophy,spares posterior parietal lobule
c.DLB—posteror parietal atrophy,hippocampi larger than AD,greater involvemet of amygdale than hippocampi
D.CJD—cortical ribboning and basal ganglia or thalamus hypointensity on diffusion or FLAIR MRI

85.Radioligand for detecting brain amyloid associated with amyloid angiopathy or neurotic plaque(H)
a.Pittsburg compound- B
b.^{18}F-AV-45
c.both
d.none

86.The neuroimaging features of normal-pressure hydrocephalus are all except(H)
a.hydrocephalus
b.little or no cortical atrophy
c.propped open sylvian fissure
d.perisylvian atrophy

87.Boxcarring is seen in(H)
a.NPH
b.aqueductal stenosis
c.Alzheimar'disease
d.CBD

88. The most common malignant paediatric brain tumour(SW)
a.medulloblastoma
b.astrocytoma
c.ependymoma
d.choroid plexus papilloma

89.The hallmark feature of Parkinson's disease are all except(H)
a. degeneration of dopaminergic neurons in

substantia nigra pars compacta

b.reduced striatal dopamine

c.leswy bodies

d.globus pallidus involvment

90.MRI features of multiple system atrophy are all except(H)

a.iron accumulation on striatum on T2 weighted scan

b.putaminal rim

c.pontine 'hot cross buns sign'

d.the'hummingbird'sign

91.The hummingbird sign in midsagittal images of MRI of brain is noted in(H)

a.Parkinson'disease

b.multiple system atrophy

c.progressive supranuclear palsy

d.corticobasal degeneration

92 Pontine 'hot cross buns sign' and putaminal rim is noted in(H)

a.Parkinson'disease

b.multiple system atrophy

c.progressive supranuclear palsy

d.corticobasal degeneration

93.Atrophy of caudate nuclei on MRI imaging is seen in(H)

a.Parkinson'disease

b.multiple system atrophy

c.progressive supranuclear palsy

d.Huntington's disease

94.CT and MRI changes in caudate,putamen and pallidum in Wilson 'disease(H)

a.hypodensity on CT and hyperintensity on T2MRI

b.hyperdensity on CT and hyperintensity on T2MRI

c.hypodensity onCT and hypointensity on T2MRI

d.hyperdensity on CT and hypointensity on T2MRI

95.Features of oligodendroglioma (H)

a.fried egg appearance on histology

b.nonenhancing

c.partially calcified

d.All

96.The most common form of hereditary ataxia is(H)

a.Friedriech ataxia

b.Spinocerebellar ataxia

c.Ataxia telangiectasia

d.none

97.MRI finding of spinal cord atrophy is noted in(H)

a.Huntington's chorea

b.Freidriech ataxia

c.SCA

d.none

98.cereballar and brainstem atrophy on MRI is noted in(H)

a.Huntington's chorea

b.Freidriech ataxia

c.SCA

d.none

99.The most common form of progressive motor neurone disease(H)

a.amytrophic lateral sclerosis

b.primary lateral sclerosis

c.progressive muscular atrophy

d.none

100.MRI finding of thinning of corticospinal tract in brain and spinal cord is noted in(H)

a.amytrophic lateral sclerosis

b.primary lateral sclerosis

c.progressive muscular atrophy

d.none

101.Crescentric blood collection in cranial trauma on CT SCAN is noted in(H)

a.Subdural haematoma

b.cpidural hematoma

c.both

d.none

102.Lenticular blood collection in cranial trauma on CT SCAN is noted in(H)

a.Subdural haematoma

b.epidural hematoma

c.both

d.none

103.The preferred diagnostic test for patients suspected of having brain tumour(H)

a.noncotrast MRI

b.contrast MRI

c.CECT

d.nuclear medicine

104.Imaging features of malignant tumour of brain are all except(H)

a.typically enhance with gadolinium

b.characteristically sorrounded by edema of the neighbouring white matter

c.both

d.none

105.All are correct regarding imaging of brain tumor except(H)

a.low grade glioma typically enhance strongly

b.low grade glioma ie best appreciated on FLAIR sequence

c.meningioma donot invade the brain

d.meningioma are dural based with dural tail

106.All are true except regarding imaging of brain tumour(H)

a.functional MRI is useful in presurgical planning and defining eloqouent motor ,sensory and language cortex

b.PET is useful in defining the metabolic activity of the lesions

c.MR perfusion provide information on blood flow

d.MR spectroscopy provide no information on tissue compostion

107. Grade iv astrocytoma is(H)

a.pilocystic astrocytoma

b.diffuse astrocytoma

c.anaplastic astrocytoma

d.glioblastoma

108.The most common brain tumour of childhood(H)

a.diffuse astrocytoma

b.pilocystic astrocytoma

c.anaplastic astrocytoma

d.glioblastoma

109.MRI finding of the cystic cerebellar lesions with enhancing mural nodule in childhood suggest(H)

a.diffuse astrocytoma

b.pilocystic astrocytoma

c.anaplastic astrocytoma

d.glioblastoma

110.All are true regarding brain tumour(H)

a.most common brain tumour is metastases rather than primary brain tumor

b.at least half of primary brain tumour is malignant in nature

c.glial tumours account for 60% of all primary brain tumour

d.only 30% of primary brain tumour is malignant in nature

111.The most common cause of malignant primary brain tumour(H)

a.metastases

b.glioblastoma

c.diffuse astrocytoma

d.anaplastic astrocytoma

112.MRI feature showing ring enhancing masses with central necrosis and surrounding edema in 6th decade suggest of(H)

a.diffuse astrocytoma

b.pilocystic astrocytoma

c.anaplastic astrocytoma

d.glioblastoma

113.Nonenhancing tumours are all except(H)

a.diffuse astrocytoma

b.oligodendroglioma

c.gliomatosis cerebri

d.glioblastoma

114.Imaging feature of primary cental nervous system lymphoma are all except(H)

a.dense tumour

b.enhancing tumour

c.basal ganglia,corpus callosum and periventricular location

d.multiple in immunocompetent patients

115.The most common malignant brain tumour of childhood(H)

a.medulloblastoma

b.lymphoma

c.glioblastoma

d.meningioma

116.The most common primary brain tumour(H)

a.meningioma

b.glioblastoma

c.lymphoma

d.medulloblastoma

117.Dural tail is found in(H)

a.meningioma

b.glioblastoma

c.lymphoma

d.medulloblastoma

118.Imaging features of meningioma are all except(H)

a.dense tumour

b.arise from dura ,dural tail

c.partially calcified

d.nonenhancing

119.imaging features on vestibular schwannomas are all except(H)

a.dense non enhancing tumor

b.enlarge internal auditory canal

c.often extend in cerebellopontine angle

d.d/d is meningioma

120. Imaging features of epidermoid cysts are all except(H)

a.usually in CP angle

b.extra-axial lesion

c.CSF like imagin characteristics

d.no restricton of diffusion

121.Imaging features of epidermoid cyst are all except(H)

a.peripheral location

b.T1 hyperintensity

c.resemble lipoma

d. both epidermal and dermal structures

122.The most common source of brain metastases(H)

a.lung

b.breast

c.GIT

d.kidney

123.which tumour has the greatest propensity to metastasize to brain(H)

a. lung

b.melanoma

c.GIT

d.kidney

124.The greatest propensity to hemorrhage in intracranial metastases are noted in all except(H)

a.melanoma

b.kidney

c.thyroid

d.prostate

125.The most common cause of hemorrhagic metastasis is(H)

a.lung

b.kidney

c.thyroid

d.prostate

126.The most common source of epidural metastases in male (H)

a.prostate

b.lung

c.kidney

d.thyroid

127.The most common source of epidural metastases in female (H)

a.breast

b.uterus

c.cervix

d.ovary

128.The best test for diagnosis of epidural metastasis(H)

a.noncontrast MRI of complete spine

b.contrast MRI of complete spine

c.CT scan of complete spine

d.nuclear scan

129.Second the most common cause of neurologic disability in early to middle childhood(H)

a.trauma

b.multiple sclerosis

c.tumour

d.nutritional deficiency

130.All are true regarding MRI imaging of multiple sclerosis except(H)

a.90% of visualized lesions are symptomatic

b.Gd enhancement serve as useful marker of inflammation

c.Gd enhancement persist for approximately one month

d.The residual MS plaque

remains visible indefinitely on T2W spin echo

131.In proper clinical setting, MRI features(FLAIR and diffusion weighted) suggestive of Cruetzfeldt Jacob disease are(H)

a.increased intensity on basal ganglia

b.cortical ribboning

c.both

d.none

132.All are true regarding lesions of multiple sclerosis except(H)

a.multifocal

b.frequently oriented perpendicular to the ventricular surface

c.lesions in anterior corpus callosum frequent in MS and rare in vascular disease

d.dark on T2

133.All are true regarding multiple sclerosis except(H)

a.total volume of T2W signal abnormality doesnot show any significant correlation with clinical disability

b.measure of brain atrophy show a significant correlation with clinical disability

c.one third of T2W lesions appear as hypointense lesions(black holes) on T1W image

d.black holes may be marker of irreversible demyelination and axonal loss

134.Imaging which may serve as a surrogate markers of clinical disability in multiple sclerosis(H)

a.magnetisation transfer ratio imaging

b.magnetic resonance spectroscopic imaging

c.both

d.none

135 which mar distinguish demyelination from edema in multiple sclerosis(H)

a.magnetisation transfer ratio imaging

b.magnetic resonance spectroscopic imaging

c.both

d.none

136.Typical locations of multiple sclerosis lesions are all exept(H)

a.periventricular and juxtacortical

b.spinal cord

c.infratentorial

d.basal ganglia

137.MRI finding that favor ADEM over MS are all except(H)

a.relatively symmetric white matter abnormalities

b.basal ganglia or cortical gray matter lesions

c.Gd enhancement of all abnormal areas

d.generally unilateral optic nerve involvement and incomplete transverse myelopathy

138.All are true regarding HSV encephalitis except(H)

a.CT is less sensitive than MRI and is normal in upto 20-35% of petients

b.lesions hypointense on T2W image

c.frontotemporal,insular and cingulate areas involvement

d.lesion sensitivity increased by addition of FLAIR/diffusion weighted image

139.All are feature of mature brain abscess on MRI imaging(H)

a.hypointense due to restricted diffusion

b.hyperintense central area of pus on T2W image

c.well defined hypointense capsule on T2W image

d.hyperintense surrounding edema on T2Wimage

140 Ring enhancing lesion with restricted diffusion of central hyperintensity on T2W image suggest of (H)

a.abscess

c.oligodendroglioma

c.HSV encephalitis

d.none

141.All are true regarding hyperperfusion syndrome of CNS except(H)

a.High T2 signal

b.primarily in occipital lobe

c. no respect of any single vascular territory

d.normal diffusion weighted image indicating cytotoxic edema

142. True regarding imaging in psychiatric disorder (H)

a.reduced metabolic or neural activity in dorsolateral prefrontal cortex in schizophrenia

b.increased activation of the amygdale by negative stimuli in depression

c.reduced activation of nucleus

accumbens by rewarding stimuli in depression

d.all

143.The thumbprint sign in lateral view of soft tissue of neck is seen in(H)

a.enlarged edematous epiglottis

b.adenoid

c.both

d.none

144.What is pragmatic choice for initial evaluation of suspected stoke /hemorrhage(H)

a.CT scan

b.MRI

c.X RAY

d.Nuclear scan

145.As per NASCET and ECST ,Carotid endaretectomy provide substantial benefit in patients with stenosis of(H)

a.=>50%

b.=>60%

c.=>70%

d=.>80%

146.All are true regarding imaging in acute strokes except(H)

a.CT may not reliably show infarction for 24-48hrs

b.CT may miss small infarct in posterior fossa and cortical surface

c.carotid diseases and intracranial vascular occlusions are readily identified by CTA

d.MRI is more sensitive than CT for detecting acute blood

147.The most common cause of recurrent aseptic viral meningitis(N)

a.herpes simplex virus

b.EBV

c.CMV

d.influenza virus

148.Brain structures showing propenisity for calcification in congenital toxoplasmosis are all except(N)

a.caudate nucleus and basal ganglia

b.chroroid plexus

c.subependyma

d.cerebellum

149.Pathognomonic sign in MRI of brain for neurocysticrcosis(N)

a.calcification

b.protoscolex in cyst

c.basialar archnoiditis

d.none

150.Single non- enhancing cyst in brain are all except(N)

a.hydatid cyst

b.arachnoid cyst

c.porencephly

d.metastases

151.Calcification in brain is noted in (N)

a.tuberous sclerosis

b.tuberculosis

c.CMV/toxoplasmosis

d.all

152.Enhancing lesions in brain is noted in(N)

a.tuberculsis

b.abscess

c.metastases

d.all

153.The most common astrocytoma in children (N)

a.fibrillary infiltration astrocytoma

b.pilocytic astrocytoma

c.pilomyxoid astrocytoma

d.malignant astrocytoma

154.The enhancing nodula within wall of cystic lesion in cerebellum of children is the classic feature of(N)

a.fibrillary infiltration astrocytoma

b.pilocytic astrocytoma

c.pilomyxoid astrocytoma

d.malignant astrocytoma

155.Calcified cortical mass in frontal lobe on CT in the patient presenting with seizure is suggestive of(N)

a.astocytoma

b.oligodendroglioma

c.ependymoma

d.medulloblastoma

156.Brain tumour associated with Li-Fraumeni syndrome (N)

a.choroid plexus tumour

b.astrocytoma

c.PNETs

d.medulloblastoma

157.Solid ,homogenous,contrast-enhancing mass in cerebellar vermis in child causing 4th ventricular obstruction and hydrocephalus is suggestive of(N)

a.choroid plexus tumour

b.ependymoma

c.PNETs

d.medulloblastoma

158.Imaging of brain of children showing a suprasellar cystic lesion with solid component and calcification suggests of (N)

a.craniopharyngioma

b.meduloblastoma

c.ependymoma

d.choroid plexus tumour

159.X-ray features of skull in chronically increased intracranial pressure are all except(N)

a.erosion of posterior clinoid processes

b.enlargement of the sella turcica

c.increased convolutional markings

d.thickening of skull bone

160.The imaging method of choice for detecting intracranial haemorrhage in infants with patent anterior fontanels(N)

a.cranial ultrasound

b. CT scan

c.MRI

d.x ray

161.The imaging method of choice for detecting periventricular leukomalacia in infants with patent anterior fontanels(N)

a.CT scan

b. cranial ultrasound

c.MRI

d.x ray

162.The imaging method of choice for detecting

hydrocephalus in infants with patent anterior fontanels(N)

a.CT scan

b. cranial ultrasound

c.MRI

d.x ray

163.All are true regarding use of CT in children except(N)

a.non-invasive

b.no radiation issue,children being less sensitive to radiation than adults

c.less useful for diagnosing acute infarct in children

d.can be used to evaluate craniofacial abnormalities or craniosynostosis

164.A noncontrast CT can demonstrate (N)

a.skull fractures/pneumocephalus

b.intracranial hemorrhage

c.impending herniation

d.all

165.Subtle signs of early infarction(<24hrs) on CT scan are all except(N)

a.sulcal effacement

b.blurring of gray white infarction

c.hyperdense middle cerebral artery

d.wedge-shaped hypodensity

166. All are true regarding hyperdense middle cerebral artery on CT scan except(N)
a.early infarction
b.often due to thrombosis
c.increased attenoution in the MCA
d. also noted in hemorrhage

167.Preferred imaging procedures in 1-24hrs old strokes in children(N)
a.MRI or MRA(head and neck) with diffusion weighted images
b.CT or CTA(head and neck)
c.USG
d.Nuclear scan

168.Preferred imaging procedures in 1-24 hrs old strokes in children who is unstable(N)
a.MRI or MRA(head and neck) with diffusion weighted images
b.CT or CTA(head and neck)
c.USG
d.Nuclear scan

169.Next investigation in children patients with infarction in the anterior circulation(detected by CT or MRI) is(N)
a.MRA

b.CTA
c.carotid USG
d.Nuclear scan

170.All are true regarding use of imagings in children except(N)
a.CT or MRI can detect infarct >24hrs.
b.MRI is preferred due to radiation issue
c.CT preferred if intraparenchymal hemorrhage<24hrs
d.MRI preferred for acute subarachnoid hemorrhage

171.The preferred imaging to detect vasospasm following subarachnoid hemorrhage in children(N)
a.CT
b.MRA
c.CTA
d.TCD(transcranial Doppler)

172. Bilateral acoustic neuromas is pathognomonic of (SW)
a.Neurofibromatosis type 1
b.Neurofibromatosis type 2
c.von hippel-Lindau syndrome
d.Sturge –Waber syndrome

173. Preferred investigation of hypoxic- ischemic brain injury in infants (N)

a. MRI

b.CT

c.USG

d.Nuclear investigation

174. Preferred investigation of metabolic disorder of brain in children(N)

a.MRI,particularly T2W and FLAIR

b.MRI,particularly T1W and diffusion-weighted image

c.noncontrast CT

d.contrast enhanced CT

175. Preferred investigation for detection of hydrocephalus in infants (N)

a.USG

b.CT

c.MRI

d.nuclear scan

176.Initial investigation in head trauma is(N)

a.CT

b.MRI

c.USG

d.none

177.MRI without and with contrast is used in all except(N)

a.multiple sclerosis

b.brain tumour

c.brain abscess

d.acute head injury

178. A noninvasive technique used to map neuronal activity during specific cognitive states/sensorimotor function is(N)

a.proton MR spectroscopy

b.functional MRI

c.SPECT

d.PET

179.Molecular imaging technique used to detect metabolites like NAA(N)

a.proton MR spectroscopy

b.functional MRI

c.SPECT

d.PET

180. Proton MR spectroscopy are useful in all except(N)

a.diagnosis of inborn error of metabolism

b.preoperative and postoperative assessment of intracranial tumour

c. in detection of cortical dysplasia

d. in detecting hypoxic-ischemic injury after 1st month day of life

181.The gold standard for diagnosing vascular disorders of the CNS(N)

a.MRA

b.CTA

c.Catheter angiography

d.none

182.SPECT radionuclide used to study regional cerebral blood flow(N)

a.Tc 99m-HMPAO

b.Tc 999m- methylene diphosphonate

c.DMSA

d.HIDA

183. SPECT of brain is particularly useful for assessing all except(N)

a.vasculitis/herpes encephalitis

b.dysplastic cortex

c.recurrent brain tumour

d.infarction

184.Spine x ray in simple spina bifida occulta shows defect in(N)

a.posterior vertebral arches and laminae

b.vertebral body

c.vertebral body and arch

d.vertebral body and lamina

185.All cases of occult spinal dysraphism is best investigated with(N)

a.CT

b.MRI

c.both

d.none

186.Imaging is indicated in all cutaneous lesions associated with occult spinal dysraphism except(N)

a.subcutaneous mass or lipoma

b.hairy patch

c.dermal sinus

d.coccygeal pits

187.Imaging is indicated in all cutaneous lesions associated with occult spinal dysraphism except(N)

a.vascular lesions – haemangioma ,telangiectasia

b.skin tags,tail-like appendages

c.scarlike lesions

d.simple dimples(deep<5mm,<25mm from anal verge)

188.All are true except(N)

a.meningocele—herniation of meninges through defect in posterior vertebral arch

b.myelomeningocele --- contain meningeal sac with spinal cord

c.encephalocele –contain meningeal sac and cerebral cortex,cerebellum or brainstem

d.anencephaly---normal

calvaria with redumentary
brain

189.Most common site of
myelomeningocele is(N)
a.cervical region
b.thoracic region
c.lumbosacral region
d.sacral region

190.MRI imaging showing
absence of cerebral
convolutions(sulci)and poorly
formed sylvian fissure giving
the appearance of 3-4 motn
fetal brain suggest of(N)
a.lissencephaly
b.heterotopia
c.schizencephaly
d.porencephaly

191.MRI study of brain
showing cerebral cleft is
suggestive of(N)
a.lissencephaly
b.heterotopia
c.schizencephaly
d.porencephaly

192.MRI study of brain
showing gray matter-like
substance within white matter
between ventricle and
cerebral cortex is suggestive
of(N)
a.lissencephaly
b.heterotopia

c.schizencephaly
d.porencephaly

193.MRI study of brain
showing single ventricle,an
absent falx and nonseprated
deep cerebral neclei is
suggestive of(N)
a.lissencephaly
b.holoprosencephaly
c.schizencephaly
d.porencephaly

194.The most common
malformation of posterior
fossa and hind brain(N)
a.Chiari malformation
b.Dandy-walker malformation
c.mega-cistena magna
d.arachnoid cysts

195.Displcement of cereballar
tonsil into cervical canal is
noted in(N)
a.Chiari malformation
b.Dandy-walker malformation
c.mega-cistena magna
d.arachnoid cysts

196.MRI imaging of brain
showing the cystic expansion
of 4th ventricle in posterior
fossa with midline cerebellar
hypoplasia is suggestive of(N)
a.Chiari malformation
b.Dandy-walker malformation
c.mega-cistena magna

d.arachnoid cysts

197.X ray feature of skull showing increased convolutinal markings(beaten-silver appearance) is noted in(N)

a.acute intracranial pressure rise

b.chronic increase of intracranial pressure

c.both

d.none

198. x ray of skull showing features of chronic increased intracranial pressures (N)

a.sepratation of sutures

b.erosion of posterior clinoid in older child

c.increased convolutional markings (silver-beaten appearance)

d.all

199 .All are features of neurofibromatosis 1 except(N)

a.sphenoid dysplasia

b.thinning of long bones

c.pseudoarthrosis

d.bilateral vestibular schwannoma

200.The characteristic brain lesion in tuberous sclerosis is(N)

a.cortical tuber

b.subependymal nodule

c.subependymal giant cell astrocytoma

d.multiple retinal hamartomas

201.Candle dripping appearance of ventricle is noted in(N)

a.Sturge –Weber syndrome

b.neurofibromatosis

c.tuberous sclerosis

d.VHL

202.The best way of identifying cortical tuber in tuberous sclerosis is(N)

a.MRI

b.CT

c.USG

d.nuclear scan

203.The imaging modality of choice for demonstrating leptomeningeal angioma in Sturge-Weber syndrome is(N)

a.MRI

b.CT

c.USG

d.nuclear scan

204. The Roach scale is related to(N)

a.Sturge –Weber syndrome

b.neurofibromatosis

c.tuberous sclerosis

d.VHL

205.Leptomeningeal angiomatosis, underlying cerebral atrophy and calcification are features of(N)

a.VHL

b.neurofibromatosis

c.tuberous sclerosis

d.Sturge –Weber syndrome

206.'Eye of the tiger sign ' (hyperentense area within hypointense area in globus pallidus) in MRI of brain is noted in(N)

a.Mcleod 's syndrome

b.Lesch- Nyhan syndrome

c.Hallervorden Spatz syndrome

d.Wilson disease

207.Which imaging technique is being used for white matter tracts in spastic diplegia(N)

a.MRI with diffusion tensor imaging

b.MRI with FLAIR

c.MRI with contrast

d.MRI with fat suppression

208.MRI finding in cerebral palsiy are all except(N)

a.periventricular leucomalacia

b.injury to thalmocortical and corticospinal pathways

c.multicystic cortical encephalomalacia

d.all

209.MRI finding in posterior reversible leucoencephalopathy are all except(N)

a.increase in signal in occipital lobes on T2W image

b.patchy lesions involving gray and white matter

c.bilateral

d.restricted diffusion as a rule

210.Criteria for MRI disseminationin space include all except(N)

a.Gadolinium enhancing lesions or 9T2 lesions

b.3 or more infratentorial lesions

c. 1 or more juxtacortical lesions

d.3 or more periventricular lesions

211.The study of choice for acute disseminated encephalitis(N)

a.CT

b.PET

c.MRI

d.USG

212.Cranial MRI features that favour ADEM is all except(N)

a.wodespresd patchy lesions

b.frequent involvement of thalamus and basal

ganglia,cortical gray-white matter junction

c.lesions of similar age,improvement in lesions on follow up MRI

d.frequent involvement of periventricular white matter and corpus callosum

213.Diffusion weighted imaging can detect acute ischemic stroke (N)

a.within minutes of strokes

b.within hrs of strokes

c.within days of strokes

d.none of above

214.Investigation that is very insensitive for cerebral sinovenousthrombosis is(N)

a.contrast CT venography

b.MR venography

c.nonenhanced CT

d.diffusion MRI

215.The most common cause of childhood subarachnoid and intraparenchymal hemorrhage is(N)

a.aneurysm

b.arteriovenous malformations

c.hematological disorder

d.cavernomas

216.Which MRI imparts black signal to blood products (N)

a.diffusion imaging

b.gradient echo imaging

c.perfusion imaging

d.tensor imaging

217.High lactate in MR spectroscopy is noted in(N)

a.MELAS

b.medulloblastoma

c.sub arachnoid hemorrhage

d.extradural hematoma

218.All are true regarding imaging of brain abscess except(N)

a.most reliable methds are CECT and MRI

b.MRI is diagnostic test of choice

c.ring enhancing lesion on CECT

d.cerebritis appears as hypardense on CECT

219.Beyand the infancy,conus medularis ends at the level of (N)

a.L1

b.L2

c.L3

d.L4

220.In congenital tethered spinal cord,the position of conus medullaris is(N)

a.L2

b.L2

c.L3

d.L4

221.MRI of spinal cord reveals two spinal cord,each with its own dural tube and seprated by a spicule of bone and cartilage.The diagnosis is (N)

a.syringomyelia

b.diastematomyelia

c.tethered cord syndrome

d.none

222.The radiologic study of choice for syringomyelia is(N)

a.MRI

b.CT

c.USG

d.Nuclear scan

223.The diagnostic study of choice for spinal cord tumours is(N)

a.MRI without contrast

b.MRI with contrast

d.CT

d.Nuclear scan

224.SCIWORA refers to(N)

a.a kind of spinal tumour

b.a kind of AVM

c.a kind of spinal cord injury

d.a kind of inflammatory lesion

225.Perinaud's syndrome may be associated with(N)

a.tumour of hypothalamus

b. a.tumour of pineal gland

c.tumour of cerebellum

d.tumour of pituitary gland

226.The anomalies of midline structures of brain with hypoplasia of optic nerves,optic chiasm,optic tracts is noted in(N)

a.Goldenhar 's syndrome

b.VHL

c.de Morsier's syndrome

d.Stargardt disease

227.The most common site fracture from blunt trauma of orbit(N)

a.orbital floor

b.medial wall

c.superior orbital fracture

d.lateral wall fracture

228.Blow-out fracture of orbit involve(N)

a.orbital floor

b.medial wall

c.superior orbital fracture

d.lateral wall fracture

229.Klippel-Trenaunay syndrome comprises all exept(N)

a.cutaneous vascular malformation

b.bony and soft tissue hypertrophy

c.venous abnormality

d.arterial aneurysm

230.In multiple pituitary harmone deficiency imaging show(N)
a.small pituitary gland
b.missing or attenuated pituitary stalk
c.ectopic posterior pituitary bright spot
d.all

231.Radiological features of congenital hypothyroidism are all except(N)
a.absent distal femoral epiphysis
b.epiphyseal dysgenesis
c.beaking of 12th thoracic ,1st,2nd lumber vertebra
d.craniosynostosis

232.Radiological features of skull of congenital hypothyroidism are all except(N)
a.large fontanels
b.wide sutures
c.wormian bones
d.often small sella turcica

233.DiGeorge syndrome is associated with(N)
a.aplasia or hypoplasia of parathyroid gland
b.aplasia or hypoplasia of parathyroid gland
c.aplasia or hypoplasia of parathyroid gland
d.aplasia or hypoplasia of parathyroid gland

234.Pancake type,cup type and ball type are types of which cranial abnormality(RUMACK)
a.ventriculomegaly
b.holoprosencephaly
c.encephalocele
d.corpus callosum agenesis

235.Lobester claw is found in(RUMACK)
a.Cornelia de Lange's syndrome
b.carpenter syndrome
c.Meckel-Gruber's syndrome
d.Proteus syndrome

236.Sandal toes is found in(RUMACK)
a.trisomy 21
b.trisomy 18
c.trisomy13
d.triploidy

237.Radial arrangement of medial sulci above the third ventricle(sunburst sign) on usg of cranium is seen in(RUMACK)
a.corpus callosum agenesis
b.spinan bifida
c.Arnold-chiari malformation
d.Dandy-Walker malformation

238.The line drawn from the lower margin of orbit to the superior border of the external auditory meatus is known as all except(GRAINGER)
a.the anthropological base line
b.Reid's line
c.Frankfurt line
d.auricular line

239.Towne's projection in skull x ray refers to(GRAINGER)
a.lateral projection
b.postero-anterior projection
c.half-axial anteroposterior projection
d.submentovertical projection

240.Physiological intracranial calcification are all except(GRAINGER)
a.pineal gland
b.habenular commissure
c.choroid plexus
d.thalamus

241.The investigation to detect site of CSF leakage(GRAINGER)
a.contrast CT
b.CT cisternography
c.xenon CT
d.none

242.True regarding magnetic resonance diffusion imaging (GRAINGER)
a.exploits the Brownian motion of water molecules
b.relatively stationary water molecules(decreased diffusion) appear bright
c.areas with decreased ADC appear dark
d.all

243.BOLD(blood oxygen dependent level) effect is used in(GRAINGER)
a.MR perfusion imaging
b.MR spectroscopy
c.PET
d.functional MRI

244.The recurrent artery of Huebner is branch of(GRAINGER)
a.anterior cerebral artery
b.middle cerebral artery
c.posterior cerebral artery
d.posterior cerebellar artery

245.The circle of Willis is formed by all except(GRAINGER)
a.the distal internal carotid artery
b.anterior cerebral artery
c.anterior communicating artery
d.posterior cerebellar atery

246.The circle of Willis is

formed by all except(GRAINGER)

a.the distal basilar artery

b.posterior cerebral arteries

c.posterior communicating arteries

d.posterior cerebellar atery

247.The great vein of Galen is formed by(GRAINGER)

a.superior sagittal sinus and inferior sagittal sinus

b.straight sinus and inferior sagittal sinus

c.basal vein of Rosenthal and septal vein

d.lateral sinus and superficial cerebral vein

248.Commonly calcified brain tumour are all except(GRAINGER)

a.oligodendroglioma

b.choroid plexus tumour

c.meningioma

d.glioblastoma multiforme

249.Most brain tumour on MRI appear(GRAINGER)

a.hypointense on T1 and hyperintense on T2W

b.hyperintense on T1 and hypointense on T2W

c.hypointense on T1 and hyporintense on T2W

d.hyperintense on T1 and hyperintense on T2W

250.Dural tail sign on CT scan of brain is noted in(GRAINGER)

a.anaplastic astrocytoma

b.oligodendroglioma

c.meningioma

d.choroid plexus tumour

251.The investigation of choice for detection of microadenoma of pituitary gland(GRAINGER)

a.CT

b.MRI

c.PET

d.USG

252.The earliest detectable change on CT in case of cerebral ischemia (GRAINGER)

a.dense artery

b.loss of gray white matter differentiation

c.wedge shaped hypodensity

d.none

253.Sylvian dot sign on CT is noted in(GRAINGER)

a.cerebral ischemia

b.intracranial haemorrhage

c.cerebral vein thrombosis

d.oligodendroglioma

254.Delta sign is noted in(GRAINGER)

a.cerebral arterial ischemia

b.cerebral venous thrombosis

c.both

d.none

255.Intracerebral hemorrhage appear on CT as(GRAINGER)

a.hypodense

b.hyperdense

c.hyperintense

d.none

256.All are true regarding brain pathology except(GRAINGER)

a.ring enhancing lesion in abscess

b.abscess centre shows low signal on diffusion and high signal on ADC

c.abnormal basal enhancement in tuberculosis

d.target sign of high central attenuation with rim enhancement in tuberculoma

257.All shows focal brain parenchymal mass lesion with enhancement in HIV-related disease except

a.toxoplasmosis(GRAINGER)

b.lymphoma

c.tuberculosis

d.cryptococcomas

258.The commonest imaging finding in HIV encephalopathy(GRAINGER)

a.cerebral atrophy

b.white matter lesions

c.both

d.none

259.Rabbit's ear configuration of frontal norn is noted in(GRAINGER)

a.unilateral subacute subdural hematoma

b.bilateral subacute subdural hematoma

c.unilateral acute extradural hematoma

d.unilateral basal ganglia hematoma

260.Tam O'Shanter deformity is noted in(GRAINGER)

a.paget's disease involving skull

b.fibrous dysplasia involving skull

c.leprosy involving skull

d.achondroplasia

261.Tarlov cyst refers to(GRAINGER)

a.perineural arachnoid cyst

b.posterior fossa arachnoid cyst

c.both

d.none

262.Cavity within the spinal cord ,lined with glial tissue and contain CSF-like fluid is known as(GRAINGER)

a.syringomyelia

b.diastematomyelia

c.myelomeningocoel

d.none

263.Bat wing appearance of fourth ventricle and molar appearance due to prominent superior cerebellar peduncle is noted in(GRAINGER)

a.Joubert's syndrome

b.Dandy-Walker syndrome

c.Arnold-Chiari syndrome

d.none

264.The most common cerebral malformation in fetus(GRAINGER)

a.cephalocele

b.anencephaly

c.Dandy-Walker syndrome

d.Arnold-Chiari syndrome

265.Lacunar skull is noted in(GRAINGER)

a.cephalocele

b.anencephaly

c.Dandy-Walker syndrome

d.Arnold-Chiari syndrome

266.'Smooth brain' is feature of(GRAINGER)

a.lissencephaly

b.pachygyria

c.schizencephaly

d.tuberous sclerosis

267.'Double cortex' in brain is noted in(GRAINGER)

a.heterotopia

b.Schizencephaly

c.lissencephaly

d.polymicrogyria

268.Harlequin deformity is noted in(GRAINGER)

a.bicoronal synostosis

b.unicoronal synostosis

c.metopic synostosis

d.none

269.Posterior fossa tumour with CT hyperdensity and T2W hypointensity is (GRAINGER)

a.medulloblastoma

b.pilocytic astrocytoma

c.meningioma

d.Schwannoma

270.Imaging in child showing suprasellar mass (solid and cystic component)with calcification and enhacement of solid component and cyst wall is suggestive of(GRAINGER)

a.craniopharyngioma

b.pilocystic astrocytoma

c.aneurysm

d.optic glioma

271.The technique of choice

for evaluation of sellar and parasellar region(GRAINGER)

a.CT

b.MRI

c.PET

d.all

272.All are features of acromegaly except(GRAINGER)

a.thickened vault

b.enlarged paranasal sinuses

c.enlarged vertebral bodies

d.small mastoid air cells

273.Radiological features of hypothyroidism are all except(GRAINGER)

a.wormian bones

b.delayed fusion and appearance of epiphyses

c.bullet shaped vertebral bodies

d.relatively small sella

274.Gelastic seizure is noted in(GRAINGER)

a.pineal gland tumour

b.hypothalmic hamartoma

c.meningioma

d.craniopharyngioma

275.The investigation of choice for staging and follow up of lymphoma(GRAINGER)

a.CT

b.MRI

c.USG

d.PET

276.Pneumocephaly refers to (SW)

a.air in thorax

a.air in abdomen

a.air in head

a.air in pericardium

277.The gold standard for evaluation of vascular pathology of the brain and spine (SW)

a.transarterial catheter- based angiography

b.MRA

c.CTA

d.none

278.On CT ,contused areas of brain appear (SW)

a.bright

b.dark

c.both

d.none

279.All are true regarding extradural haematoma excep(SW)

a.blood between skull and dura

b.hyperdense on CT

c.lunate(crescentric)

d.Usually respect cranial suture line

280. 'Dumbbell shape ' tumour refers to(SW)

a.neurofibroma
b.schwannoma
c.meningioma
d.ependymoma

281.A true chronic subdural haematoma ,on CT appear as (SW)
a.as dark as CSF(hypodense)
b.bright(hyperdense)
c.mixed hypersense with hypodense
d.none

282.Indication for open craniotomy for evacuation of acute subdural haematoma(SW)
a.lesion thickness >1cm
b.midline shift >5mm
c.GCS drop by two points from time of injury to hospitalization
d.all

283.indication of conservative management of epidural hematoma (SW)
a.clot volume<30 cm^3
b.maximum thickness <1.5cm
c.GCS score >8
d.all

284.indication of surgical treatment of chronic subdural hematoma (SW)

a.thickness >1cm
b.any symptomatic SDH
c.both
d.none

285.Indications for craniotomy for intraparenchymal haemorrhag(SW)
a.clot volume>50 cm^3
b.clot volume >30 cm^{3}with GCS 6-8 and associated midline shift>5mm
c.basal cistern compression
d.all

286.Angiographic features of arterial dissection are (SW)
a.string sign(stenosis of true lumen)
b.visible intimal flap
c.both
d.none

287.Bursting fracture of the ring of C1 due due to compression forces is known as (SW)
a.Jefferson's fractures
b.Hangman's fracture
c.odontoid fracture
d.Bennet's fracture

288.Hangman's fracture refers to (SW)
a.bilateral C2 pars interarticularis fracture
b.C1 ring fracture

c.odantoid fracture

d.jumped facets

289.Most common location of cerebral aneurysm (SW)

a.anterior communicating artery

b.posterior communicating artery

c.middle cerebral artery bifurcation

d.basilar artery

290. The most common intramedullary tumour of cord in adult(SW)

a.ependymoma

b.astrocytoma

c.haemangioblastoma

d.teratomas

291.The gold standard for assessing cerebral vasculature (SW)

a.catheter angiography

b.MRA

c.CTA

d.none

292.On MRI ,Multiple sclerosis is characterized by all except

a.involvement of white matter

b.Dawson's fingers

c.'lesion within lesion' appearance

d.ovoid high signal on T1W image

293.The most common location of intracranial haemorrhage in hypertension is

a.basal ganglia

b.cerebellum

c.brainstem

d.subarachnoid space

294.Diffuse axonal injuries is characterized by all except

a.No loss of consciousness at the time of impact

b.small petechial hemorrhages

c.grey-white matter junction and corpus callosum typical site

d.the most significant cause of morbidity in traumatic brain injury

295.Imaging of Meningioma of the brain is characterized by all except

a.parasagittal location in 25%

b.hyperdense in 70-80% cases

c.strong enhancement

d.hemorrhage very common

296.Causes of basal ganglia calcification are all exept

a.hyporarathyroidism

b.Fahr's syndrome

c.post natal hypoxia

d.wilson'disease

297. The least useful investigation for multiple myeloma is
a.bone scan
b.x ray
c.bone marrow biopsy
d.CT

298. Caudal regression syndrome is associated with
a.PIH
b.cardiac disease
c.respiratory disease
d.gestational diabetes

299.Vein of Galen malformation is characterized by all except
a.high output congestive failure
b.hydrocephalus
c.sonolucent posterior third centricular mass on USG
d.vein of Galen formed by internal cerebral vein and vein of Labbe

300.MRI features of mesial temporal sclerosis are all except
a.atrophy of hippocampus
b.atrophy of mammilary body
c.atrophy of fornix
d.blurring of grey –white matter junction

301.All are true regarding Ossified posterior longitudinal ligament (OPLL) except
a.thoracic spine is most common site
b.MRI is best for diagnosis
c.low signal intensity on all sequences
d.gradient echo overestimate the canal stenosis

302.The earliest CT and MRI feature of communicating hydrocephalus is
a.dilatation and rounding of the temporal horns
b.enlargement and rounding of the frontal horns
c.enlargement and ballooning of the temporal horns
d.enlargement of fourth ventricle

303.Bracket calcification in x ray skull is found in
a.aneurysm
b.lipoma
c.habenular commissure calcification
d.falx calcification

NERVOUS SYSTEM(ANSWERS)

1.a--Diffusion MR sequence is sensitive to the microscopic motion of water(H)

2.b—Diffusion is the most sensitive technique for detecting acute ischemic stroke (H)

3.d---CT scan is pragmatic choice for initial evaluation of (H) acute changes in mental status,suspected stroke/heamorrhage,intrcranial/spinal trauma

4.a---CT scan is pragmatic choice for initial evaluation of intracranial trauma/spinal trauma(H)

5.a---Regarding role of MRI and CT:(H)In general,MRI is more sensitive than CT for lesions of CNS,MRI is more sensitive than CT for lesions of spinal cord,cranial nerves posterior fossa structures,CT is more sensitive than MRI for fine osseos detail,CT is indicated in iniatial evalution of conducting hearing loss

6.d---MRI with contrast is recommended technique for (H) neoplasm(primary/metastatic),infection /abscess,ranial neuropathy/menineal disease

7.a---MRI with coronal T2 imaging is recommended in(H) partial complex/refractory seizure

8.a---Recommended technique for subacute /chronic hemorrhage is(H) MRI

9.c---Recommended technique for acute parenchymal hemorrhage is(H) CT,MRI

10.d---Recommended technique for subarachmoid hemorrhage are (H) CT and CTA,lumbar puncture,Angiography

11.a---Recommended technique for aneurysm is (H)
Angiography

12.c---Recommended technique for hemorrhagic infarction is
(H)CT,MRI

13.a---Recommended technique for vertebral /carotid
dissection is (H) MRI/MRA

14.d--CTA is recommended in (H)subachnoid
hemorrhage,vertebral basilar insufficiency,carotid stenosis

15.c---MRI+gradient echo imaging is recommended in(H) shear
injury/chronic hemorrhage

16.d---MRI is recommended technique for(H) vascular
malformation/dementia,white matter diseases,demyelinating
disease

17.c--Regarding cysticerci in brain parenchyma: size 5-20mm in
diameter,round

18.a---On CT scan bone appears as(H) an area of high density
due to greater x ray attenuation

19.a---Advantages of MDCT are (H) reduced patient and organ
motion,CT perfusion study,CT angiography study

20.d--- Regarding iodinated contrast CT scan :(H)identify
vascular structures,detect defect in blood- brain-
barrier,pituitary gland,chroid plexux,dura normally enhance
after contrast,low risk of allergic reactions

21.d---CT scan is the primary study of choice in the evaluation
of(H)subacute /chronic hemorrhage

22.d---CT is complimentary to MR in evaluation of(H) the skull
base,orbit,osseous structures of spine

23.d--- CT cisternography : (H) Indicated in CSF fistula ,evaluate
intracranial cisterns,involve intrathecal contrast injection

24.b---Cortical tuber,subependymal nodule and giant cell
astrocytoma are features of tuberous sclerosis

25c---.'Tram track ' gyriform calcification is feature of Sturge –
Weber syndrome

26. a--- Intraconal orbital mass lesion is optic nerve glioma/meningioma

27.a---Intradural spinal mass is (C) meningioma

28.a---Percentage of retinoblastoma showing calcification on CT(C) over 90%

29.b---Tram track sign is noted in which orbital lesion(C) optic nerve meningioma

30.a----The most common type of cranial herniation is(H) transtentorial herniation

31.b---Kernohan-Waltman sign is seen in (H)uncal herniation

32.d---MRI abnormalities in mesial temporal lobes are seen in paraneoplastic encephalitis,autoimmune encephalitis,HHV-6 encephalitis

33.b---Meningeal involvement in tuberculous meningitis is pronounced at base of brain

34.a----more than 50 % of cases of tuberculous meningitis has evidence of old pulmonary lesions or of milliary pattern

35.d---Causes of ring enhancing lesion in brain in HIV infected patients are toxoplasmosis ,CNS lymphoma,TB/Fungal/bacterial abscess

36.d---Neuro imaging finding suggestive of nerocysticercosis cystic lesions with or without enhancement,one or more nodular calcifactions,focal enhancing lesions

37.b---Imaging modality of choice in patients with acute strokes(H) noncontrast CT of head

38.d----True about T2-weighted signal are (H) use of longer TE and TR,Csf and edema produce high signal,more sensitive to demyelination,infarction and chronic hemorrhage,Csf has longT1 and T2 relaxation time

39 a---

	CSF	FAT	EDEMA
T1W	low	high	low

40.a---Fat produces high signal on T1W images(H)

41.d---Edema produces bright Signal on T2W images (H)

42. a—CSF produces low signal on FLAIR images (H)

43.d----True about MRI sequence :(H),In FLAIR, csf signal is suppressed,FLAIR is more sensitive to edema or water containing lesions than standard spin echo,susceptibility weighted imaging is indicated in lesions with microhemorrhages,Gradient echo imaging is more sensitive to magnetic susceptibility generated by blood,calcium and air

44.b---The most common intramedullary tumour of cord in children(SW)astrocytoma

45.c---Insular ribbon sign is a finding of Middle cerebral artery infarction

46.c---Empty delta sign is a feature of acute venous infarction

47.c---Multiple arteriovenous malformations are noted in Osler-Weber-Rendu syndrome and Wyburn-Mason syndrome

48.c---MRI of brain showing a central pop-corn core of high T1W with surrounding rim of hemosiderin(very lowT2W signal) is suggestive of cavernous angioma

49.c---Rasmussen 's encephalitis is characterized by atrophy localized to one cerebral hemisphere

50.d----All are hyperdense leions of brain on CT meningioma,lymphoma,colloid cyst

51.C-shaped calcification in brain is due to habenular commissure calcification

52.a---Sharply defined CSF-containing structures that surround small arteries as they penetrate the brain is known asVirchow-Robin space

53.c---The standard technique for extracranial vascular MRA(H) contrast –enhanced MRA

54.b--- The most common primary CNS neoplasm(SW)astrocytoma

55.a---Gray matter contain 10—15%more water than white matter(H)

56.d--- Echoplanar MR imaging is basis of a(H) diffusion imaging and tractography,perfusion imaging,functional imaging

57.b--Regarding Diffusion weighted imaging:(H) assess microscopic motion of water,restricted motion of water appear as high signal ,infarcted tissue reduces water motion within cells and interstitial tissue,sensitive to infarction,encephalitis,abscess

58.a---The most sensitive technique for detection of acute cerebral infarction of <7days(H) diffusion weighted imaging

59.D---Typical finding of infarction on perfusion imaging is(H)delay in mean transit time,reduction in cerebral blood volume,reduction in cerebral blood flow

60.a----Imaging that assess the microscopic motion of water along white matter tracts (H) diffusion tensor imaging

61.d---EPI technique that localizes regions of activity in brain following task activation(H) functional imaging

62.d---Regarding magnetic nerve neurography :(H) indicated in rediculopathy with normal conventional MR study of spine,suspected peripheral nerve entrapement,peripheral nerve trauma,T2weighted image

63.a---PET finding in Alzheimer's diseases(H) is a lower activity of FDG in the parietal lobes

64.d---Present indications of conventional plan-film myelography are(H)suspected meningeal or arachnoid cyst,localisation of spinal dural arteriovenous ,localisation of spinal CSF fistula

65.d---Myelography should be prformed with caution in(H) elevated intracranial pressure,evidence of spinal block,history of allergic reactions to intrathecal contrast

66.a--- The most commonly used route for angiography (H) femoral route

67.a---The most feared complication of cerebral angiography(H) is stroke

68.a---Prior to aortic artery aneurysm,spinal angiography is done to identify(H) the artery of Adamkiewicz

69.d---Correct matching of interventinal therapy are (H) carebral aneurysm—detachable coils,arteriovenous malformation—particulate or liquid adhesive emboisation,carotid-cavernous fistula—balloon occlusion

70.a---The most common syndrome associated with focal seizure with dyscognitive features(H) .medial temporal lobe sclerosis

71.d---High resolution MRI finding of medial temporal lobe sclerosis are (H) small hippocampus ,small temporal lobe,enlarged temporal horn,high signal on T2 weighted image

72.c---imaging in seizures:(H)almost all patients with new- onset seizure should have brain imaging,MRI is superior to CT for detection of lesions associated with epilepsy,Hippocampal sclerosis is associated with medial temporal lobe sclerosis,PET and SPECT is used to evaluate some of patients with medical refractory seizures

73.b---Eligibility criteria for use of IV rtPA are :(H)<3 hr time window, no hemorrhage or edema of >1/3 of MCA territory on CT,age = >18yrs,clinical diagnosis of stroke

74. c---Drop metastases is noted (SW)epedymoma

75.a---Puff of smoke appearance on conventional x ray angiography is noted in(H) moyamoya disease

76.a---Notch-3 mutation is noted in(H)CADASIL

77.d---Role MRI in strokes are (H) reliably document infarction in posterior fossa and cortical surface,DWI is more sensitive for early brain infarction than standard MRI sequences,Brain regions showing poor perfusion but no abnormality on diffusion are equivalent measure of ischemic penumbra,MR angiography is sensitive for stenosis of extracranial internal crotd arteries and of large intracranial cessels

78.a---The Gold standard for identifying and quantifying atherosclerotic stenoses of cerebral arteries is(H)conventional x ray cerebral angiography

79. d---Conventional x- ray cerebral angiography is gold standard for identifying and characterizing(H) aneurysm,vasospasm,intraluminal thrombus

80.d--- Conventional x- ray cerebral angiography is gold standard for identifying and characterizing(H) fibromuscular dysplasia,arteriovenous fistula,vasculitis

81.b---Investigation that can quantify cerebral blood flow (H) xenon-CT,PET

82.a---The most common type of intracranial hemorrhage (H) ICH

83.b---probably the most common cause of lobar hemorrhage in the elderly(H).cerebral amyloid angiopathy

84.d---Neuroimaging feature suggestive of dementia :(H)Alzheimer's disease---hippocampal atrophy and posterior dominant cortical atrophy,FTD—frontal,insular and or temporal atrophy,spares posterior parietal lobule,DLB—posteror parietal atrophy,hippocampi larger than AD,greater involvemet of amygdale than hippocampi,CJD—cortical ribboning and basal ganglia or thalamus hyperintensity on diffusion or FLAIR MRI

85.c---Radioligand for detecting brain amyloid associated with amyloid angiopathy or neurotic plaque(H) Pittsburg compound-B,^{18}F-AV-45

86.d---The neuroimaging features of normal-pressure hydrocephalus are (H)hydrocephalus,little or no cortical atrophy,propped open sylvian fissure

87.a---Boxcarring is seen in(H) NPH

88.a--- The most common malignant paediatric brain tumour(SW) medulloblastoma

89.d---The hallmark feature of Parkinson's disease are (H) degeneration of dopaminergic neurons in substantia nigra pars compacta,reduced striatal dopamine,lewy bodies

90.d--MRI features of multiple system atrophy are (H) iron accumulation on striatum on T2 weighted scan,putaminal rim,pontine 'hot cross buns sign',The'hummingbird'sign is noted in progressive supranuclear palsy

91.c---The hummingbird sign in midsagittal images of MRI of brain is noted in(H) progressive supranuclear palsy

92.b--- Pontine 'hot cross buns sign' and putaminal rim is noted in(H) multiple system atrophy

93.d---Atrophy of caudate nuclei on MRI imaging is seen in(H) Huntington's disease

94.a----CT and MRI changes in caudate,putamen and pallidum in Wilson 'disease is (H) hypodensity on CT and hyperintensity on T2MRI

95.D--Features of oligodendroglioma :(H)fried egg appearance on histology,nonenhancing,partially calcified

96.a---The most common form of hereditary ataxia is(H) Friedriech ataxia

97.b---MRI finding of spinal cord atrophy is noted in(H) Freidriech ataxia

98.c---cereballar and brainstem atrophy on MRI is noted in(H) SCA

99.a---The most common form of progressive motor neurone disease(H) amytrophic lateral sclerosis

100.a---MRI finding of thinning of corticospinal tract in brain and spinal cord is noted in(H) amytrophic lateral sclerosis

101.a---Crescentric blood collection in cranial trauma on CT SCAN is noted in(H) Subdural haematoma

102.b---Lenticular blood collection in cranial trauma on CT SCAN is noted in(H) epidural hematoma

103.b----The preferred diagnostic test for patients suspected of having brain tumour(H)contrast MR

104.c---Imaging features of malignant tumour of brain are (H) typically enhance with gadolinium,characteristically sorrounded by edema of the neighbouring white matter

105.a---Regarding imaging of brain tumor:(H) low grade glioma typically doesnot enhance,low grade glioma ie best appreciated on FLAIR sequence,meningioma donot invade the brain,meningioma are dural based with dural tail

106.d----Regarding imaging of brain tumour:(H) functional MRI is useful in presurgical planning and defining eloqouent motor ,sensory and language cortex,PET is useful in defining the metabolic activity of the lesions,MR perfusion provide information on blood flow

107. a---Grade iv astrocytoma is(H) pilocystic astrocytoma

108.b----The most common brain tumour of childhood(H) pilocystic astrocytoma

109.b----MRI finding of the cystic cerebellar lesions with enhancing mural nodule in childhood suggest(H) pilocystic astrocytoma

110.d---Regarding brain tumour:(H)most common brain tumour is metastases rather than primary brain tumor,at least half of primary brain tumour is malignant in nature,glial tumours account for 60% of all primary brain tumour

111.b---The most common cause of malignant primary brain tumour(H) glioblastoma

112.d---MRI feature showing ring enhancing masses with central necrosis and surrounding edema in 6th decade suggest of(H) glioblastoma

113.d---Nonenhancing tumours are all except(H)glioblastoma

114.d---Imaging feature of primary cental nervous system lymphoma are (H)dense tumour ,enhancing tumour,basal ganglia,corpus callosum and periventricular location

115.a---The most common malignant brain tumour of childhood(H) medulloblastoma

116.a---The most common primary brain tumour(H) meningioma

117.a---Dural tail is found in(H) meningioma

118.d---Imaging features of meningioma are (H) dense tumour,arise from dura ,dural tail,partially calcified,enhancing

119.a---imaging features on vestibular schwannomas are (H) enhancing tumor,enlarge internal auditory canal,often extend in cerebellopontine angle,d/d is meningioma

120. d---Imaging features of epidermoid cysts are (H) usually in CP angle,extra-axial lesion,CSF like imagin characteristics, restricton of diffusion

121.a--Imaging features of epidermoid cyst are (H)midline location,T1 hyperintensity,resemble lipoma,both epidermal and dermal structures

122.a----The most common source of brain metastases(H)lung

123.b---Melanoma has the greatest propensity to metastasize to brain(H)melanoma

124.d---The greatest propensity to hemorrhage in intracranial metastases are noted in (H) melanoma,kidney,thyroid

125.a---The most common cause of hemorrhagic metastasis is(H) lung

126.a---The most common source of epidural metastases in male (H) prostate

127.b----The most common source of epidural metastases in female (H)breast

128.a---The best test for diagnosis of epidural metastasis(H)noncontrast MRI of complete spine

129.b---Second the most common cause of neurologic disability in early to middle childhood(H) multiple sclerosis

130.a---Regarding MRI imaging of multiple sclerosis :(H)90% of visualized lesions are asymptomatic,Gd enhancement serve as useful marker of inflammation,Gd enhancement persist for approximately one month,The residual MS plaque remains visible indefinitely on T2W spin echo

131.c---In proper clinical setting, MRI features(FLAIR and diffusion weighted) suggestive of Cruetzfeldt Jacob disease are(H) increased intensity on basal ganglia,cortical ribboning

132.d---Regarding lesions of multiple sclerosis :(H)multifocal,frequently oriented perpendicular to the ventricular surface,lesions in anterior corpus callosum frequent in MS and rare in vascular disease,bright on T2

133.a---Regarding multiple sclerosis (H)total volume of T2W signal abnormality shows any significant correlation with clinical disability,measure of brain atrophy show a significant correlation with clinical disability,one third of T2W lesions appear as hypointense lesions(black holes) on T1W image,black holes may be marker of irreversible demyelination and axonal loss

134.c---Imaging which may serve as a surrogate markers of clinical disability in multiple sclerosis(H) magnetisation transfer ratio imaging,magnetic resonance spectroscopic imaging

135. A--- magnetisation transfer ratio imaging distinguish demyelination from edema in multiple sclerosis(H)

136.D--Typical locations of multiple sclerosis lesions are (H)periventricular and juxtacortical ,spinal cord,infratentorial

137.D---MRI finding that favor ADEM over MS are (H)relatively symmetric white matter abnormalities,basal ganglia or cortical gray matter lesions,Gd enhancement of all abnormal areas

138.b--Regarding HSV encephalitis (H)CT is less sensitive than MRI and is normal in upto 20-35% of petients,frontotemporal,insular and cingulate areas involvement,lesion sensitivity increased by addition of FLAIR/diffusion weighted image

139.a---Feature of mature brain abscess on MRI imaging:(H) hyperintense central area of pus on T2W image,well defined hypointense capsule on T2W image,hyperintense surrounding edema on T2Wimage

140 .a---Ring enhancing lesion with restricted diffusion of central hyperintensity on T2W image suggest of (H) abscess

141.d---Regarding hyperperfusion syndrome of CNS :(H) High T2 signal ,primarily in occipital lobe, no respect of any single vascular territory

142. d---Regarding imaging in psychiatric disorder (H)reduced metabolic or neural activity in dorsolateral prefrontal cortex in schizophrenia,increased activation of the amygdale by negative stimuli in depression,reduced activation of nucleus accumbens by rewarding stimuli in depression

143.a---The thumbprint sign in lateral view of soft tissue of neck is seen in(H) enlarged edematous epiglottis

144.a---CT is pragmatic choice for initial evaluation of suspected stoke /hemorrhage(H)

145.c---As per NASCET and ECST ,Carotid endaretectomy provide substantial benefit in patients with stenosis of(H)=>70%

146.d---Regarding imaging in acute strokes (H) CT may not reliably show infarction for 24-48hrs,CT may miss small infarct in posterior fossa and cortical surface,carotid diseases and intracranial vascular occlusions are readily identified by CTA,CT is more sensitive than MRI for detecting acute blood

147.a---The most common cause of recurrent aseptic viral meningitis(N)herpes simplex virus

148.d---Brain structures showing propenisity for calcification in congenital toxoplasmosis are caudate nucleus and basal ganglia,chroroid plexus ,subependyma

149. b---Pathognomonic sign in MRI of brain for neurocysticrcosis(N) protoscolex in cyst

150.d--- non- enhancing cyst in brain are (N)hydatid cyst,arachnoid cyst,porencephly

151.d---Calcification in brain is noted in (N) tuberous sclerosis,tuberculosis,CMV/toxoplasmosis

152.d---Enhancing lesions in brain is noted in(N)tuberculosis,abscess,metastases

153.b---The most common astrocytoma in children (N) pilocytic astrocytoma

154.b---The enhancing nodula within wall of cystic lesion in cerebellum of children is the classic feature of(N)pilocytic astrocytoma

155.b---Calcified cortical mass in frontal lobe on CT in the patient presenting with seizure is suggestive of(N)oligodendroglioma

156.a---Brain tumour associated with Li-Fraumeni syndrome (N) choroid plexus tumour

157.d---Solid ,homogenous,contrast-enhancing mass in cerebellar vermis in child causing 4th ventricular obstruction and hydrocephalus is suggestive of(N)medulloblastoma

158.a---Imaging of brain of children showing a suprasellar cystic lesion with solid component and calcification suggests of (N) craniopharyngioma

159.d---X-ray features of skull in chronically increased intracranial pressure are (N)erosion of posterior clinoid processes,enlargement of the sella turcica,increased convolutional markings

160.a---The imaging method of choice for detecting intracranial haemorrhage in infants with patent anterior fontanels(N)cranial ultrasound

161.b----The imaging method of choice for detecting periventricular leukomalacia in infants with patent anterior fontanels(N)cranial ultrasound

162.b----The imaging method of choice for detecting hydrocephalus in infants with patent anterior fontanels(N)cranial ultrasound

163.b---Regarding use of CT in children (N)non-invasive,radiation issue,children being more sensitive to radiation than adults,less useful for diagnosing acute infarct in children,can be used to evaluate craniofacial abnormalities or craniosynostosis

164.d---A noncontrast CT can demonstrate (N),skull fractures/pneumocephalus,intracranial hemorrhage,impending herniation

165.d---Subtle signs of early infarction(<24hrs) on CT scan are (N)sulcal effacement,blurring of gray white infarction,hyperdense middle cerebral artery

166. d---Regarding hyperdense middle cerebral artery on CT scan: (N)early infarction,often due to thrombosis,increased attenoution in the MCA

167.a---Preferred imaging procedures in 1-24hrs old strokes in children(N) MRI or MRA(head and neck) with diffusion weighted images

168.b---Preferred imaging procedures in 1-24 hrs old strokes in children who is unstable(N) is CT or CTA(head and neck)

169.c---Next investigation in children patients with infarction in the anterior circulation(detected by CT or MRI) is(N)carotid USG

170.d---Regarding use of imagings in children :(N)CT or MRI can detect infarct >24hrs.MRI is preferred due to radiation issue,CT preferred if intraparenchymal hemorrhage<24hrs

171.d---The preferred imaging to detect vasospasm following subarachnoid hemorrhage in children(N)TCD(transcranial Doppler)

172.b--- Bilateral acoustic neuromas is pathognomonic of (SW) Neurofibromatosis type 2

173.a--- Preferred investigation of hypoxic- ischemic brain injury in infants (N) MRI

174. a---Preferred investigation of metabolic disorder of brain in children(N) MRI,particularly T2W and FLAIR

175.a--- Preferred investigation for detection of hydrocephalus in infants (N)USG

176.a---Initial investigation in head trauma is(N)CT

177.d---MRI without and with contrast is used in(N) multiple sclerosis.brain tumour,brain abscess

178.b--- A noninvasive technique used to map neuronal activity during specific cognitive states/sensorimotor function is(N)functional MRI

179.a---Molecular imaging technique used to detect metabolites like NAA(N)proton MR spectroscopy

180.d--- Proton MR spectroscopy are useful in (N) diagnosis of inborn error of metabolism,preoperative and postoperative assessment of intracranial tumour, in detection of cortical dysplasia

181.c---The gold standard for diagnosing vascular disorders of the CNS(N) Catheter angiography

182.a---SPECT radionuclide used to study regional cerebral blood flow(N) Tc 99m-HMPAO

183. d---SPECT of brain is particularly useful for assessing (N)vasculitis/herpes encephalitis,dysplastic cortex,recurrent brain tumour

184.a---Spine x ray in simple spina bifida occulta shows defect in(N)posterior vertebral arches and laminae

185.b---All cases of occult spinal dysraphism is best investigated with(N)MRI

186.d---Imaging indicated in all cutaneous lesions associated with occult spinal dysraphism are (N) subcutaneous mass or lipoma,hairy patch,dermal sinus

187.d---Imaging is indicated in all cutaneous lesions associated with occult spinal dysraphism (N) vascular lesions – haemangioma ,telangiectasia,skin tags,tail-like appendages,scarlike lesions

188.d---(N)meningocele—herniation of meninges through defect in posterior vertebral arch,myelomeningocele ---contain meningeal sac with spinal cord.encephalocele –contain meningeal sac and cerebral cortex,cerebellum or brainstem,anencephaly---absent calvaria with redumentary brain

189.c---Most common site of myelomeningocele is(N) lumbosacral region

190.a---MRI imaging showing absence of cerebral convolutions(sulci)and poorly formed sylvian fissure giving the appearance of 3-4 motn fetal brain suggest of(N) Lissencephaly

191.c---MRI study of brain showing cerebral cleft is suggestive of(N)schizencephaly

192.b---MRI study of brain showing gray matter-like substance within white matter between ventricle and cerebral cortex is suggestive of(N)heterotopia

193.c---MRI study of brain showing single ventricle,an absent falx and nonseprated deep cerebral neclei is suggestive of(N)holoprosencephaly

194.a---The most common malformation of posterior fossa and hind brain(N) Chiari malformation

195.a---Displcement of cereballar tonsil into cervical canal is noted in(N)Chiari malformation

196.b---MRI imaging of brain showing the cystic expansion of 4th ventricle in posterior fossa with midline cerebellar hypoplasia is suggestive of(N)Dandy-walker malformation

197.b---X ray feature of skull showing increased convolutinal markings(beaten-silver appearance) is noted in(N)chronic increase of intracranial pressure

198.d--- x ray of skull showing features of chronic increased intracranial pressures (N)sepratation of sutures,erosion of posterior clinoid in older child,increased convolutional markings (silver-beaten appearance)

199 .d---Features of neurofibromatosis 1 :(N)sphenoid dysplasia,thinning of long bones,pseudoarthrosis

200.a----The characteristic brain lesion in tuberous sclerosis is(N) cortical tuber

201.c---Candle dripping appearance of ventricle is noted in(N)tuberous sclerosis

202.a---The best way of identifying cortical tuber in tuberous sclerosis is(N)MRI

203.a---The imaging modality of choice for demonstrating leptomeningeal angioma in Sturge-Weber syndrome is(N) MRI

204. a---The Roach scale is related to(N)Sturge –Weber syndrome

205.d---Leptomeningeal angiomatosis, underlying cerebral atrophy and calcification are features of(N) Sturge –Weber syndrome

206.c---'Eye of the tiger sign ' (hyperentense area within hypointense area in globus pallidus) in MRI of brain is noted in(N)Hallervorden Spatz syndrome(pantothenate kinase associated neurodegeneration)

207.a---Which imaging technique is being used for white matter tracts in spastic diplegia(N)MRI with diffusion tensor imaging

208.d---MRI finding in cerebral palsiy are (N)periventricular leucomalacia,injury to thalmocortical and corticospinal pathways,multicystic cortical encephalomalacia

209.d---MRI finding in posterior reversible leucoencephalopathy are (N)increase in signal in occipital lobes on T2W image,patchy lesions involving gray and white matter,bilateral

210.b---Criteria for MRI dissemination in space include (N)Gadolinium enhancing lesions or 9T2 lesions,1 or more juxtacortical lesions,3 or more periventricular lesions

211.c---The study of choice for acute disseminated encephalitis(N)MRI

212.d---Cranial MRI features that favour ADEM are (N)wodespresd patchy lesions,frequent involvement of thalamus and basal ganglia,cortical gray-white matter junction,lesions of similar age,improvement in lesions on follow up MRI

213.a---Diffusion weighted imaging can detect acute ischemic stroke (N) within minutes of strokes

214.c----Investigation that is very insensitive for cerebral sinovenousthrombosis is(N) nonenhanced CT

215.b---The most common cause of childhood subarachnoid and intraparenchymal hemorrhage is(N) arteriovenous malformations

216.b-- MRI that imparts black signal to blood products (N) gradient echo imaging

217.a--High lactate in MR spectroscopy is noted in(N)MELAS

218.d---Regarding imaging of brain abscess :(N)most reliable methds are CECT and MRI,MRI is diagnostic test of choice,ring enhancing lesion on CECT

219.a---Beyand the infancy,conus medularis ends at the level of (N) L1

220.a---In congenital tethered spinal cord,the position of conus medullaris is(N) L2

221.b---MRI of spinal cord reveals two spinal cord,each with its own dural tube and seprated by a spicule of bone and cartilage.The diagnosis is (N) diastematomyelia

222.a---The radiologic study of choice for syringomyelia is(N) MRI

223.b---The diagnostic study of choice for spinal cord tumours is(N) MRI with contrast

224.c---SCIWORA refers to(N)a kind of spinal cord injury

225.b---Perinaud's syndrome may be associated with(N) a.tumour of pineal gland

226.c---The anomalies of midline structures of brain with hypoplasia of optic nerves,optic chiasm,optic tracts is noted in(N)de Morsier's syndrome

227.a---The most common site fracture from blunt trauma of orbit(N) orbital floor

228.a---Blow-out fracture of orbit involve(N) a orbital floor229.d---Klippel-Trenaunay syndrome comprises (N)cutaneous vascular malformation,bony and soft tissue hypertrophy,venous abnormality

230.d---In multiple pituitary harmone deficiency imaging show(N) small pituitary gland,missing or attenuated pituitary stalk,ectopic posterior pituitary bright spot

231d---.Radiological features of congenital hypothyroidism are (N)absent distal femoral epiphysis,epiphyseal dysgenesis,beaking of 12th thoracic ,1st,2nd lumber vertebra

232.d---Radiological features of skull of congenital hypothyroidism are (N)large fontanels,wide sutures,wormian bones

233.a---DiGeorge syndrome is associated with(N) aplasia or hypoplasia of parathyroid gland

234.b---Pancake type,cup type and ball type are types of which cranial abnormality(RUMACK) holoprosencephaly

235.a---Lobester claw is found in(RUMACK)Cornelia de Lange's syndrome

236.a---Sandal toes is found in(RUMACK) trisomy 21

237.a----Radial arrangement of medial sulci above the third ventricle(sunburst sign) on usg of cranium is seen in(RUMACK) corpus callosum agenesis

238.a----The line drawn from the lower margin of orbit to the superior border of the external auditory meatus is known as all except(GRAINGER) auricular line

239.c---Towne's projection in skull x ray refers to(GRAINGER).half-axial anteroposterior projection

240.d---Physiological intracranial calcification seen in (GRAINGER)pineal gland,habenular commissure,choroid plexus

241.b---The investigation to detect site of CSF leakage(GRAINGER)CT cisternography

242.d---True regarding magnetic resonance diffusion imaging (GRAINGER) exploits the Brownian motion of water molecules,relatively stationary water molecules(decreased diffusion) appear bright,areas with decreased ADC appear dark

243.d---BOLD(blood oxygen dependent level) effect is used in(GRAINGER)functional MRI

244.a---The recurrent artery of Huebner is branch of(GRAINGER) anterior cerebral artery

245.d---The circle of Willis is formed by (GRAINGER)the distal internal carotid artery,anterior cerebral artery,anterior communicating artery

246.d---The circle of Willis is formed by (GRAINGER)the distal basilar artery,posterior cerebral arteries,posterior communicating arteries

247.a---The great vein of Galen is formed by(GRAINGER) superior sagittal sinus and inferior sagittal sinus

248.d---Commonly calcified brain tumour are (GRAINGER)oligodendroglioma,choroid plexus tumour,meningioma

249.a---Most brain tumour on MRI appear(GRAINGER) hypointense on T1 and hyperintense on T2W

250.c---Dural tail sign on CT scan of brain is noted in(GRAINGER)meningioma

251.b---The investigation of choice for detection of microadenoma of pituitary gland(GRAINGER) MRI

252.a---The earliest detectable change on CT in case of cerebral ischemia (GRAINGER) dense artery

253.a---Sylvian dot sign on CT is noted in(GRAINGER)cerebral ischemia

254.b---Delta sign is noted in(GRAINGER) cerebral venous thrombosis

255.b---Intracerebral hemorrhage appear on CT as(GRAINGER) hyperdense

256.b---Regarding brain pathology (GRAINGER)ring enhancing lesion in abscess,abnormal basal enhancement in tuberculosis,target sign of high central attenuation with rim enhancement in tuberculoma

257.d ---All shows focal brain parenchymal mass lesion with enhancement in HIV-related disease toxoplasmosis,lymphoma,tuberculosis

258.a---The commonest imaging finding in HIV encephalopathy(GRAINGER) cerebral atrophy

259.b---Rabbit's ear configuration of frontal norn is noted in(GRAINGER)bilateral subacute subdural hematoma

260.a---Tam O'Shanter deformity is noted in(GRAINGER) paget's disease involving skull

261.a---Tarlov cyst refers to(GRAINGER) perineural arachnoid cyst

262.a---Cavity within the spinal cord ,lined with glial tissue and contain CSF-like fluid is known as(GRAINGER) syringomyelia

263.a---Bat wing appearance of fourth ventricle and molar appearance due to prominent superior cerebellar peduncle is noted in(GRAINGER) Joubert's syndrome

264.b---The most common cerebral malformation in fetus(GRAINGER) anencephaly

265.d---Lacunar skull is noted in(GRAINGER) Arnold-Chiari syndrome

266.a---'Smooth brain' is feature of(GRAINGER) lissencephaly

267.a---'Double cortex' in brain is noted in(GRAINGER).heterotopia

268.a---Harlequin deformity is noted in(GRAINGER) bicoronal synostosis

269.a---Posterior fossa tumour with CT hyperdensity and T2W hypointensity is (GRAINGER) medulloblastoma

270.a---Imaging in child showing suprasellar mass (solid and cystic component)with calcification and enhacement of solid component and cyst wall is suggestive of(GRAINGER)craniopharyngioma

271.b---The technique of choice for evaluation of sellar and parasellar region(GRAINGER) MRI

272.d---Features of acromegaly (GRAINGER) thickened vault,enlarged paranasal sinuses,enlarged vertebral bodies

273.D----Radiological features of hypothyroidism are (GRAINGER)wormian bones,delayed fusion and appearance of epiphyses,bullet shaped vertebral bodies

274.b---Gelastic seizure is noted in(GRAINGER) hypothalmic hamartoma

275.a---The investigation of choice for staging and follow up of lymphoma(GRAINGER) CT

276.a---Pneumocephaly refers to (SW) air in head

277.a---The gold standard for evaluation of vascular pathology of the brain and spine (SW) transarterial catheter- based angiography

278.a---On CT ,contused areas of brain appear (SW).bright

279.c---Regarding extradural haematoma (SW)blood between skull and dura,hyperdense on CT,Usually respect cranial suture line

280. b---'Dumbbell shape ' tumour refers to(SW) schwannoma

281.a---A true chronic subdural haematoma ,on CT appear as (SW) as dark as CSF(hypodense)

282.d---Indication for open craniotomy for evacuation of acute subdural haematoma(SW)lesion thickness >1cm,midline shift >5mm.GCS drop by two points from time of injury to hospitalization

283.d---indication of conservative management of epidural hematoma (SW)clot volume<30 cm^3,maximum thickness <1.5cm,GCS score >8

284.c---indication of surgical treatment of chronic subdural hematoma (SW)thickness >1cm,any symptomatic SDH

285.d---Indications for craniotomy for intraparenchymal haemorrhag(SW) clot volume>50 cm^3,clot volume >30 cm^{3}with GCS 6-8 and associated midline shift>5mm,basal cistern compression

286.c---Angiographic features of arterial dissection are (SW)string sign(stenosis of true lumen),visible intimal flap

287.a---Bursting fracture of the ring of C1 due due to compression forces is known as (SW)Jefferson's fractures

288.a---Hangman's fracture refers t(SW)bilateral C2 pars interarticularis fracture

289.a---Most common location of cerebral aneurysm (SW)anterior communicating artery

290.A--- The most common intramedullary tumour of cord in adult(SW) ependymoma

291.a---The gold standard for assessing cerebral vasculature (SW)catheter angiography

292.d---On MRI ,Multiple sclerosis is characterized by all involvement of white matter,Dawson's fingers,'lesion within lesion' appearance,ovoid high signal on T2W image

293.a---The most common location of intracranial haemorrhage in hypertension is basal ganglia

294.a---Diffuse axonal injuries is characterized by loss of consciousness at the time of impact,small petechial hemorrhages,grey-white matter junction and corpus callosum typical site,the most significant cause of morbidity in traumatic brain injury

295.d--Imaging of Meningioma of the brain is characterized by parasagittal location in 25%,hyperdense in 70-80% cases,strong enhancement

296.d---Causes of basal ganglia calcification are hyporarathyroidism,Fahr's syndrome,post natal hypoxia

297. a---The least useful investigation for multiple myeloma is bone scan

298. d---Caudal regression syndrome is associated with gestational diabetes

299.d---Vein of Galen malformation is characterized by high output congestive failure,hydrocephalus,sonolucent posterior third centricular mass on US,vein of Galen formed by internal cerebral vein and basal vein of Rosenthal

300.d---MRI features of mesial temporal sclerosis are blurring of grey –white matter junction

301.a---Regarding Ossified posterior longitudinal ligament (OPLL) :MRI is best for diagnosis,low signal intensity on all sequences,gradient echo overestimate the canal stenosis

302.a---The earliest CT and MRI feature of communicating hydrocephalus is dilatation and rounding of the temporal horns

303.b---Bracket calcification in x ray skull is found in lipoma

b.MRI

c.USG

d.PET

3.The radiological hallmark of antrochonal polyp is(GRAINGER)

a.hazy maxilla

c.deviated septum

 b.enlarged ostia

d.all

4.The most common site of osteoma in PNS(GRAINGER)

a.frontal sinus

b.maxillary sinus

c.sphenoid sinus

d.ethmoidal sinus

5.The presence of nasal mass with widened pterygoplatine fissure in HRCT of face in adolescent boys suggest of(GRAINGER)

a.inverting papilloma

b.juvenile angiofibroma

c.paranasal granuloma

d.none

6.Common multilocular radiolucent lesions of jaw are all except(GRAINGER)

a.odontogenic keratocyst

b.central giant cell granuloma

c.ameloblastoma

d.hypercementosis

ENT

1. Feature of sinus aspergilloma is

a.hypoattenuation on CT

b.decreased signal on T2W image

c.both

d.none

2.The investigation of choice for congental malformation of ear(GRAINGER)

a.HRCT

7.Common unilocular radiolucent lesions of jaw are all except(GRAINGER)
a.alveolar abscess
b.radicular cyst
c.dentigerous cyst
d.ameloblastoma

8.Correctly matched are all except(GRAINGER)
a.radicular cysts are derived from the cell rests of Malassez
b.dentigerous cyst is associated with unerupted teeth
c.odontogenic cysts lack the more ballooning characteristics of odontogenic cysts
d.multiple radicular cysts are noted in Gorlin-Goltz syndrome

9.Stafne cyst is noted in(GRAINGER)
a.jaw
b.humerous
c.femur
d.calcaneum

10.The imaging of choice for temporal bone lesions
a.CT
b.MRI
c.x ray
d.USG

11.All are x ray view for temporal bone except(DHINGRA)
a.Law 's view
b.Schuller 's view
c.Stenver's view
d.Water's view

12.Schuller 's view of temporal bone is taken for all except(DHINGRA)
a.to see extent of pneumatisation
b.destruction of intercellular septa
c.cholesteatoma
d.transeverse fracture of petrous pyramid

13.Law's view shows all except(DHINGRA)
a.attic,aditus,and antrum
b.mastoid air cells
c.tegmen
d.lateral sinus plate

14.Schuller's view shows all except(DHINGRA)
a.mastoid air cells
b.tegmen and lateral sinus plate
c.antrum and upper part of attic
d.cochlea

15.Stenver view shows all except(DHINGRA)

a.entire petrous pyramid

b.internal auditory meatus

c.labyrinth with its vestibule and chochlea

d.mastoid antrum and attic

16.Which view of temporal bone shows the petrous pyramid bilaterally(DHINGRA)

a.Law 's view

b.Schuller 's view

c.Stenver's view

d.Towne's view

17.Which view shows both petrous pyramid (DHINGRA)

a.Towne's view

b.Transorbital view

c.both

d.none

18.Which view is usually taken for acoustic neuroma and apical petrositis(DHINGRA)

a.Law 's view

b.Schuller 's view

c.Stenver's view

d.Towne's view

19.Water's view of PNS shows all except(DHINGRA)

a.Frontal sinuses

b.maxillary sinuses

c.sphenoid sinuses

d.ethmoid sinuses

20.Maxillary sinuses are best seen in which view(DHINGRA)

a.Caldwell view

b.Water's view

c.Towne's view

d.Basal view

21.Caldwell's view shows all except(DHINGRA)

a.Frontal sinuses

b.maxillary sinuse

c.sphenoid sinuses

d.ethmoid sinuses

22.Frontal sinuses are best seen in which view(DHINGRA)

a.Caldwell view

b.Water's view

c.Towne's view

d.Basal view

23. Sphenoid sinuses are best seen in which view(DHINGRA)

a.Caldwell view

b.Water's view

c.Towne's view

d.Basal view

24.X ray for nasal fractures are all except(DHINGRA)

a.lateral view

b.occlusal view

c.Water's view

d.Caldwell vi

25.X ray view taken to differentiate a foreign body of

the airway from that of food passage is(DHINGRA)

a.lateral view of neck

b.AP view of neck

c.Water's view

d.Caldwell's view

26.X ray view taken to differentiate a foreign body of the larynx from that of esophagus is(DHINGRA)

a.lateral view of neck

b.AP view of neck

c.Water's view

d.Caldwell's view

27.Lyre sign on angiogram is noted in(DHINGRA)

a.carotid body tumour of neck

b.angiofibroma

c.Subclavian steal syndrome

d.All

28.The gold standard for diagnosis of acoustic neuroma is(DHINGRA)

a.MRI

b.MRI with contrast

c.CT scan

d.x ray

29.Investigation of choice for intracanalicular acoustic neuroma (DHINGRA)

a.MRI

b.MRI with contrast

c.CT scan

d.x ray

30.Tripod fracture is noted in(DHINGRA)

a.zygoma fracture

b.mandibular fracture

c.maxillary fracture

d.nasal bone fracture

31.Craniofacial dysjunction is noted in(DHINGRA)

a.Le Fort I fracture

b. a.Le Fort II fracture

c.Le Fort III fracture

d.Le Fort IV fracture

32.All are true regarding PNS except(DHINGRA)

a.maxillary and ethmoid sinuses are present at birth

b.Frontal and ethmoid sinuses are not present at birth

c.Frontal sinus begins to develop at age of 4yrs

d.maxillary sinus reaches adult size by 5yrs

33.All are true regarding age of first radiologic evidence of PNS except(DHINGRA)

a.maxillary sinus at 4-5 months after birth

b.ethmoid sinus at 1yrs

c.frontal sinus 6yrs

d.sphenoid sinus at 10 yrs

34.Antral sign on CT scan of

head is pathognomonic
of(DHINGRA)

a.juvenile nasophayngeal
angiofibroma
b.maxillary carcinoma
c.adenoid
d.antrochoanal polyp
35.Reinke edema is noted
in(DHINGRA)

a.lung
b.vocal cord
c.trachea
d.hila

ENT(ANSWERS)

1. b---Feature of sinus aspergilloma :decreased signal on T2W image

2.b--The investigation of choice for congental malformation of ear(GRAINGER) MRI

3.b---The radiological hallmark of antrochonal polyp is(GRAINGER) enlarged ostia

4.a---The most common site of osteoma in PNS(GRAINGER) frontal sinus

5.b---The presence of nasal mass with widened pterygoplatine fissure in HRCT of face in adolescent boys suggest of(GRAINGER) juvenile angiofibroma

6.d---Common multilocular radiolucent lesions of jaw are (GRAINGER)odontogenic keratocyst,central giant cell granuloma,ameloblastoma

7.d---Common unilocular radiolucent lesions of jaw are (GRAINGER) ameloblastoma

8.d---Correctly matched are (GRAINGER)radicular cysts are derived from the cell rests of Malassez,dentigerous cyst is associated with unerupted teeth,odontogenic cysts lack the more ballooning characteristics of odontogenic cysts,multiple odontogenic keratocyte are noted in Gorlin-Goltz syndrome

9.a---Stafne cyst is noted in(GRAINGER) jaw

10.a---The imaging of choice for temporal bone lesions CT

11.d---X ray view for temporal bone (DHINGRA) Law 's view,Schuller 's view,Stenver's view

12.d---Schuller 's view of temporal bone is taken for (DHINGRA) to see extent of pneumatisation,destruction of intercellular septa,cholesteatoma,longitudinal fracture of petrous pyramid

13.a---Law's view shows (DHINGRA)mastoid air cells,tegmen,lateral sinus plate

14.d---Schuller's view shows (DHINGRA) mastoid air cells,tegmen and lateral sinus plate,antrum and upper part of attic

15.d---Stenver view shows (DHINGRA)entire petrous pyramid,internal auditory meatus,labyrinth with its vestibule and chochlea

16.d---Towne view of temporal bone shows the petrous pyramid bilaterally(DHINGRA)

17.c---Towne's viewand Transorbital view both shows petrous pyramid (DHINGRA)

18.d---Which view is usually taken for acoustic neuroma and apical petrositis(DHINGRA)Towne's view

19.d---Water's view of PNS shows (DHINGRA)Frontal sinuses,maxillary sinuses,sphenoid sinuses

20.b---Maxillary sinuses are best seen in which view(DHINGRA) Water's view

21.c---Caldwell's view shows (DHINGRA)Frontal sinuses,maxillary sinuses,ethmoid sinuses

22.a----Frontal sinuses are best seen in which view(DHINGRA)Caldwell view

23. d---Sphenoid sinuses are best seen in which view(DHINGRA) Basal view

24.d---X ray view for nasal fractures are (DHINGRA)lateral view,occlusal view,Water's view

25.a----X ray view taken to differentiate a foreign body of the airway from that of food passage is(DHINGRA) lateral view of neck

26.b---X ray view taken to differentiate a foreign body of the larynx from that of esophagus is(DHINGRA) AP view of neck

27.a---Lyre sign on angiogram is noted in(DHINGRA) carotid body tumour of neck

28.b---The gold standard for diagnosis of acoustic neuroma is(DHINGRA) MRI with contrast

29.b---Investigation of choice for intracanalicular acoustic neuroma (DHINGRA) MRI with contrast

30.a---Tripod fracture is noted in(DHINGRA) zygoma fracture

31.c---Craniofacial dysjunction is noted in(DHINGRA) Le Fort III fracture

32.d---- Regarding PNS :(DHINGRA) maxillary and ethmoid sinuses are present at birth,Frontal and ethmoid sinuses are not present at birth,Frontal sinus begins to develop at age of 4yrs,maxillary sinus reaches adult size by 15yrs

33.d---Regarding age of first radiologic evidence of PNS :(DHINGRA) maxillary sinus at 4-5 months after birth,ethmoid sinus at 1yrs,frontal sinus 6yrs,sphenoid sinus at 4yrs c

34.a---Antral sign on CT scan of head is pathognomonic of(DHINGRA)juvenile nasophayngeal angiofibroma

35.b--Reinke edema is noted in (DHINGRA) vocal cord

EYE

1.The preferred imaging for child with leukokoria(GRAINGER)
a.MRI
b.CT
c.USG
d.PET

2.CT of orbit shows calcification in intraocular mass in child less than 3yrs .The most likely diagnosis(GRAINGER)

a.retinoblastoma
b.optic nerve glioma
c.meningioma
d.haemangioblastoma

3.All are true regarding retinoblastoma except(GRAINGER)
a.most common tumour of globe in children
b.75% unilateral unifocal
c.calcification in 95% cases
d.CT best for showing extention along optic nerve

4.All are true regarding uveal melanoma except(GRAINGER)
a.most common intra-ocular malignancy in adults
b.hypodense on CT
c.hyperintense on T1W
d.hypointense on T2W

5.Intra-ocular mass giving appearance of 'Mushroom cloud' on CT/MRI is (GRAINGER)
a.retinoblastoma
b.optic nerve glioma
c.meningioma
d.uveal melanoma

6.The commonest cause of intra-orbital mass lesion in adults(GRAINGER)
a. pseudotumour
b.optic nerve glioma

c.meningioma

d.uveal melanoma

7.All are true regarding pseudotumour except(GRAINGER)

a.usually bilateral

b.involve tendon

c.hypointense to fat on T2

d.idioathic nflammatury condition

8.Imaging shows bilateral enhancing orbital mass moulding to contour of orbit without bone destruction.The lesion is hypointense onT1W and hyperintense on T2W.the most likely diagnosis is(GRAINGER)

a. pseudotumour

b.lymphoma

c.meningioma

d.uveal melanoma

9.'Tram track' sign on axial image and 'doughnut sign' on coronal image of orbit is seen in(GRAINGER)

a.optic nerve meningioma

b.optic nerve glioma

c.retinoblastoma

d.uveal melanoma

NEUROLOGY

10. Which is intraconal orbital mass lesion

a.optic nerve glioma/meningioma

b.rhabdomyosarcoma

c.orbital cellulitis

d.dermoid

11.Percentage of retinoblastoma showing calcification on CT(C)

a.over 90%

b.over 70%

c.over60%

d.over50%

12.Tram track sign is noted in which orbital lesion(C)

a.optic nerve glioma

b.optic nerve meningioma

c.retinoblastoma

d.toxocariasis

13.The anomalies of midline structures of brain with hypoplasia of optic nerves,optic chiasm,optic tracts is noted in(N)

a.Goldenhar 's syndrome

b.VHL

c.de Morsier's syndrome

d.Stargardt disease

14.The most common site fracture from blunt trauma of orbit(N)

a.orbital floor

b.medial wall

c.superior orbital fracture

d.lateral wall fracture

15.Blow-out fracture of orbit involve(N)

a.orbital floor

b.medial wall

c.superior orbital fracture

d.lateral wall fracture

16.All are true regarding Graves ophthalmopathy except

a.fusiform enlargement of extra-ocular muscle

b.tendinous involvement

c.inferior rectus muscle most commonly affected

d.retro-orbital fat infiltration by inflammatory cells

17.The investigation of choice in evaluation of vision loss or suspected cranial nerve dysfunction(SUTTON)

a.CT

b.MRI

c.USG

d.PET

18.The most common orbital mass in adult is(SUTTON)

a.Idiopathic inflammatory pseudotumour

b.malignant melanoma

c.lymphoma

d.rhabdomyosarcoma

19.The most common primary orbital malignancy in the pediatric age group(SUTTON)

a. lymphoma

b.malignant melanoma

c.retinoblastoma

d.rhabdomyosarcoma

20.The most common benign orbital tumours in adult(SUTTON)

a. lymphoma

b.malignant melanoma

c.cavernous hemangioma

d.lymphangioma

21.The diagnostic procedure of choice for carotid cavernous fistula(SUTTON)

a..MRI

b.CT

c.angiography

d.USG

EYE(ANSWERS)

1.b---The preferred imaging for child with leukokoria(GRAINGER) CT

2.a---CT of orbit shows calcification in intraocular mass in child less than 3yrs .The most likely diagnosis(GRAINGER) retinoblastoma

3.d---Regarding retinoblastoma :(GRAINGER) most common tumour of globe in children,75% unilateral unifocal,calcification in 95% cases,MRI best for showing extention along optic nerve

4.b---Regarding uveal melanoma :(GRAINGER) most common intra-ocular malignancy in adults,hyperdense on CT,hyperintense on T1W,hypointense on T2W

5.d---Intra-ocular mass giving appearance of 'Mushroom cloud' on CT/MRI is (GRAINGER) uveal melanoma

6.a---The commonest cause of intra-orbital mass lesion in adults(GRAINGER) pseudotumour

7.a--Regarding pseudotumour: (GRAINGER)usually unilateral,involve tendon,hypointense to fat on T2,idioathic inflammatury condition

8.b---Imaging shows bilateral enhancing orbital mass moulding to contour of orbit without bone destruction.The lesion is hypointense onT1W and hyperintense on T2W.the most likely diagnosis is(GRAINGER) lymphoma

9.a---'Tram track' sign on axial image and 'doughnut sign' on coronal image of orbit is seen in(GRAINGER) optic nerve meningioma

10.a--- Which is intraconal orbital mass lesion optic nerve glioma/meningioma

11.a---Percentage of retinoblastoma showing calcification on CT(C) over 90

12.b---Tram track sign is noted in which orbital lesion(C) optic nerve meningioma

13.c---The anomalies of midline structures of brain with hypoplasia of optic nerves,optic chiasm,optic tracts is noted in(N) de Morsier's syndrome

14.a---The most common site fracture from blunt trauma of orbit(N) orbital floor

15.a---Blow-out fracture of orbit involves(N) orbital floor

16.b---Regarding Graves ophthalmopathy :fusiform enlargement of extra-ocular muscle,no tendinous involvement,inferior rectus muscle most commonly affected,retro-orbital fat infiltration by inflammatory cells

17.b---The investigation of choice in evaluation of vision loss or suspected cranial nerve dysfunction(SUTTON) MRI

18.a---The most common orbital mass in adult is(SUTTON) Idiopathic inflammatory pseudotumour

19.d---The most common primary orbital malignancy in the pediatric age group(SUTTON)rhabdomyosarcoma

20.c---The most common benign orbital tumours in adult(SUTTON) cavernous hemangioma

21.c---The diagnostic procedure of choice for carotid cavernous fistula(SUTTON) angiography b.Lateral view

c.Lateral decubitus view

d.Apical lordotic view

3.Limitations of portable chest films are all except(H)

a.PA View

b.magnification of cardiac silhouette

c.lack of edge sharness

d.loss of fine detail

4.True regarding portable chest radiographraphy are all except (H)

a.often used for acutely ill patients

b.variability in under- and over exposure of film

c.use of shorter focal spot-film distance

d.No change in cardiac silhouette

5.Most frequent mass of middle mediastinum(SW)

a.cyst

b.lymph node

c.nerve tumour

d.none

6.Chest x ray features in ARDS are all except typically shows(H)

a.bilateral

b.interstitial and alveolar opacities

RESPIRATORY SYSTEM

1.The chest view which is often useful to determine whether pleural abnormalties represent freely flowing fluids(H)

a.The PA view

b. The lateral view

c.Lateral decubitus view

d.Apical lordotic view

2. For better visualization of diseases of lung apices,which view of chest is preferred(H)

a. PA View

c.involve at least three-quarters of lung field

d.pleural effusion

7.CT of chest is particularly valuable in (H)

a.assessing hilar and mediastinal diseases

b.diseases adjacent to spine or chest wall

c. pleural diseases

d.all

8.Role of contast CT of chest are all except(H)

a.to indentify fat or calcification in pulmonary nodule

b.to distinguish lymph nodes and masses from vascular structures in mediastinum

c. pulmonary embolism

d.bronchogenic carcinoma

9.In HRCT,the thickness of individual cross-sectional images is(H)

a.1-2mm

b.3-4mm

c.5-7mm

d.7-10mm

10.Disease/s which shows characteristic pattern on HRCT is/are(H)

a.lymphagitic carcinomatosa

b.idiopathic pulmonary fibrosis

c.sarcoidosis

d.all

11.HRCT scan allows better recognition of all except(H)

a.subtle parenchymal and airway disease

b.thickened interlobular septa

c.abnormally thickened or airways (bronchiectasis)

d.large nodules

12.Overall, most common malignancy of the mediastinum (SW)

a.neuroblastoma

b.lymphoma

c.thymoma

d.ganglioneuroma

13.The most common mediastinal tumours in children(SW)

a.lymphoma

b.neurogenic tumour

c.germ-cell tumour

d.thymoma

14. Which feature of anterior mediastinal multilocular cyst on CT scan suggest of mature teartoma

a.combination of fluid soft tissue,calcium or fat(SW)

b.only soft tissue

c.only calcium

d.only fat

15.Most common site of primary mediastinal cyst(SW)
a.anterior
b.middle
c.posterior
d.equally distributed

16 All are true regarding CT pulmonary angiography(CTPA) except(H)
a.detect segmental and subsegmental emboli
b.equal in accuracy to pulmonary angiography
c. test of choice for the evaluation of pulmonary embolism for many clinicians
d.more associated risks than pulmonary angiography

17.Albumin macroaggregates labeled with ^{99m}Tc is used in(H)
a.MDCT
b.MRA
c.PET SCAN
d.ventilation-perfusion scan

18.Functional-anatomical maping make use of(H)
a.PET SCAN only
b.CT scan only
c.PET +CT SCAN
D.MRI

19.The most frequently encountered neoplasm of anterior mediastinum in adult(SW)
a.lymphoma
b.thymoma
c.cyst
d.thyroid

20.The most common extracranial solid malignancy in paediartic patients(SW)
a.neuroblastoma
b.neurilemoma
c.neurofibroma
d.ganglioneuroma

21.The most common intrathoracic malignancy of childhood(SW)
a.neuroblastoma
b.lymphoma
c.thymoma
d.ganglioneuroma

22. all are true regarding PET scan except(H)
a.used in evaluation of solitary pulmonary nodule.
b.used in staging of lung cancer
c.uses FDG
d.unstable ^{18}F emits alpha particle

23.All of followings shows false negative finding in PET scan except(H)
a.carcinoid tumour

b.bronchioalveolar cell carcinoma

c.malignant lesions <1 cm

d.granulomatus lesions

24. Indications of pulmonary angiography are(H)

a.pulmonary embolism

b.pulmonary arteriovenous malformation

c.assessment of pulmonary arterial invasion by tumour

d.all

25. Vertual bronchoscopy shows airways down to(H)

 a.sixth to seventh generation of airways

b.four to five genetation of airways

c.two to three generation of airways

d. no limitation

26.X- ray finding in mycoplasm pneumonia are all except(N)

a.interstitial or brochopneumonic

b.hilar lymphadenopathy

c.unilateral ,central dense in lung

d.very common significant pleural effusion

27.Radiological features of invasive pulmonary aspergillosis (N)

a.halo sign on CT(hemorrhagic nodule surrounded by ischemia)

B.air crescent on CT(due to lung necroses around fungal mass)

c.target sign on MRI(a nodule with lower central signal)

d.central dot sign on CT

28.'Buckshot calcifiaction' involving lung and spleen is noted in(N)

a.histoplasmosis

b.aspergillosis

c.candidiasis

d.tuberculosis

29.Rope sign (acute angulation between chin and larynx caused by weekness of the hyoid muscle) is noted in(N)

a.poliomyelitis

b.diptheria

c.botulinism

d.none

30.Which pneumatised sinus is present at birth(N)

a.maxillary sinus

b.ethmoidal sinus

c.frontal sinus

d.sphenoid sinus

31.All are true regarding paranasal sinuses except(N)

a.maxillary and ethmoidal sinuses are present at birth

b.maxillary sinuses are not pneumatised until 4yrs of birth

c.sphenoid sinuses are present by 5yrs of birth

d.frontal sinuses begin to develop by 2yrs and is completed by adolescence

32.Lemiere disease involive(N)

a.internal jugular vein

b.cephalic vein

c.femoral vein

d.IVC

33.Subglottic narrowing(steeple sign) on PA view of neck is mainly found in(N)

a.acute epiglottitis

b.croup(laryngotracheobronchitis)

c.acute infectious laryngitis

d.bacterial tracheitis

34.Thumb sign on lateral neck radiograph is noted in(N)

a.acute epiglottitis

b.croup(laryngotracheobronchitis)

c.acute infectious laryngitis

d.bacterial tracheitis

35. Foreign body that may be radiopaque is

a.grapes

b.nuts

c.fish bone

d.meat

36.The 'sandstorm' appearance on chest x ray is noted in(N)

a.pulmonary alveolar micolithiasis

b.bronchiolitis obliterans

c.follicular bronchitis

d.primary pulmonary hemosiderosis

37.Radiographic feature that favours pulmonary edema are except(N)

a.peribronchial cuffing/septal lines

b.pleural effusion

c.balanced or inverted vascular distribution

d.peripheral edema

38.Radiographic feature that favours cardiogenic pulmonary edema are all except(N)

a.cardiomegaly

b.increase in vascular pedicle width

c.peripheral or patchy edema

d.pleural effusion

39.Butterfly pattern of interstitial or alveolar infiltrates is noted in(N)

a.pulmonary edema

b.bronchogenic carcinoma

c.Chronic pulmonary eosinophilia

d.sequestration

40. Peripheral infiltrates with central sparing(photographic negative of pulmonary edema) on chest x ray is seen in(N)

a.pulmonary edema

b.bronchogenic carcinoma

c.Chronic pulmonary eosinophilia

d.sequestration

41.Confluent lobar consolidation on chest x ray is noted in(N)

a.viral pneumonia

b.pneumococcal pneumonia

c.streptococcal pneumonia

d.eosinophilic pneumonia

42.The gold standard test for bronchiectasis is(N)

a.HRCT

b.x ray

c.conventional CT

d.MRI

43.HRCT finding of bronchiectasis are all except(N)

a.'tram lines'/'signet ring' appearance

b.bronchi with 'beaded' contour

c.cysts in 'strings and clusters'

d.halo sign

44.X ray showing parenchymal inflammation with a cavity containing air fluid level is noted in(N)

a.pulmonary abscess

b pneumatocele

c.empyema

d.none

45.The diagnostic test of choice for detecting pulmonary embolism(N)

a.spiral CT with contrast

b.NECT

d.V/Q scan

d.x ray

46.Gold standard for diagnosing pulmonary embolism (N)

a.spiral CT with contrast

b.NECT

d.V/Q scan

d.pulmonary embolism

47.The typical finding of atelectasis are all except(N)

a.volume loss

b.displement of fissures

c.displacement of mediastinal structures and heart

d.widening of intercostal spaces

48.The most common form of pulmonary malignancy in children(N)

a.metastatic lesions

b.bronchial carcinoids

c.adenoid cystic carcinoma

d.mucoepidermoid carcinoma

49.Which view of lung is preferred for pneumothorax(N)

a.inspiratory

b.expiratory

c.mid –expiratory

d.none

50.All are sonographic sign of pleural fluid except(RUMACK)

a.diaphragm sign

b.displaced crus sign

c.bare –area sign

d.cog wheel sign

51.All are true regarding view of chest x ray except(GRAINGER)

a.lateral decubitus view is used to show pleural effusion not visible on PA view

b.expiratory film useful in showing air trapping,particularly in childeren

c.expiratory film useful in showing small pneumothorax

d.lateral decubitus view is not useful in small subpulmonic view

52.Which post precessing technique is used to highlight regions of emphesyma or air trapping(GRAINGER)

a.maximumintensity projection

b.minimum intensity projection

c.shaded surface time

d.volume rendering

53.All are true regarding high resolution CT except(GRAINGER)

a.thin collimation ,usually 1-2mm

b.high frequency algorithm reconstruction

c.used in suspected interstitial lung disease

d.more radition exposure than volumetric CT

54.Which is used for perfusion scintigraphy(GRAINGER)

a.$_{99m}$Tc labelled protein microparticles

b.$_{81m}$Kr

c.$_{133}$Xe

d.$_{99m}$Tc DMSA

55.Radionuclide used for

ventilation imaging are all except(GRAINGER)

a. $_{99m}$Tc DTPA

b.$_{133}$ Xe

c.$_{99mTc}$- technegas

d.$_{99m}$Tc MAG3

56.The ideal agent of choice for ventilation imaging(GRAINGER)

a.$_{81m}$Kr

b. $_{99m}$Tc DTPA

c.$_{133}$ Xe

d.$_{99mTc}$- technegas

57.True regarding dome of diaphragm(GRAINGER)

a.right dome is 1.5 to 2.5 cm higher than left

b.right dome is 1.5 to 2.5 cm lower than left

c.left dome is never higher than left

d.the normal excursion diaphragm is less than <1.5cm

58.Approximate pleural effusion to blent CP angle on PA view(GRAINGER)

a.<100 cc

b.<100 to 200 ml

c.200 to 500 ml

d.>500ml

59.The most common cause of pneumothorax in adult(GRAINGER)

a.primary spontaneous pneumothorax

b.airway obstruction

c.diffuse lung disease

d.pulmonary infection

60.'Double diaphragm sign ' is noted in(GRAINGER)

a.subpulmonic effusion

b.pneumothorax

c.hydrothorax

d.diaphragmatic palsy

61.All are sign of diaphragmatic injury except(GRAINGER)

a.dependent viscera sig

b.thick crus sign

c.collar sign

d.crescent sign

62.The most useful investigation of madiastinal mass(GRAINGER)

a.MDCT

b.MRI

c.x ray

d.USG

63.The most common primary tumour of anterior mediastinumin adult(GRAINGER)

a.thymomas

b.germ cell tumour

c.lymphoma

d.thymus

64. The most common tumour to arise in posterior mediastinum(GRAINGER)
a.germ cell tumour
b.lymphoma
c.neurogenic tumour
d.none

65.Continous diaphragm sign is noted in(GRAINGER)
a.pnuemothorax
b.pneumomediastinum
c.bilateral pleural effusion
d.pneumopericardium

66.Flask or water bottle cardiac configuration is noted on(GRAINGER)
a.pericardial effusion
b.constrictive pericarditis
c.cardiomyopathy
d.restrictive pericarditis

67.Epicardial fat pad sign noted in lateral x ray of chest is seen in(GRAINGER)
a.pericardial effusion
b.pericardial thickenig
c.both
d.none

68.Hallmark of pericardial constriction (GRAINGER)
a.pericardial thickening
b.pericardial thickening
c.both
d.none

69.The most common manifestation of primary tubarculosis in children(GRAINGER)
a.unilateral hilar lymphadenopathy
b.pleural effusion
c.pneumonia
d.bilateral hilar lymphadenopathy

70.Ghon lesion or focus refers to(GRAINGER)
a. pneumonia of primary tuberculosis
b.residual opacity following primary tuberculosis
c.cavitatory lesion of tuberculosis
d.none

71.True regarding Ranke's comple(GRAINGER)
a.Ghon lesion +ipsilateral hilar lymph node calcification
b.reflects prior pulmonary tuberculosis
c.does not imply activity of disease
d.all

72.Rasmussen aneurysm in lung is noted in(GRAINGER)
a.cavitary tuberculosis
b.cavitatory bronchogenic carcinoma

c.pulmonary abscess

c.hydatid cyst

73.All are feature of complex cavitary lesions of hydatid cyst of lung except(GRAINGER)

a.a floating membrane (water lily sign,camalote sign)

b.a dry cyst with crumpled membrane(rising sun sign ,serpent sign)

c.a cyst with all contents expectorated(empty cyst sign)

d.collar sign

74.all are sign of hydatid cyst except(GRAINGER)

a.camalote sign

b.rising sun sign

c.air bubble sign

d.sun set sign

75.Typical chest xray of pneumocystitis carnii is(GRAINGER)

a.diffuse or focal military nodules

b.homogenous opacities/nodules

c.lymphadenopathy

d.bilateral diffuse ,symmetrical ,fine to moderate reticular opacities

76.All are features of pulmonary tuberculosis in advanced HIV disease except(GRAINGER)

a.diffuse bilateral coarse reticulonodular opacities

b.hilar and or mediastinal lymphadenopathy

c.mid or loer lobe predominance

d.multiple cavities

77.Sabre-sheath trachea is noted in(GRAINGER)

a.congenital syphilis

b.COPD

c.intrathoracic thyroid

d.sequelae of tracheostomy

78.Tracheobronchomegaly is also known as(GRAINGER)

a.Mounier-Kuhn disease

b.Kartagener syndrome

c.Treitz 's disease

d.Wegener's disease

79.The tracheal appearance in tracheomalacia is(GRAINGER)

a.circular

b.elliptical

c.lunate

d.oval

80.Routine use of MRI in lung cancer is reserved for all except(SW)

a.history of contrast allergy

b.suspected madiastinal and vascularinvasion

c.suspected vertebral body invasion

d.all

81.The most effective noninvasive method to assess mediastinal and hilar lymphnode enlargement(SW)

a.chest x ray

b.MRI

c.CT scan

d.PET scan

82.Mediastinal and hilar lymph node is said to be enlarged on CT (SW)

a.size>2cm

b a.size>3cm

c.size>1cm

d.size>4cm

83.All are true regarding PET imaging of lung cancer except (SW)

a.PET uses ^{18}F-FDG

b.image whole body after single injection

c.more accuracy than CT in assessing mediastinal lymph node staging

d.based on metabolic activity of fructose of cancer cells

84.Which imaging has recently emerged as a method of staging in NSCLC(SW)

a.CT scan

b.MRI

c.Endoesophageal ultrasound(EUS)

d.PET scan

85.Primary tool for diagnosing pulmonary abscess(SW)

a.chest x-ray

b.CT scan

c.USG

d.none

86.Possible differential diagnosis of pulmonary lung abscess are all except(SW)

a.loculated or interlobar emyema

b.cavtating lung carcinoma

c.hamartoma

d.wegenar's granulomatosis

87.The current gold standard of diagnosis of bronchectasis is(SW)

a. chest x-ray

b.PET scan

c.CT scan

d.MRI

88.Solid mass within a cavity surrounded by a rim of air between the mass and cavity wall in chest x ray of aspergilloma is known as(SW)

a.monad's sign

b.ghon focus

c.McBurney sign

d.none

89.The most common primary chest wall malignancies(SW)

a.Chondrosarcoma

b.osteosarcoma

c.Ewing's tumour

d.none

90.Cardinal sign of bronchectasis on HRCT is(GRAINGER)

a.lack of tapering of bronchial lumena

b.signet ring sign

c.visualisation of bronchi within 1cm of the costal pleura

d.mucous filled dialted bronchi

91.The internal bronchial diameter greater than that of adjacent pulmonary artery noted in bronchectasis, on HRCT of lung is known as(GRAINGER)

a.signet ring sign

b.dot sign

c.tram track sign

d.racemose sign

92.Small centrilobular nodular and linear branching opacities (tree-in-bud sign) on HRCT is characteristic of (GRAINGER)

a.inflammatory and infectious bronchiolitis

b.cystic fibrosis

c.bronchectasis

d. aspergillosis

93.The technique of choice for detection and assessment of the extent of bronchectasis is(GRAINGER)

a.HRCT

b.MDCT with thin collimation

c. X ray

d.PET

94.Various shapes of opacities of bronchoceles in ABPA are(GRAINGER)

a.gloved finger opacities/toothpaste opacities

b.band shaped opacities that point to the hilum

c.V-and-Y shaped opacities

d.star shaped

95. Broncholithiasis is noted in(GRAINGER)

a.hyperparathyroidism

b.pneumocyctis carnii

c.mycobacterium tuberculosis

d.ABPA

96.Overinflation with alterations in lung vessels suggest of(GRAINGER)

a.emphysema

b.chronic bronchitis

c.bronchectasis

d.cystic fibrosis

97.Size of bulla(GRAINGER)
a.>1cm
b.>2cm
c.>3cm
d.>4cm

98.The cardinal radiographic features of lobar collapse are all except(GRAINGER)
a.increased opacity of affected lobe
b.volume loss
c.both
d.none

99.All are direct sign of volume loss except(GRAINGER)
a.displacements of fissure
b.crowding of vessels and bronchi
c.ipsilateral pull of hila in upper lobe collapse
d.compensatory hyperinflation

100.Shifting granuloma sign is a feature of(GRAINGER)
a.healing of granuloma
b.lung collapse
c.malignant change in the lesion
d pulmoary embolism

101.Paramediastinal translucency(Luftischel's sign) is typically seen in(GRAINGER)
a.left upper lobe collapse
b.left lower lobe collapse
c.right lower lobe collapse
d.right middle lobe collapse

102.Juxtaphrenic peak of diaphragm is noted in(GRAINGER)
a.lung collaspse
b.consolidation
c.pleural effusion
d.emphysema

103.The radiographic sign resulting from right upper lobar collapse due to central obstructing bronchogenic carcinoma is(GRAINGER)
a.Luftischel 's sign
b.Golden's S sign
c.signet ring sign
d.crescentric sign

104.CT mucous bronchogram sign suggest of(GRAINGER)
a.obstructive lesion causing lung collapse
b.pnuemonia
c.pleural effusion
d.emphysema

105.the loss of silhouette of right cardiac border is feature of(GRAINGER)
a.right upper lobe collapse
b.left lower lobe collapse
c.right middle lobe collapse
d.right lower lobe collapse

106.Middle lobe syndrome is due to(GRAINGER)

a.tuberculous infection

b.measles infection

c.pertussis infection

d.klebsiella infection

107.Superior triangle sign is seen in (GRAINGER)

a.right upper lobe collapse

b.left lower lobe collapse

c.right middle lobe collapse

d.right lower lobe collapse

108.Flat waist sign is seen in(GRAINGER)

a.right upper lobe collapse

b.left lower lobe collapse

c.right middle lobe collapse

d.right lower lobe collapse

109.Iceberg lesions are noted in(GRAINGER)

a.bronchogenic carcinoma

b.carcinoid tumour

c.hamartoma

d.pulmonary AVM

110.Popcorn calcification is noted in(GRAINGER)

a.hamartoma

b.chondrosarcoma

c.both

d.none

111.All are true rgrading solitary pulmonary nodule except(GRAINGER)

a.fat in lesion is virtually diagnostic of hamartoma

b.a lack of enhancement (<15HU)following iv contrast indicative of benign nature

c.presence of central or concentric calcification is in favor of malignancy

d.a lesion unchanged over 2yrs is more likely benign in nature

112.HRCT feature showing multiple cavitary lesions of bizarre shape and sparing extremes of lung bases and anterior lips of middle lobe and lingual suggest of(GRAINGER)

a.Langerhans cell histiocytosis

b.lymphangioleomyomatosis

c.rheumatoid arthritis

d.cystic fibrosis

113.HRCT features that favor lymphangioleomyomatosis overLangerhans cell histiocytosis are all except(GRAINGER)

a.more diffuse distribution of cysts

b.sparing of bases

c.more regularly shaped cyst

d.normal intervening lung parenchyma

114.Comet tail sign on chest x ray or CT scan is noted in(GRAINGER)

a.round atelectasis

b.round pneumonia

c.metastases

d.sarcoidosis

115.Deep sulcus sign is a sign noted in supine x ray of(GRAINGER)

a.pneumothorax

b.hydrothorax

c.pleural effusuin

d.subpulmonic effusin

116.The collar sign and dependent viscera sign on CT of thorax is noted in(GRAINGER)

a.rupture of esophagus

b.rupture of trachea

c.rupture of diaphragm

d.lung contusion

117.The Macklin effect is related to (GRAINGER)

a.production of x ray in x ray tube

b. heat producing effect of radlofrequency on tissue

c.an effect producing pneumomediastinum

d.an effect producing pleural effusion

118.Fallen lung sign is noted in(GRAINGER)

a.complete rupture of mainstem bronchus

b.complete rupture of pulmonary vessel

c.complete rupture of diaphragm

d.complete rupture of trachea

119.All radiological features favor cardiac cause of pulmonary edema except(GRAINGER)

a.cardiomegaly

b.vascular redistribution

c.wedened vascular pedicle

d.patcy peripheral air space opacification

120.Sign seen in pulmonary embolism(GRAINGER)

a.peripheral area of wedge shaped consolidation(Hampton's hump)

b.regional oligemia(Westermark sign)

c.both

d.none

121.Double bronchial wall sign is feature of (GRAINGER)

a.pneumomediastinum

b.pnuemothorax

c.pneumopericardium

d.none

122.Optimum location of tip of endotracheal tube is(GRAINGER)

a.2-5cm above carina

b.3-8cm above carina

c.4-10cm above carina

d.5-15cm above carina

123.All are radiological features of emphysema except (GRAINGER)

a.flattened,depressed ,hemidiaphragms

b.increased retosternal space

c.hyper-transradiancy

d.prominent vessels

124.'Crazy-paving' pattern is noted in except(GRAINGER)

a.alveolar proteinosis

b.mucinous bronchiolo-alveolar carcinoma

c.exogenous lipid pneumonia

d.cystic fibrosis

125.Black bronchus sign on CT is noted in(GRAINGER)

a.subtle ground- glass opacification

b.bronchectasis

c.overt ground –glass opacification

d.bronchogenic carcinoma

126.Feature of interstitial edema are all except(GRAINGER)

a.Kerley'B and A lines

b.peribronchial cuffing

c.thickening of interlobar fissures

d.Pleural effusion

127.Multifocal areas of ground glass opacification with a surrounding rim of consolidation(reverse halo sign) is noted in(GRAINGER)

a.Wgener's granulomatosis

b.cryptogenic organizing pneumonia

c.pulmonary heamorrhage

c.eosinophilic granuloma

128.Mean wedge pulmonary arterial pulmonary pressure is(GRAINGER)

a.5mmHg

b.8mmHg

c.15mmHg

 d.20mmHg

129.The first recognized radiological sign of pulmonary venous hypertention(GRAINGER)

a.Kerley's B lines

b.upper lobe venous diversion

c.perihilar haze

d.peribronchial cuffing

130.All are true regarding Kerley A lines except(GRAINGER)

a.approx. 4cmm in length,reaches pleura

b.most conspicuous in upper and mid portion of lung

c.deep septal lines(lymphatic channel) radiating from hila

d.reflect acute or severe degree of oedema

131.All are true regarding Kerley B line except(GRAINGER)

a.<=1cm in length,interlobular septal lines

b.located in peripherally in upper zone

c.parallel to ech other

d.at right angles to pleural surface

132. All are cause of persistent septal lines except(GRAINGER)

a.idiopathic interstitial fibrosis

b.lymphangitis carcinomatosa

c.pneumoconiosis

d.acute pulmonary enous hypertention

133.Perihilar batwing's pattern of airspace consolidation is seen in(GRAINGER)

a.left ventricular failure

b.renal failure

c.both

d.none

134.interstitial edema (peribronchial cuffing and Kerley lines) develop when pulmonary capillary wedge pressure is(GRAINGER)

a.8-12mmHg

b.12-18mmHg

c.19-25mmHg

d.>25mmHg

135.Pulmonary arterial hypertention is defined as elevation in mean arterial pulmonary pressure above (GRAINGER)

a.30mmHg at exercise and 25mmHg at rest

b.20mmHg at exercise and 25mmHg at rest

c.25mmHg at exercise and 30mmHg at rest

d.30mmHg at exercise and 220mmHg at rest

136.All are radiographic features of pulmonary arterial hyperttention except(GRAINGER)

a.cardiac enlargement(right atrial and ventricular enlargement)

b.enlargement of main pulmonary artery and its

branches down to segmental branches

c.tappering of peripheral arterial branches beyond segmental branches (peripheral pruning)

d.perihilar haze

137.Pulomonary arterial size is said to be enlarged when transeverse diameter of right descending pulmonary artery is greater than(GRAINGER)

a.15mm

a.17mm

c.19mm

d.13mm

138.Perfusion (pulmonary) scintigraphy uses all except(GRAINGER)

a.krypton-81m

b.$_{99m}$Tc DTPA

c. technegas

d.$_{99m}$Tc MAA

139.'Tram track' appearance on pulmonary angiography is noted in(GRAINGER)

a.bronchogenic carcinoma

b.pulmonary embolism

c.pulmonary arterial hypertention

d.bronchectasis

140.Scimitar syndrome is characterized by all except(GRAINGER)

a.small ipsilateral lung

b.mediastinal shift away from lesion side

c.an abnormal vessel usually drainig down and enlarging towards diaphragm

d.the lung is normally connected to bronchial tree

141.The most common subglottic soft tissue mass in infancy(CHAPMAN)

a.subglottic haemangioma

b.respiratory papillomatosis

c.subglottic cyst

d.none

142.Unilateral congenital absence of pectoral muscles is ssen in(CHAPMAN)

a.Poland's syndrome

b.Apert 's syndrome

c.Mcleod's syndrome

d.none

143.Mcleod's syndrome is characterized by all except(CHAPMAN)

a.unilateral hypertransradiant hemithorax

b.small lung

c.small main and peripheral arteries

d.no air trapping

144. No mediastinal displacement is seen in (CHAPMAN)

a.pleural effusion

b.collapse

c.consolidation

d.none

145.'Spring water'cyst refers to(CHAPMAN)

a.pericardial cyst

b.bronchogenic cyst

c.oesophageal duplication cyst

d.none

146.Size of solitary pulmonary nodule (SW)

a.<3cm

b.<4cm

c.<5cm

d.<6cm

147.Most common cause of benign solitary pulmonary nodule(SW)

a.infectious nodule

b.hamartomas

c.AVM

d.none

148.Upto what % of solitary pulmonary nodule on chest x ray shows multiple nodule on CT scan(SW)

a.20%

b.30%

c.40%

d.50%

149.Highly specific cancer sign in solitary pulmonary nodule(SW)

a.size>3cm

b.irregular edge

c.corona radiate/speculated edge

d.lobulated edge

150.four patterns of benign calcification in nodule are all except(SW)

a.stippled

b.diffuse

c.central

d.laminated

151.Pattern of calcification usually associated with cancer in solitary pulmonary nodule are all except(SW)

a.stippled

b.amorphous

c.eccentric

d.popcorn

152.Volume doubling time of lung cancer is(SW)

a.20-400 days

b.400-600 days

c.600-800 days

d.none

153.Tracer used in PET scan (SW)

a.^{17}F-FDG

b.^{16}F-FDG

c.^{19}F-FDG

d.^{18}F-FDG

154.False negative PET scanof lungs is noted in all except(SW)

a.bronchoalveolar carcinoma

b.carcinoids

c.tumours<1 cm

d.adenocarcinoma

155.Consolidation with buling of fissures is noted in(CHAPMAN)

a.staphylococcus aureus

b.Klebsiella pneumoniae

c.streptococcus pyogenes

d.none

156.Bronchiectasis with immotile cilia syndrome is noted in(CHAPMAN)

a.Kartagener's syndrome

b.Williams-Campbell syndrome

c.Chediak-Higashi syndrome

d.none

157.Bronchiectasis is noted in(CHAPMAN)

a.Kartagener's syndrome

b.Williams-Campbell syndrome

c.Chediak-Higashi syndrome

d.all

158.Bronchiectasis due to bronchial cartilage deficiency is noted in(CHAPMAN)

a.Kartagener's syndrome

b.Williams-Campbell syndrome

c.Chediak-Higashi syndrome

d.none

159.Bronchiectasis due to immune deficiency states is noted in(CHAPMAN)

a.Kartagener's syndrome

b.Williams-Campbell syndrome

c.Chediak-Higashi syndrome

d.none

160.Aspiration pneumonia is known as(CHAPMAN)

a.Kartagener's syndrome

b.Williams-Campbell syndrome

c.Chediak-Higashi syndrome

d.Mendelson's syndrome

161.Honeycombing is noted in all except(CHAPMAN)

a.rhematoid arthritis

b.extrinsic allergic alveolitis

c.sarcoidosis

d.bronchogenic carcinoma

162.Solitary pulmonary nodule may be seen in (CHAPMAN)

a.tuberculosis

b.bronchogenic carcinoma

c.hamartoma

d.all

163. Solitary pulmonary nodule may be seen in (CHAPMAN)

a.Hydatid cyst

b.Sequestration

c.bronchogenic cyst

d.all

164.Chest x ray suggesting malignancy in solitary pulmonary nodules are all except(CHAPMAN)

a.lesion crosses fissure

b.umblicated or notched margin

c.corona radiate/spiculation

d. abundant calcification

165.Water lily sign is seen in (CHAPMAN)

a.hydatid cyst

b.carcinoids

c.bronchogenic cyst

d.Sequestration

166.Most common site of pulmonary sequestration(CHAPMAN)

a.left lower lobe

b.right lower lobe

c.right upper lobe

d.left upper lobe

167.Diagnosis of pulmonary sequestration is confirmed by(CHAPMAN)

a.bronchography

b.aortography

c.both

d.none

168.Opacity with air bronchogram (CHAPMAN)

a.pneumonia

b.lymphoma

c.alveolar cell carcinoma

d.all

169.Solitary calcifying /ossifying metastasis is noted in all except(CHAPMAN)

a.osteosarcoma/chondrosarcoma

b.papillary carcinoma of thyroid

c.mucinous adenocarcinoma of colon/breast

d.all

170. Bilateral symmetrical hilar lymphadenopathy is noted in(CHAPMAN)

a.lymphoma

b.primary tuberculosis

c.sarcoidosis

d.carcinoma of bronchus

171.'Egg-shell' calcification of lymph node are noted in all except(CHAPMAN)

a.silicosis

b.coal mlner's calcification

c.sarcoidosis

d.pulmonary tuberculosis

172.Pleural calcification is noted in all except(CHAPMAN)

a.old empyema

b.asbestosis

c.silicosis

d.sarcoidosis

173.most common cause of rib destruction(CHAPMAN)

a.tuberculosis

b.bronchogenic carcinoma

d.multiple myeloma

d.metastases

174.Radiological feature of hyaline membrane disease is all except(CHAPMAN)

a.pleural effusion

b.maximum findings at 12-14hrs

c.fine granular pattern throughout both lungs

d.may be complete 'white-out'

175.Mikity-Wilson syndrome is characterized by all except(CHAPMAN)

a.streaky opacities radiating from both hila

b.small bubbly areas throughout both lungs

c.moderate hyperinflation

d.seen in full term normal delivery child

176.The most common lobe involved in Congenotal lobar emphysema is(CHAPMAN)

a.left upper lobe

b.right upper lobe

c.right middle lobe

d.left lower lobe

177.All are radiological signs that aid in diagnosis of thymus except(CHAPMAN)

a. sail sign

b.wave sign

c.notch sign

d.interruptd bronchus sign

178.All are anterior mediastinal masses in children except(CHAPMAN)

a.thymus

b.lymphoma

c.germ cell tumour

d.ganglion cell tumour

179.All are true regarding imaging in lung cancer except

a.PET-CT improve accuracy of staging in non-small cell carcinoma

b.PET-CT is superior in identifying pathologically enlarged mediastinal lymph nodes and extrathoracic metastases

c.Standardized uptake value (SUV) >2.5 on PET is highly suspicious of malignancy

d.CT is done to rule out brachial plexus involvement in superior sulcus syndrome

180. 204. Features of chest x ray in Kaposi's sarcoma
a.bilateral lower lobe infiltrates
b.pleural effusions
c.both
d.none

181.Classic finding on chest x-ray of pnuemocystis infection
a.bilateral diffuse infiltrates
b.infiltrates begin in peripheral region
c.pneumothorax
d.ground glass opacification on HRCT in early astage

182.Lack of growth of solitary pulmonary nodule over what period of----yrs predict of its benign nature
a.2yrs
b.1yrs
c.3yrs
d.4yrs

183.Pattern of calcification highly suggestive of benign nature of solitary pulmonary nodule are all except
a.a dense central nidus
b.multiple punctuate foci
c.'bull's eye' and 'popcorn ball'calcification
d.asymmetric calcification

184.All feature are associated with high risk of malignancy in solitary pulmonary nodule except
a.size=>3.2cm
b.age >60yrsyrs
c.current smokers>20cigarettes /day
d.margin—corona radiate/speculated

185.'Bull's eye' calcification is noted in
a.granuloma
b.hamartoma
c.carcinoid
d.AVM

186.'Popcorn ball' calcification is noted in
a.granuloma
b.hamartoma
c.carcinoid
d.AVM

187.Classical radiological appearance of pneumococcal pneumonia is
a.lobar or segmental consolidation
b.patcy consolidation
c.both
d.none

188.In children,Round pneumonia is caused by
a.pneumoccocus

b.streptococcus

c.E.coli

d.pseudomonas

189.The most common focal complication of pneumococcal pneumonia

a.parapneumonic effusion

b.empyema

c.parenchymal effusion

d.none

190.Pneumatoceles is noted in

a.pneumococcus

b.staphylococcus

c.pseudomonas

d.E.coli

191.Complete clearing of infiltrates in legionella requires

a.1-2weeks

b.4-6weeks

c.1-4months

d.<2weeks

192 .X-ray features with mass lesions/pneumonia suggestive of actinomycosis are all except

a.donot cross fissure or pleura

b.involve mediastinum

c.involve contiguous bone

d.involve chest wall

193.All are true regarding the Ghon focus except

a.initial parenchymal infection

b.usually central location

c. accompanied by transient hilar or paratracheal lymphadenopathy

d.most of lesions hael spontaneously

194.Ghon complex consists of all except

a.The Ghon focus with or without pleural reaction

b.thickening

c.regional lymphadenopathy

d.cavitaion

195.All are true regarding postprimary(adult-type)/reactivation/secondary TB

a.usually localized to apical and posterior segments of upper lobe

b.superior segments of lower lobes are also more frequently involved

c. cavity formation rare

d.caseating pneumonia,fibrosis,calcificatio n

196.Rasmussen's aneurysm is found in

a.Pulmonary tuberculosis

b.bronchogenic carcinoma

c.both

d.none

197.The most common site for extrapulmonary TB
a.lymphnodes
b.Pleura
c.Genitourinary tract
d.bones

198.All are true of miliary tuberculosis except
a.due to hematogenous spread of tuberculosis
b.granuloma size 4-5mm
c.choroidal tubercles pathognomonic
d.tubarcles more easily seen on underpenetrated film

199.All are true regarding HIV-associated TB except
a.prmary –TB like pattern
b.diffuse interstitial or miliary pattern
c.pronounced cavitation
d.intrathoracic lymphadenopathy

200.CT changes in chest highly consistent with nontubarculous mycobacterial infections are
a.tree-in bud appearance
b.involvement of lingual and right middle lobe
c.bronchectasis and cavity formation in more advanced disease
d.All

201.Which is the earliest feature of pulmonary venous hypertention on chest x ray
a.pleural effusion
b.cephalisation of pulmonary vessel
c.pulmonar edema
d.Kerley B lines

202.investigation of choice for ILD
a.HRCT
b.MRI
c.x ray
d.V/Q scan

203.Prunning of pulmonary arteries is seen in
a.pneumonia
b.chronic bronchitis
c.pulmonary hypertension
d.pulmonary transplant

204.The aortic knuckle is obliterated on chest x ray in consolidation of
a.right upper lobe
b.left upper lobe posterior part
c.lingular lobe
d.apex of lower lobe

205.CT halo sign on chest is noted in (Hagga)
a.wegner granulomatosis

b.invasive pulmonary aspergillosis

c.round pneumonia

d.bronchiectasis

206.Commet tail or vacuum cleaner sign on CT of chest is noted in(Hagga)

a.wegner granulomatosis

b.invasive pulmonary aspergillosis

c.round atelectasis

d.bronchiectasis

207.Beaded septum sign on CT chest is noted in(Hagga)

a. a.wegner granulomatosis

b.invasive pulmonary aspergillosis

c.round atelectasis

d.lymphangitic carcinomatosis

208.Simon focus is noted in(Hagga)

a.healed tuberculosis in lower lobe

b.healed tuberculosis in middle lobe

c.healed tuberculosis in lingular lobe

d.healed tuberculosis at apices

RESPIRATORY SYSTEM (ANSWERS)

1.c---The chest view which is often useful to determine whether pleural abnormalties represent freely flowing fluids(H)Lateral decubitus view

2. d---For better visualization of diseases of lung apices,view of chest preferred is(H) Apical lordotic view

3.a--Limitations of portable chest films are (H)magnification of cardiac silhouette,lack of edge sharness,loss of fine detail

4.d---Regarding portable chest radiographraphy are (H)often used for acutely ill patients,variability in under- and over exposure of film,use of shorter focal spot-film distance

5.A---Most frequent mass of middle mediastinum(SW) cyst

6.d---Chest x ray features in ARDS are (H)bilateral ,interstitial and alveolar opacities,involve at least three-quarters of lung field there is no pleural effusion

7.d---CT of chest is particularly valuable in (H)assessing hilar and mediastinal diseases,diseases adjacent to spine or chest wall ,pleural diseases

8.d---Role of contast CT of chest are (H)to distinguish lymph nodes and masses from vascular structures in mediastinum,pulmonary embolism

9.a---In HRCT,the thickness of individual cross-sectional images are(H) 1-2mm

10.d---Diseases which shows characteristic pattern on HRCT are(H)lymphagitic carcinomatosa,idiopathic pulmonary fibrosis,sarcoidosis

11.d---HRCT scan allows better recognition of (H)subtle parenchymal and airway dise ase,thickened interlobular septa,abnormally thickened or airways (bronchiectasis)

12.b----Overall, most common malignancy of the mediastinum (SW) lymphoma

13.b---The most common mediastinal tumours in children(SW) neurogenic tumour

14. a--Features of anterior mediastinal multilocular cyst on CT scan that suggest of mature teartoma is combination of fluid soft tissue,calcium or fat (SW)

15.b---Most common site of primary mediastinal cyst(SW) middle

16. d---Regarding CT pulmonary angiography(CTPA) :(H) detect segmental and subsegmental emboli,equal in accuracy to pulmonary angiography,test of choice for the evaluation of pulmonary embolism for many clinicians ,less associated risks than pulmonary angiography

17.d---Albumin macroaggregates labeled with ^{99m}Tc is used in(H) ventilation-perfusion scan

18.c---Functional-anatomical maping make use of(H) PET +CT SCAN

19.b---The most frequently encountered neoplasm of anterior mediastinum in adult(SW)thymoma

20.a---The most common extracranial solid malignancy in paediartic patients(SW) neuroblastoma

21.a---The most common intrathoracic malignancy of childhood(SW) neuroblastoma

22. d---Regarding PET scan :(H) used in evaluation of solitary pulmonary nodule.,used in staging of lung cancer,uses FDG,unstable ^{18}F emits positron particle

23.d---- False negative finding in PET scan: (H)carcinoid tumour,bronchioalveolar cell carcinoma,malignant lesions <1 cm

24.d--- Indications of pulmonary angiography are(H) pulmonary embolism,pulmonary arteriovenous malformation,assessment of pulmonary arterial invasion by tumour

25. a---Vertual bronchoscopy shows airways down to(H) sixth to seventh generation of airways

26.d---X- ray finding in mycoplasm pneumonia are (N)interstitial or brochopneumonic unilateral ,central dense lesion,hilar lymphadenopathy

27.d---Radiological features of invasive pulmonary aspergillosis (N) halo sign on CT(hemorrhagic nodule surrounded by ischemia).air crescent on CT(due to lung necroses around fungal mass),target sign on MRI(a nodule with lower central signal)

28.a---'Buckshot calcifiaction' involving lung and spleen is noted in(N) histoplasmosis

29.a---Rope sign (acute angulation between chin and larynx caused by weekness of the hyoid muscle) is noted in(N) poliomyelitis

30.b--- Pneumatised sinus present at birth:(N) ethmoidal sinus

31.d---Regarding paranasal sinuses :(N)maxillary and ethmoidal sinuses are present at birth,maxillary sinuses are not pneumatised until 4yrs of birth,sphenoid sinuses are present by 5yrs of birth,frontal sinuses begin to develop at 7-8yrs and are not completely developed until adolescence .

32.a---Lemiere disease involive(N) internal jugular vein

33.b---Subglottic narrowing(steeple sign) on PA view of neck is mainly found in(N) .croup(laryngotracheobronchitis)

34.a---Thumb sign on lateral neck radiograph is noted in(N) acute epiglottitis

35.c---Radiopaque foreign body may be (N) fish bone

36.a---The 'sandstorm' appearance on chest x ray is noted in(N) pulmonary alveolar micolithiasis

37.d---Radiographic feature that favours pulmonary edema are (N)peribronchial cuffing/septal lines,pleural effusion,balanced or inverted vascular distribution

38.c---Radiographic feature that favours cardiogenic pulmonary edema are (N) cardiomegaly,increase in vascular pedicle width,pleural effusion

39.c---Butterfly pattern of interstitial or alveolar infiltrates is noted in(N)pulmonary edema

40.c--- Peripheral infiltrates with central sparing(photographic negative of pulmonary edema) on chest x ray is seen in(N) chronic pulmonary eosinophilia

41.b---Confluent lobar consolidation on chest x ray is noted in(N) pneumococcal pneumonia

42.a---The gold standard test for bronchiectasis is(N) HRCT

43.d---HRCT finding of bronchiectasis are 'tram lines'/'signet ring' appearance,bronchi with 'beaded' contour,cysts in 'strings and clusters'

44.a---X ray showing parenchymal inflammation with a cavity containing air fluid level is noted in(N) pulmonary abscess

45.a---The diagnostic test of choice for detecting pulmonary embolism(N)spiral CT with contrast

46.d---Gold standard for diagnosing pulmonary embolism (N) pulmonary embolism

47.d---The typical finding of atelectasis are (N) volume loss,displement of fissures,displacement of mediastinal structures and heart,crowding of intercostal spaces

48.a---The most common form of pulmonary malignancy in children(N).metastatic lesions

49.b---expiroatory view of lung is preferred for pneumothorax(N)

50.d---Sonographic sign of pleural fluid (RUMACK) diaphragm sign,displaced crus sign,bare –area sign

51.d---Regarding view of chest x ray: (GRAINGER)lateral decubitus view is used to show pleural effusion not visible on PA view,expiratory film useful in showing air trapping,particularly in children,expiratory film useful in showing small pneumothorax,lateral decubitus view is useful in small subpulmonic view

52.b--- Post precessing technique is used to highlight regions of emphesyma or air trapping(GRAINGER) minimum intensity projection

53.d---Regarding high resolution CT :(GRAINGER) thin collimation ,usually 1-2mm,high frequency algorithm reconstruction,used in suspected interstitial lung disease,less radition exposure than volumetric CT

54.a---$_{99m}$Tc labelled protein microparticles is used for perfusion scintigraphy(GRAINGER)

55.d---Radionuclide used for ventilation imaging are (GRAINGER) $_{99m}$Tc DTPA,$_{133}$ Xe,$_{99mTc}$- technegas

56.a---The ideal agent of choice for ventilation imaging(GRAINGER) $_{81m}$Kr

57.a---Regarding dome of diaphragm(GRAINGER) right dome is 1.5 to 2.5 cm higher than left

58.c---Approximate pleural effusion to blunt CP angle on PA view(GRAINGER) 200 to 500 ml

59.a---The most common cause of pneumothorax in adult(GRAINGER) primary spontaneous pneumothorax

60.b---'Double diaphragm sign ' is noted in(GRAINGER) pneumothorax

61.d---Sign of diaphragmatic injury are (GRAINGER) dependent viscera sig,thick crus sign,collar sign

62.a---The most useful investigation of madiastinal mass(GRAINGER) MDCT

63.a----The most common primary tumour of anterior medlastinum in adult(GRAINGER) thymomas

64.c--- The most common tumour to arise in posterior mediastinum:(GRAINGER) neurogenic tumour

65.b---Continous diaphragm sign is noted in(GRAINGER) pneumomediastinum

66.a----Flask or water bottle cardiac configuration is noted on(GRAINGER) pericardial effusion

67.c---Epicardial fat pad sign noted in lateral x ray of chest is seen in(GRAINGER) pericardial effusion,pericardial thickenig

68.c---Hallmark of pericardial constriction (GRAINGER) pericardial thickening,pericardial thickening

69.a---The most common manifestation of primary tubarculosis in children(GRAINGER) unilateral hilar lymphadenopathy

70.b---Ghon lesion or focus refers to(GRAINGER)residual opacity following primary tuberculosis

71.d---True regarding Ranke's complex:(GRAINGER)Ghon lesion +ipsilateral hilar lymph node calcification,reflects prior pulmonary tuberculosis,does not imply activity of disease

72.a---Rasmussen aneurysm in lung is noted in(GRAINGER) cavitary tuberculosis

73.d---All are feature of complex cavitary lesions of hydatid cyst of lung (GRAINGER) a floating membrane (water lily sign,camalote sign),a dry cyst with crumpled membrane(rising sun sign ,serpent sign),a cyst with all contents expectorated(empty cyst sign)

74.d---Sign of hydatid cyst (GRAINGER) camalote sign,rising sun sign,air bubble sign

75.d---Typical chest xray of pneumocystitis carnii is(GRAINGER) bilateral diffuse ,symmetrical ,fine to moderate reticular opacities

76.d---Features of pulmonary tuberculosis in advanced HIV disease are (GRAINGER) diffuse bilateral coarse reticulonodular opacities,hilar and or mediastinal lymphadenopathy,mid or lower lobe predominance

77.b---=Sabre-sheath trachea is noted in(GRAINGER) COPD

78.a---Tracheobronchomegaly is also known as(GRAINGER) Mounier-Kuhn disease

79.c---The tracheal appearance in tracheomalacia is(GRAINGER).lunate

80.d---Routine use of MRI in lung cancer is reserved for (SW) history of contrast allergy,suspected madiastinal and vascularinvasion,suspected vertebral body invasion

81.c---The most effective noninvasive method to assess mediastinal and hilar lymph node enlargement(SW) CT scan

82.c---Mediastinal and hilar lymph node is said to be enlarged on CT (SW) when size>1cm

83.d---Regarding PET imaging of lung cancer : (SW) uses^{18}F-FDG ,image whole body after single injection,.more accuracy than CT in assessing mediastinal lymph node staging,based on metabolic activity of glucose of cancer cells

84.c--Imaging has recently emerged as a method of staging in NSCLC(SW) Endoesophageal ultrasound(EUS)

85.a---Primary tool for diagnosing pulmonary abscess(SW) chest x-ray

86.c---Possible differential diagnosis of pulmonary lung abscess are (SW) loculated or interlobar emyema,cavtating lung carcinoma,wegenar's granulomatosis

87.c---The current gold standard of diagnosis of bronchectasis is(SW) CT scan

88.a---Solid mass within a cavity surrounded by a rim of air between the mass and cavity wall in chest x ray of aspergilloma is known as(SW) monad's sign

89.a---The most common primary chest wall malignancies(SW) Chondrosarcoma

90.a---Cardinal sign of bronchectasis on HRCT is(GRAINGER) lack of tapering of bronchial lumena

91.a---The internal bronchial diameter greater than that of adjacent pulmonary artery noted in bronchectasis, on HRCT of lung is known as(GRAINGER) signet ring sign

92.d---Small centrilobular nodular and linear branching opacities (tree-in-bud sign) on HRCT is characteristic of (GRAINGER) inflammatory and infectious bronchiolitis

93.b---The technique of choice for detection and assessment of the extent of bronchectasis is(GRAINGER) MDCT with thin collimation

94.d---Various shapes of opacities of bronchoceles in ABPA are(GRAINGER)gloved finger opacities/toothpaste opacities,band shaped opacities that point to the hilum,V-and-Y shaped opacities

95.c--- Broncholithiasis is noted in(GRAINGER) mycobacterium tuberculosis

96.a---Overinflation with alterations in lung vessels suggest of(GRAINGER)emphysema

97.a---size of bulla(GRAINGER) >1cm

98.c---The cardinal radiographic features of lobar collapse are (GRAINGER) increased opacity of affected lobe,volume loss

99.d---Direct sign of volume loss :(GRAINGER) displacements of fissure,crowding of vessels and bronchi,ipsilateral pull of hila in upper lobe collapse

100.Shifting granuloma sign is a feature of(GRAINGER) lung collapse

101.a----Paramediastinal translucency(Luftischel's sign) is typically seen in(GRAINGER) left upper lobe collapse

102.a---Juxtaphrenic peak of diaphragm is noted in(GRAINGER) lung collaspse

103.b---The radiographic sign resulting from right upper lobar collapse due to central obstructing bronchogenic carcinoma is(GRAINGER) Golden's S sign

104.a---CT mucous bronchogram sign suggest of(GRAINGER)obstructive lesion causing lung collapse

105.a----the loss of silhouette of right cardiac border is feature of(GRAINGER) right middle lobe collapse

106.a---Middle lobe syndrome is due to(GRAINGER) tuberculous infection

107.d---Superior triangle sign is seen in (GRAINGER) right lower lobe collapse

108.b---Flat waist sign is seen in(GRAINGER)left lower lobe collapse

109.b---Iceberg lesions are noted in(GRAINGER) carcinoid tumour

110.c---Popcorn calcification is noted in(GRAINGER) hamartoma,chondrosarcoma

111.c---Regrading solitary pulmonary nodule :(GRAINGER)fat in lesion is virtually diagnostic of hamartoma,a lack of enhancement (<15HU)following iv contrast indicative of benign nature,presence of central or concentric calcification is in favor of benign lesion,a lesion unchanged over 2yrs is more likely benign in nature

112.a---HRCT feature showing multiple cavitary lesions of bizarre shape and sparing extremes of lung bases and anterior lips of middle lobe and lingual suggest of(GRAINGER) Langerhans cell histiocytosis

113.b----HRCT features that favor lymphangioleomyomatosis over Langerhans cell histiocytosis are :(GRAINGER)more diffuse distribution of cysts,more regularly shaped cyst,normal intervening lung parenchyma

114.a---Comet tail sign on chest x ray or CT scan is noted in(GRAINGER) round atelectasis

115.a---Deep sulcus sign is a sign noted in supine x ray of(GRAINGER) pneumothorax

116.c---The collar sign and dependent viscera sign on CT of thorax is noted in(GRAINGER) rupture of diaphragm

117.c---The Macklin effect is related to (GRAINGER)an effect producing pneumomediastinum

118.a---Fallen lung sign is noted in(GRAINGER)complete rupture of mainstem bronchus

119.d---Radiological features that favor cardiac cause of pulmonary edema are (GRAINGER) cardiomegaly,vascular redistribution,widened vascular pedicle

120.c---Sign seen in pulmonary embolism(GRAINGER) peripheral area of wedge shaped consolidation(Hampton's hump) and regional oligemia(Westermark sign)

121.a---Double bronchial wall sign is feature of (GRAINGER) pneumomediastinum

122.b---Optimum location of tip of endotracheal tube is(GRAINGER) 3-8cm above carina

123.d---Radiological features of emphysema are (GRAINGER) flattened,depressed ,hemidiaphragms,increased retosternal space,hyper-transradiancy

124.d---'Crazy-paving' pattern is noted in(GRAINGER)alveolar proteinosis,mucinous bronchiolo-alveolar carcinoma,exogenous lipid pneumonia

125.a---Black bronchus sign on CT is noted in(GRAINGER) subtle ground- glass opacification

126.d----Feature of interstitial edema are (GRAINGER) Kerley'B and A lines,peribronchial cuffing,thickening of interlobar fissures

127.b---Multifocal areas of ground glass opacification with a surrounding rim of consolidation(reverse halo sign) is noted in(GRAINGER) cryptogenic organizing pneumonia

128.a---Mean wedge pulmonary arterial pulmonary pressure is(GRAINGER) 5mmHg

129.b---The first recognized radiological sign of pulmonary venous hypertention(GRAINGER) upper lobe venous diversion

130.a---Regarding Kerley A lines (GRAINGER)most conspicuous in upper and mid portion of lung,deep septal lines(lymphatic channel) radiating from hila ,reflect acute or severe degree of oedema

131.b---Regarding Kerley B line :(GRAINGER) <=1cm in length,interlobular septal lines,located in peripherally in lower zone ,parallel to ech other,at right angles to pleural surface

132. d----Cause of persistent septal lines (GRAINGER)idiopathic interstitial fibrosis,lymphangitis carcinomatosa,pneumoconiosis

133.b---Perihilar batwing's pattern of airspace consolidation is seen in(GRAINGER) left ventricular failure,renal failure

134.c---interstitial edema (peribronchial cuffing and Kerley lines) develop when pulmonary capillary wedge pressure is(GRAINGER) 19-25mmHg

135.a----Pulmonary arterial hypertention is defined as elevation in mean arterial pulmonary pressure above (GRAINGER) 30mmHg at exercise and 25mmHg at rest

136.d---Radiographic features of pulmonary arterial hyperttention are(GRAINGER)cardiac enlargement(right atrial and ventricular enlargement),enlargement of main pulmonary artery and its branches down to segmental branches,tappering of peripheral arterial branches beyond segmental branches (peripheral pruning)

137.a---Pulomonary arterial size is said to be enlarged when transeverse diameter of right descending pulmonary artery is greater than(GRAINGER) 17mm

138.d---Perfusion (pulmonary) scintigraphy uses (GRAINGER)krypton-81m,$_{99m}$Tc DTPA, technegas

139.b---'Tram track' appearance on pulmonary angiography is noted in(GRAINGER) pulmonary embolism

140.b---Scimitar syndrome is characterized by (GRAINGER)small ipsilateral lung,mediastinal shift towards lesion side,an abnormal vessel usually drainig down and enlarging towards diaphragm,the lung is normally connected to bronchial tree

141.a---The most common subglottic soft tissue mass in infancy(CHAPMAN) subglottic haemangioma

142.a---Unilateral congenital absence of pectoral muscles is seen in(CHAPMAN) Poland's syndrome

143.d---Mcleod's syndrome is characterized by (CHAPMAN) unilateral hypertransradiant hemithorax,small lung,small main and peripheral arteries, air trapping

144. c---No mediastinal displacement is seen in (CHAPMAN) consolidation

145.a---'Spring water'cyst refers to(CHAPMAN) pericardial cyst

146.a---Size of solitary pulmonary nodule (SW) <3cm

147.a---Most common cause of benign solitary pulmonary nodule(SW) infectious nodule

148.d---Upto 50 % of solitary pulmonary nodule on chest x ray shows multiple nodule on CT scan(SW)

149.c---Highly specific cancer sign in solitary pulmonary nodule(SW) corona radiate/speculated edge

150.a---four patterns of benign calcification in nodule are (SW)diffuse,central,laminated

151.d---Pattern of calcification usually associated with cancer in solitary pulmonary nodule are (SW) stippled,amorphous,eccentric

152.a---Volume doubling time of lung cancer is(SW) 20-400 days

153.d---Tracer used in PET scan (SW) ^{18}F-FDG

154.d---False negative PET scan of lungs is noted in (SW) bronchoalveolar carcinoma,carcinoids,tumours<1 cm

155.b---Consolidation with buling of fissures is noted in(CHAPMAN) Klebsiella pneumoniae

156.a---Bronchiectasis with immotile cilia syndrome is noted in(CHAPMAN) Kartagener's syndrome

157.d---Bronchiectasis is noted in(CHAPMAN) Kartagener's syndrome,Williams-Campbell syndrome,Chediak-Higashi syndrome

158.b---Bronchiectasis due to bronchial cartilage deficiency is noted in(CHAPMAN)Williams-Campbell syndrome

159.c---Bronchiectasis due to immune deficiency states is noted in(CHAPMAN)Chediak-Higashi syndrome

160.d---Aspiration pneumonia is known as(CHAPMAN) Mendelson's syndrome

161.d---Honeycombing is noted in all except(CHAPMAN) bronchogenic carcinoma

162.d---Solitary pulmonary nodule may be seen in (CHAPMAN) tuberculosis,bronchogenic carcinoma,hamartoma

163. d---Solitary pulmonary nodule may be seen in (CHAPMAN)Hydatid cyst,Sequestration,bronchogenic cyst

164.d---Chest x ray suggesting malignancy in solitary pulmonary nodules are (CHAPMAN)lesion crosses fissure,umblicated or notched margin,corona radiate/spiculation

165.a---Water lily sign is seen in (CHAPMAN) hydatid cyst

166.a---Most common site of pulmonary sequestration(CHAPMAN)left lower lobe

167.b---Diagnosis of pulmonary sequestration is confirmed by(CHAPMAN)aortography

168d---.Opacity with air bronchogram (CHAPMAN) pneumonia,lymphoma,alveolar cell carcinoma

169.d---Solitary calcifying /ossifying metastasis Is noted in (CHAPMAN) osteosarcoma/chondrosarcoma,papillary carcinoma of thyroid,mucinous adenocarcinoma of colon/breast

170.c--- Bilateral symmetrical hilar lymphadenopathy is noted in(CHAPMAN) sarcoidosis

171.d---'Egg-shell' calcification of lymph node are noted in (CHAPMAN) silicosis,coal miner's calcification,sarcoidosis

172.d---Pleural calcification is noted in (CHAPMAN)old empyema,asbestosis,silicosis

173.b---most common cause of rib destruction(CHAPMAN) bronchogenic carcinoma

174.a---Radiological feature of hyaline membrane disease is (CHAPMAN)maximum findings at 12-14hrs ,fine granular pattern throughout both lungs,may be complete 'white-out'

175.d--Mikity-Wilson syndrome is characterized by (CHAPMAN) streaky opacities radiating from both hila,small bubbly areas throughout both lungs,moderate hyperinflation

176.a---The most common lobe involved in Congenotal lobar emphysema is(CHAPMAN) left upper lobe

177.d---All are radiological signs that aid in diagnosis of thymus (CHAPMAN)sail sign,wave sign,notch sign

178.d---All are anterior mediastinal masses in children (CHAPMAN)thymus,lymphoma,germ cell tumour

179.d---Regarding imaging in lung cancer:PET-CT improve accuracy of staging in non-small cell carcinoma,PET-CT is superior in identifying pathologically enlarged mediastinal lymph nodes and extrathoracic metastases,Standardized uptake value (SUV) >2.5 on PET is highly suspicious of malignancy,MRI is done to rule out brachial plexus involvement in superior sulcus syndrome

180. c---Features of chest x ray in Kaposi's sarcoma :bilateral lower lobe infiltrates,pleural effusions

181.b---Classic finding on chest x-ray of pnuemocystis infection,infiltrates begin in peripheral region

182.a---Lack of growth of solitary pulmonary nodule over what period of—2yrs--yrs predict of its benign nature

183.d---Pattern of calcification highly suggestive of benign nature of solitary pulmonary nodule are a dense central nidus,multiple punctuate foci,'bull's eye' and 'popcorn ball'calcification

184.a---Feature associated with high risk of malignancy in solitary pulmonary nodular are age >60yrsyrs,current smokers>20cigarettes /day,margin—corona radiate/speculated

185.a---'Bull's eye' calcification is noted in granuloma

186.b---'Popcorn ball' calcification is noted in hamartoma

187.a---Classical radiological appearance of pneumococcal pneumonia is lobar or segmental consolidation

188.a---In children,Round pneumonia is caused by pneumoccocus

189.a---The most common focal complication of pneumococcal pneumonia is parapneumonic effusion

190.b---Pneumatoceles is noted in staphylococcus

191.c---Complete clearing of infiltrates in legionella requires 1-4months

192 .a----X-ray features with mass lesions/pneumonia suggestive of actinomycosis are cross fissure or pleura,involve mediastinum,involve contiguous bone,involve chest wall

193.b---.Regarding the Ghon focus: initial parenchymal infection ,usually peripheral location,accompanied by transient hilar or paratracheal lymphadenopathy,most of lesions hael spontaneously

194.d---Ghon complex consists of the Ghon focus with or without pleural reaction,thickening,regional lymphadenopathy

195.c---Regarding postprimary(adult-type)/reactivation/secondary TBusually localized to apical and posterior segments of upper lobe,superior segments of lower lobes are also more frequently involved,cavity formation ,caseating pneumonia,fibrosis,calcification

196.a---Rasmussen's aneurysm is found in Pulmonary tuberculosis

197.a---The most common site for extrapulmonary TB lymphnodes

198.b---.Regarding miliary tuberculosis: due to hematogenous spread of tuberculosis,granuloma size mm,choroidal tubercles pathognomonic ,tubarcles more easily seen on underpenetrated film

199.c---Regarding HIV- associated TB:prmary –TB like pattern,diffuse interstitial or miliary pattern,pronounced cavitation

200.d---CT changes in chest highly consistent with nontubarculous mycobacterial infections are tree-in bud appearance,involvement of lingual and right middle lobe,bronchectasis and cavity formation in more advanced disease

201.b---Which is the earliest feature of pulmonary venous hypertention on chest x ray :cephalisation of pulmonary vessel

202.a---Investigation of choice for ILD HRCT

203.c---Prunning of pulmonary arteries is seen in pulmonary hypertension

204.b---The aortic knuckle is obliterated on chest x ray in consolidation of left upper lobe posterior part

205.b---CT halo sign on chest is noted in (Hagga) invasive pulmonary aspergillosis

206.c---Commet tail or vacuum cleaner sign on CT of chest is noted in(Hagga) round atelectasis

207.d---Beaded septum sign on CT chest is noted in(Hagga) lymphangitic carcinomatosis

208.d---Simon focus is noted in (Hagga)healed tuberculosis at apices

CARDIOVASCULAR SYSTEM

1.2-D Echocardiography uses(H)
a.ultrasound
b.x ray
c.radiofrequency
d.radionuclide

2.2-D Echo is used to assess all except(H)
a.chamber size
b.morphology and motion of valve
c.pericardium
d.valve stenosis (gradient and area)

3.Which kind of echo is used to assess myocardial ischemia(H)
a.2-D echo
b.stress echo
c.doppler
d.TFF

4.An ideal imaging modality in cardiac emergencies is(H)
a.ECHO
b.CT
c.PET SCAN
d.MRI

5.An ideal imaging modality for assessing left ventricular size and function is(H)
a.2-D echo
b.doppler
c.stress echo
d.Nuclear scan

6.The imaging modality of choice for diagnosing hypertrophic cardiomyopathy(H)
a.2-D echo
b.doppler
c.stress echo
d.nuclear scan

7.The gold standard for imaging valve morphology and motion is(H)
a.2-D echo
b.doppler
c.stress echo
d.nuclear scan

8.The gold standard for diagnosis of mitral valve stenosis is(H)
a.2-D echo
b.doppler
c.stress echo
d.nuclear scan

9.The imaging modality of choice for the detection of pericardial effusion is(H)

a.stress echo

b.doppler

c.2-D echo

d.nuclear scan

10.Isotopes are used in which imaging modality(H)

a.SPECT

b.PET

c.CT

d.SPECT and PET

11.SPECT perfusion tracers are(H)

a.thalium-201 and^{99m}Tc isonitriles

b.thallium-201 and rubidium-82

c.rubidum-82 and ^{13}N ammonia

d.^{99m}Tc isonitriles and ^{13}N ammonia

12.PET tracers are

a.thalium-201 and^{99m}Tc isonitriles

b.thallium-201 and rubidium-82

c.rubidum-82 and ^{13}N ammonia

d.^{99m}Tc isonitriles and ^{13}N ammonia

13 In nuclear scan,myocardial ischemia is indicated by presence of(H)

a.relatively preserved or improved tracer uptake in resting image

b.reduced tracer uptake in stress image

c.both ,combination of a+ b

d improved tracer uptake in stress image

14 In comparison to thallium 201,true about ^{99m}Tc SPECT are all except(H)

A shorter half-life and shorter scan time

b.more radiation exposure

c.better image quality

d.acute imaging in myocardial infarction and unstable angina

15.Which is used for detection of resting ischemia(hibernating myocardium) (H)

a.SPECT thallium 201

b.SPECT ^{99m}Tc

c.PET Rubidium

d.PET N-13 ammonia

16.All are true regarding PET myocardial perfusion imaging in comparison to SPECT except(H)

a.higher accuracy

b.higher sensitivity

c.higher specificity

d.poorer resolution

17.The gold standard technique for the assessment of myocardial viability is(H)

a.PET

b.SPECT

c.MRI

d.CT

18.LV function and volume can be assessed by(H)

a.PET

b.SPECT

c.MUGA

d.all

19.Finding on chest x ray suggestive of descending thoracic aortic tear are all except(SW)

a.widened mediastinum

b.abnormal aortic contour

c.left apical cap

d.depression of right main bronchus

20.An ideal imaging modality for diagnosing cardiomyopathy is(H)

a.CT

b.USG

c.MRI

d.PET

21.Delayed enhancement in myocardium in MRI indicate(H)

a.nonviable or infracted myocardium

b.viable myocardium

c.hybernating myocardium

d.none

22. Diagnosis of pericardial temponade is best achieved by(SW)

a.USG

b.x- ray

c.both

d.none

23. Examination of choice for in the evaluation of patients suspected with pulmonary embolism is(H)

a.CT angiography

b.MR angiography

c.catheter angiography

d.V/Q SCAN

24.An attracting technique for imaging patients suspected with arrythmogenic right ventricular dysplasia(H)

a.CT scan

b.MRI

c.PET scan

d.SPECT

25.Role of CT scan in cardiology involves(H)

a.detection of pericardial calcification

b.imaging aorta and great vessels

c.in coronary calcium scoring

d.all

26.Initial modality of choice for LV size/function and valve disease is(H)

a.nuclear scan

b.ECHO

c.MRI

d.CT

27.Primary imaging modality for assessment of LV cavity size,systolic function and wall thicknes(H)

a.nuclear scan

b.ECHO

c.MRI

d.CT

28.The first imaging modality of choice in suspected pericardial effusion and temponade(H)

a.ECHO

b.SPECT

c.MRI

d.CT

29.Imaging modalities of choice for evaluation of stable patients with suspected aortic aneurysm or aortic dissection(H)

a.CT

b.MRI

c.both

d.none

30.The gold standard in the assessment of the anatomy and physiology of the heart and associated vasculature is(H)

a.diagnostic cardiac catheterization and coronary angiography

b.MDCT

c.MRI

d.SPECT

31.Who demonstrated the feasibility of cardiac catheterization in humans(H)

a.Cournand

b.Richards

c.Frossman

d.Sones

32.Who inadverdently performed first selective coronary angiography(H)

a.Cournand

b.Richards

c.Frossman

d.Sones

33.Physcians awarded Nobel Prize in 1956 for cardiac catheterization are(H)

a. Cournand ,Richards and Frossman

b.Sones

c.Judkins

d.Bloch and Purcell

34.Indications of cardiac catheterization and coronary angiography are all except(H)

a.for reperfusion in acute MI

b.stable angina

c.suspected valve disease in symptomatic patients

d.hypertrophic cardiomyopathy with angina

35.The risk associated with elective cardiac catheterization is(H)

a 0.05%-0.14%

b.0.25%

c.0.5%

d.1.0%

36.The most common complication of cardiac catheterization is(H)

a.tachyarrhythmias

b.acute renal failure

c.vascular access-site bleeding

d.bradyarrhythmias

37.All are true regarding lymphography except(SW)

a.colored dye is used first to visualise the lymphatics

b.oil based dye is injected in the lymphatics

c.dye is injected as fast as possible

d.indicated in lymphagiectasia or lymphatic fistula

38.Massive hemothorax is defined as(SW)

a.500 ml of blood

a.1000 ml of blood

a.1500 ml of blood

a.2000 ml of blood

39. The preferred access site for cardiac catheterization is(H)

a.femoral artery and vein

b.brachial artery

c.radial artery

d.Internal jugular vein

40.Brockenbrough-Braunwald sign noted during cardiac catheterization is seen in(H)

a.aortic stenosis

b.hypertrophic obstructive cardiomyopathy

c.mitral stenosis

d.pericarditis

41.Correct maching are all except(H)

a.mean right atrial pressure(10 to 15mmHg)

b.mean pulmonary artery pressure(9 to 19 mmHg)

c.mean pulmonary artery wedge pressure(4 to 12 mmHg)

d.cardiac index(2.8 to 4.2 L-min/m^2)

42. Square root sign is noted in(H)

a.cardiac tempnade

b.constrictive pericarditis

c.restrictive cardiomyopathy

d.mitral stenosis

43.Methods of cardiac output measurement are (H)

a.Fick method

b.thermodilution method

c.use of left ventricular angiography

d.all

44.Gorlin formula is used to calculate(H)

a. valve area

b.cardiac output

c. degree of intracadic shunt

d. vascular resistance

45.The gold standard for assessing LV mass and volume(H)

a.ECHO

b.MRI

c.SPECT

d.CT

46.Investigation best suited for diagnosis of chronic thromboembolic disease is(H)

a.V/Q SCAN

b.SPECT

c.PET SCAN

d.CT SCAN

47. The pathognomonic sign of the coarctation of aorta is(H)

a.dilated left subclavian artery

b.dilated descending aorta

c.inferior notching of ribs

d.the '3' sign

48.The indentation of aorta at the site of coarctation and pre-and poststenotic dilation is known as(H)

a.the '3' sign

b.Palla sign

c.Braunwaldsign

d.Romanus sign

49. All are x ray features of the coarctation of aorta except(H)

a.dilated left subclavian artery

b.dilated descending aorta

c.superior notching of ribs

d.the '3' sign

50. True regarding rib notching noted in the coarctation of aorta

a.inferior notching

b.third to ninth rib

c.due to development of collaterals

d.ALL

51.All are components of the tetralogy of Fallot except(H)

a.malaligned VSD

b.obstruction to right RV outflow

c.aortic override of the VSD

d.LV hypertrophy

52.Boot shaped heart (Coeur en sabot) is feature of(H)

a.TOF

b.TAPVD

c.TGA

d.hypertrophic cardiomyopathy

53.Radiological finding notes in TOF are all except(H)

a.normal sized heart

b.prominent right ventricle and concavity in region of pulmonary conus

c.increased pulmonary vascular markings

d. right sided aortic arch and knob

54.Chest x ray finding in mitral stenosis are all except(H)

a. straightening of upper left border of cardiac silhouette

b.promonence of main pulmonary arteries

c.dilataion of upper lobe pulmonary vein

d.anterior displacement of oesophagus

55.All are true about Kerley B lines in mitral stenosis except(H)

a.horizontal lines

b.most prominent in lower and mid lung fields

c.due to distension of interlobular septae and lymphatics

d.resting mean LA pressure <20mmHg

56. Calcification of the mitral annulus is particularly seen on which view of chest(H)

a.PA view

b.lateral view

c.lordotic view

d.swimmer's view

57.Systolic anterior motion of mitral valve is the classical finding on ECHO of(H)

a.dilated cardiomyopathy

b.restrictive cardiomyopathy

c.hypertrophic cardiomyopathy

d.myocarditis

58.normal amount of pericardial fluid is(H)

a.15-50 ml

b.0-10 ml

c.50-75 ml

d.about 100ml

59.Water- bottle configuration of cardiac silhouette on chest x ray is noted in(H)

a.pericardial effusion

b.cardiomyopathy

c.mitral stenosis

d.aortic stenosis

60.On ECHO Small pericardial effusion appears as relatively echo free space between(H)

a.posterior pericardium and left ventricular epicardium

b.anterior right ventricle and parietal pericardium

c. anterior pericardium and left ventricular epicardium

b.anterior left ventricle and parietal pericardium

61.The investigations that are key in distinguishing restrictive cardiomyopathy and chronic constrictive pericarditis(H)

a.CE CT and MRI

b.SPECT

c.PET

d.ECHO

62.Most common primary tumour in all age group(H)

a.myxoma

b.rhabdomyoma

c.fibroma

d.lymphoma

63.Most common cause of myocardial ischemia is(H)

a.atherosclerotic disease of coronary artery

b.hypertesion

c.metabolic disorder

d.Spasm

64.Cold spot on myocardial perfusion scanning with[201] thallium indicate(H)

a.acute infarct

b.chronic scar

c.both

d.none

65.All are true regarding cardiac MRI imaging in STEMI except(H)

a.use of Gadolinium

b.use of early enhacement technique

c bright signal in infarct area

d.dark areas in normal myocardium

66.Who first introduced PTCA as an alternative to CABG(H)

a.Andreas Gruentzig

b.Charles Dotter

c. Frossman

d. Sones

67.Second generation drug eluting stents use all except(H)

a.everolimus

b.biolimus

c.zotarolimus

d.sirolimus

68.The gold standard for evaluation of renal artery stenosis is(H)

a.contrast atreriography

b.MRI

c.CECT

d. nuclear scan

69.The diameter of descending aorta in abdomen in adult is(H)

a. 3cm

B .2.5cm

c.1.8 to 2cm

d.4cm

70.Sensitive and specific tests for assessment of aneurysms of thoracic aorta are all except(H)

a.CECT

b.MRI

c.conventional aortography

d.chest x ray

71.Tests used for screening of patients at risk for abdominal aortic aneurysm(H)

a.USG

b.x ray

c.MRI

d.CECT

72.USG screening is recommended for abdominal aortic aneurysm for all except(H)

a.men ,65-75yrs of age with history of smoke

b.siblings or offspring of persons with abdominal aortic aneurysm

c.individuals with thoracic aortic aneurysm or peripheral arterial aneurysm

d.men ,50-60yrs of age

73.The investigation that provides most reliable view of mediastinal anatomy(H)

a.CT

b.x ray

c.SPECT

d.PET

74.Lymphangioscintigraphy uses(SW)

a.technetium 99m sulphur colloid

b.indium

c.iodine

c.thallium

75.Heart is usually enlarged when cardiothoracic ratio (H)

a.>40%

b.>50%

c.>55%

d.>60%

76.The Left border of cardiac shadow comprises all except(H)

a.the aortic knob

b.the main and left pulmonary arteries

c.left ventricle

d.outflow tract of right ventricle

77.Structures contributing to the right border of cardiac silhouette are all except(H)

a.superior vena cava

b.the ascending aorta

c.the right atrium

d.the right ventricle

78.All are true except(H)

a.the right sided aortic arch is found in TOF

b.normal hilar shadows is due to lymphnodes

c.pulmonary overcrculation is mainly associated with L-R shunt lesions

d.pulmonary undercirculation is associated with obstruction of outflow tract of right ventricle

79.Erlenmeyer flask type of cardiac contour is noted in(H)

a.pericardial effusion

b.cardiomyopathy

c.restrictive pericarditis

d.TOF

80.The most common pediatric cardiac tumour(H)

a.fibroma

b.myxoma

c.rhabdomyoma

d.lipoma

81.The most common cardiac tumour in adult(H)

a.fibroma

b.myxoma

c.rhabdomyoma

d.lipoma

82.All are acynotic shunts except(GRAINGER)

a.ASD/VSD

b.TOF

c.PDA

d.APW

83.Central cyanosis present within few hrs of birth may be due to(GRAINGER)

a.UTGA

b.TOF

c.PS with ER

d.TS with ER

84.Increased pulmonary perfusion (plethora) is seen in(GRAINGER)

a.ASD

b.VSD

c.PDA

d.TOF

85.Pulmonary plethro is recognized by (GRAINGER)

a.enlarged central pulmonary and peripheral arteries in all zones

b a.enlarged central pulmonary and peripheral veins in all zones

c.enlarged central pulmonary and peripheral arteries and veins in all zones

d.enlarged central pulmonary and and smaller peripheral arteries in all zones

86.In Eisenmenger reaction or syndrome shows(GRAINGER)

a.enlarged central pulmonary and peripheral arteries in all zones

b a.enlarged central pulmonary and peripheral veins in all zones

c.enlarged central pulmonary and peripheral arteries and veins in all zones

d.enlarged central pulmonary and and smaller peripheral arteries in all zones

87.Increased bronchial circulation is noted in(GRAINGER)

a.ASD

b.VSD

c.TOF

d.PDA

88.A vascular pedicle narrow in the frontal view and wide on lateral view is seen in(GRAINGER)

a.TOF

b.PDA

c.uncorrected transposition

d.tricuspid atresia

89.A very long convexity on the left upper mediastinal contour of ascending aorta is noted in(GRAINGER)

a.congenitally corrected transposition

b.TOF

c.coarctaion of aorta

d.PDA

90.The feature that distinguish high cervical arch(pseudocoarctation) from coarctation of aorta is(GRAINGER)

a.deformed high aortic knuckle

b.indented aortic arch left border

c.figure of 3 indentaion deformity of left border of esophagus

d.rib notching

91.All are true regarding rib notching in aortic coarctation except(GRAINGER)

a.involve lower margin of 3rd to 8th rib

b.usually bilaterally symmetrical

c. due to enlarged tortuous intercostals arteries

d. usually seen in infancy

92.3D imaging investigation of choice of heart (GRAINGER)

a.MDCT

b.MRI

c.PET

d.none

93.The most common cyanotic congenital heart disease(GRAINGER)

a.TOF

b.uncorrected transposition of heart

c.ebstein anomaly

d.PS

94.The imaging modality of choice for initial diagnosis and assessment of TOF(GRAINGER)

a.x ray

b.MRI

c.Trans thoracic usg

d.MDCT

95.Boot-shaped heart, small hila and pulmonary oligemia are x ray features of(GRAINGER)

a.uncorrected transposion of heart

b.TOF

c.PA

d.TS

96. In what percentage of case of TOF, right-sided aortic arch is noted (GRAINGER)

a.5%

b.10%

c.20%

d.30%

97.The 2nd most common cyanotic CHD in first year of life (GRAINGER)

a.transposition of great arteries

b.TOF

c.double outlet right ventricle

d.truncus arteriosus

98.In cardiomegaly ,the cardiothoracicview in PA view exceed(GRAINGER)

a.35%

b.40%

c.45%

d.50%

99.Double density through the heart on PA view is seen in (GRAINGER)

a.left atrial enlargement

b.right atrial enlargement
c.left ventricular enlargemet
d.right ventricular enlargement
100.Appearance of mitral annulus calcification is(GRAINGER)
a.C –shaped
b.J-shaped
c.both
d.none
101.In which anomaly,insertion of the septal cusp of the tricuspid valve is displaced towards the apex of right ventricle(GRAINGER)
a.lutembacher's syndrome
b.Ebstein 's anomaly
c.Uhl 's disease
d.Kugel's anomaly
102.Agatston calcium score is done for(GRAINGER)
a.coronary artery calcification
b.carotid artery calcification
c.aortic artery calcification
d.femoral artery calcification
103.ACC/AHA guideline for coronary angiography are all except(GRAINGER)
a.severe resting left ventricular dysfunction(LVEF<35%)

b.high risk treademill score(score=>11)
c.severe execrcise left ventricular dysfunction(exercise LVEF<35%)
d.stress induced perfusion defect of any size
104.Kugel's anomaly is related to(GRAINGER)
a.pulmonary vasculature
c.coronary artery circulation
c.hepatic vasculature
d.brain parenchymal circulation
105.The Kommerell diverticulum refers to(GRAINGER)
a.nonresorbed element of the left fourth aortic arch
b.bronchial artery diverticulum
c. a kind of esophageal diverticulum
d.a kind of ureteric diverticulum
106.'3' sign in coarctation of aorta is due to(GRAINGER)
a.enlargemenl of right subclavian artery above the coarctation
b. a.enlargement of left subclavian artery above the coarctation

a.enlargement of common carotid artery above the coarctation

a.enlargement of left vertebral above the coarctation

107.The imaging technique of choice for coarctation of aorta(GRAINGER)

a.MDCT

b.MRI

c.X ray

d.PET

108.All are related to aortic dissection classification except(GRAINGER)

a.Crawford

b.DeBakey

c.Stanford

d.Todani

109.Situs inversus is noted in(CHAPMAN)

a.Kartagener's syndrome

b.Williams-Campbell syndrome

c.Chediak-Higashi syndrome

d.none

110.Small heart is noted in all except(CHAPMAN)

a.emphysema

b.addition disease

c.constrictive pericarditis

d.cardiomyopathy

111.Uhl's disease involve (CHAPMAN)

a.right atrium

b.right ventricle

c.left atrium

d.left ventricle

112.Radiological feature of enlarged left atrium are all except(CHAPMAN)

a.prominent left atrial appendage

b.'Double' left heart border

c.splying of carina

d.elevated left main bronchus

113.Right sided aortic arch is found in all except(CHAPMAN)

a.TOF

b.truncus arteriosus

c.double outlet left ventricle

d.pulmonary atresia with VSD

114.All are ture regarding thallium 201 scan except(SW)

a.initial uptake in myocardial cell is dependent on myocardial perfusion

b delayed uptake myocardial cell is dependent on myocardial viability

c.fixed defect suggest nonviable myocardium

d.reversible defect suggest of nonviable myocardium

115.The best overall test to detect myocardial ischemia(SW)

a.thallium scan

b.exercise thallium scan

c.MRI

d.ECHO

116.Drug used to provoke in thallium scan is(SW)

a.dipyridamole

b.nitroprusside

c.metopropalol

d.nifedipine

117.Calcium scoring is done using(SW)

a.CT scan

b.MRI

c.PET

d.none

118.Transmyocardial laser revascularistion is done by(SW)

a.high powered CO_2 laser

b.holmium:yttrium-aluminium-garnet laser

c.both

d.none

119.The straightening of left heart border is noted in (SW)

a.Mitral stenosis

b.aortic stenosis

c.mitral regurgitation

c.VSD

120.The propenisity to atrial fibrillation is greatly increased when left atrial size(SW)

a.>6-6.5 cm

a.>6.5-7.0cm

a.>4.5-5.0cm

a.>5-5.50cm

121.'Coeur de stein' in which the entire visceral surface of heart is covered with an armour like calcification is noted in(SW)

a.restrictive cardiomyopathy

b.constrictive pericarditis

c.rheumatic pericarditis

d.TOF

122.Characteristic catheterization finding in constrictive pericarditis are(SW)

a.square root sign

b.equalization of pressure

c.both

d.none

123.Chest x ray finding in ascending aortic aneurysm (SW)

a.convex shadow to right of cardiac shilhouette

b.loss of retrosternal space

c.both

d.none

124.The most common imaging modality for evaluating thoracic aortic aneurysm(SW) a.CECT

b.MRI

c.USG

d.PET

125.Which investigation should now be considered as gold standard for thoracic aortic disease(SW)

a.USG

b.catheter angiography

c.CT and MRA

d.none

126.On CECT ,the double lumen aorta is classic diagnostic feature of(SW)

a. aortic dissection

b.aortic aneurysm

c.both

d.none

127.The diagnostic modality of choice in hemodynamically unstable patients with suspected aortic dissection(SW)

a.TEE

b.CECT

c.MRI

d.USG

128.Contrast used for MRI angiography(SW)

a.iodine

b.barium

c.gadolinium

d.manganese

129.Gold standard in vascular imaging(SW)

a.CECT

b.MRI

c.catheter angiography

d.none

130.The most widely used screening tool to evaluate for atherosclerotic plaque and stenosis of extracranial carotid artery(SW)

a.CT

b.MRI

c.USG

d.catheter angiography

131.All are true regarding USG of carotid artery except(SW)

a.normal internal carotid artery(ICA) has low resistance flow

b.normal external carotid artery(ECA) has high resistance flow

c.flow pattern in CCA resemble that in ECA

d.the peak systolic velocity is increased at the site of vessel stenosis

132. Normal parameter of carotid artery on Doppler study (SW)

a.ICA peak systolic velocity <125cm/s

b.ICA end diastolic velocity >40cm/s

c.ICA/CCA peak systiloic ratio>4

d.none

133.All except one is Doppler criteria to diagnose carotid artery stenosis>70% but less near occlusion

a.ICA peak systolic velocity >230cm/s

b.ICA end diastolic velocity >100/s

c.ICA/CCA peak systiloic ratio 2-4

d.plaque estimate (diameter reduction)=>50%

134.Carotid stenting should be avoided in following carotid angiographic appearance except(SW)

a.extensive carotid calcification

b.polypoid or globular carotid lesions

c.severe tortuosity of common carotid artery

d.long segment stenoses(>3cm in length)

135.Carotid stenting should be avoided in following carotid angiographic appearance except(SW)

a.carotid artery occlusion

b.severe intraluminal thrombus

c.extensive posterior cerebral artery thrombosis

d.exctensive carotid calcification

136.The most common lacation of abdominal aortic aneurysm is(SW)

a.supra-renal aorta

b.infrarenal aorta

c.juxtarenal

d.equally distributed

137.All are true regarding abdominal aortic aneurysm except(SW)

a.normal size of aorta is 2-3 cm

b.the average aggregate growth of aneurysm is 3-4mm/year

c.rupture risk is quite low for aneurysm< 5.5 cm

d.estimated annual risk of rupture is >10% for aneurysm size of 6-7cm

138.In abdominal aortic aneurysm size of aorta is(SW)

a.>30mm

b.1.5 times the adjacent diameter of the normal aorta

c.both
d.none
139.The screening modality of choice for abdominal aortic aneurysm(SW)
a.CECT
B.MRI
c.USG
d.DSA
140.The gold standard for determination of anatomic eligibility for endovascular repair is(SW)
a.CECT
B.MRI
c.USG
d.DSA
141.The inferior mesenteric artery provide collateral flow to the superior mesenteric artery through(SW)
a.the marginal artery of Drummond
b.arc of Riolan
c.maendering mesenteric arteries
d.all
142.Most common radiographic appearance of acute mesenteric ischemia (SW)
a.adynaic ileus
b.gasless abdomen

c.both
d.none
143.Which investigation is contraindicated in mesentric ischemia(SW)
a.Barium
b.CECT
c.MRI
d.USG
144.The defintive diagnosis of mesenteric vascular ischemia is(SW)
a CECT
c.MRA
C.USG
d.biplanar arteriography
145.Dolichostenomelia is a feature of(SW)
a.Down syndrome
b.achodroplasia
c.cretinsm
d.Marfan syndrome
146. Scimitar sign on angiography is found in
a.FMD
b.adventiatial cystic disease of popliteal artery
c.popliteal artery entrapment syndrome
d.none
147.The vein of Giacomini is related to(SW)
a.small saphenous vein

b.great saphenous vein

c.common femoral vein

d.superficial femoral vein

148.All are true about perforators in lower legs(SW)

a.the Cokett perforator veins drain the medial lower leg

b.the Cokett perforator connect the posterior arch vein (a tributary to great saphenous vein) and posterior tibial vein

c.the Boyd perforator veins connect the great saphenous vein to deep veins

d.the Boyd perforator lies approximately 5cm below the knee

149.The most commonly performed test for detection of deep vein thrombosis(SW)

a.duplex USG

b.CT

c .MRI

d.venography

150.The primary method of detection of deep venous thrombosis is(SW)

a.lack of coaptation

b.lack of spontaneous flow

c.loss of respiratory flow variation

d.venous distention

151.All are Duplex usg features of lower limb DVT(SW)except

a.inability to compress the vein

b.lack of spontaneous flow

c.loss of respiratory flow variation

d.color filling of the lumen on color Doppler

152.Iodine 125 fibrinogen uptake investigation is meant for (SW)

a.detection of DVT

b.detection of thyroid nodule

c.detection of adrenal mass

d.detection of ovarian malignancy

153.The most definitive test for diagnosis of DVT in both symptomatic and asymptomatic patients (SW)

a.duplex USG

b.CT

c.MRI

d.venography

154.The gold standard test for DVT(SW)

a.duplex USG

b.CT

c.venography

d.MRI

155.Earliest sign of left atrial enlargement is

a.elevation of left bronchus

b.double shadow of right border

c.posterior displacement of esophagus

d.widening of carinal angle

156.Egg-on –side appearance is noted in

a.TOF

b.TAPVC

c.TGA

d.tricuspid atresia

CARDIOVASCULAR SYSTEM(ANSWERS)

1.a---2-D Echocardiography uses(H)ultrasound

2.d---2-D Echo is used to assess (H)chamber size,morphology and motion of valve,pericardium,but not valve stenosis (gradient and area)

3.b---Stresss echo is used to assess myocardial ischemia(H)

4.a---An ideal imaging modality in cardiac emergencies is(H) ECHO

5.a---An ideal imaging modality for assessing left ventricular size and function is(H) 2-D echo

6.a---The imaging modality of choice for diagnosing hypertrophic cardiomyopathy(H) 2-D echo

7.a---The gold standard for imaging valve morphology and motion is(H) 2-D echo

8.a---The gold standard for diagnosis of mitral valve stenosis is(H) 2-D echo

9.c---The imaging modality of choice for the detection of pericardial effusion is(H) 2-D echo

10.d----Isotopes are used (H)SPECT and PET

11.a---SPECT perfusion tracers are(H) thalium-201 and^{99m}Tc isonitriles

12.c---PET tracers are rubidum-82 and ^{13}N ammonia

13 c----In nuclear scan,myocardial ischemia is indicated by presence of(H) combination of relatively preserved or improved tracer uptake in resting image and reduced tracer uptake in stress image

14b--- In comparison to thallium 201, ^{99m}Tc SPECT has(H)shorter half-life and shorter scan time,lass radiation exposure,better image quality,acute imaging role in myocardial infarction and unstable angina

15.a---SPECT thallium 201 is used for detection of resting ischemia(hibernating myocardium) (H)

SPECT thallium 201

16.d---PET myocardial perfusion imaging has higher accuracy ,higher sensitivity ,higher specificity and better resolution in comparison to SPECT (H)

17.a---The gold standard technique for the assessment of myocardial viability is(H) PET

18.d---LV function and volume can be assessed by(H)PET,SPECT,MUGA

19.d--Finding on chest x ray suggestive of descending thoracic aortic tear are (SW) widened mediastinum,abnormal aortic contour,left apical cap

20.c---An ideal imaging modality for diagnosing cardiomyopathy is(H)MRI

21.a---Delayed enhancement in myocardium in MRI indicate(H)nonviable or infracted myocardium

22.a--- Diagnosis of pericardial temponade is best achieved by(SW)USG

23. a---Examination of choice for in the evaluation of patients suspected with pulmonary embolism is(H) CT angiography

24.a----An attracting technique for imaging patients suspected with arrythmogenic right ventricular dysplasia(H)CT scan

25.d---Role of CT scan in cardiology involves(H) detection of pericardial calcification,imaging aorta and great vessels,in coronary calcium scoring

26.b---Initial modality of choice for LV size/function and valve disease is(H) ECHO

27.b---Primary imaging modality for assessment of LV cavity size,systolic function and wall thicknes(H) ECHO

28.a---The first imaging modality of choice in suspected pericardial effusion and temponade(H) ECHO

29.c---Imaging modalities of choice for evaluation of stable patients with suspected aortic aneurysm or aortic dissection(H) is CT,MRI

30.a----The gold standard for the assessment of the anatomy and physiology of the heart and associated vasculature is(H) is diagnostic cardiac catheterization and coronary angiography

31.c---Frossman demonstrated the feasibility of cardiac catheterization in humans(H)

32.d---Sones inadverdently performed first selective coronary angiography(H)

33.a---Physcians awarded Nobel Prize in 1956 for cardiac catheterization are(H) Cournand ,Richards and Frossman

34.b---Indications of cardiac catheterization and coronary angiography are (H) for reperfusion in acute MI,suspected valve disease in symptomatic patients,hypertrophic cardiomyopathy with angina

35.a---The risk associated with elective cardiac catheterization is(H) 0.05%-0.14%

36.c---The most common complication of cardiac catheterization is(H) vascular access-site bleeding

37.c--- In lymphography (SW) colored dye is used first to visualise the lymphatics,oil based dye is injected in the lymphatics very slowly,indicated in lymphagiectasia or lymphatic fistula

38.c--Massive hemothorax is defined as(SW) 1500 ml of blood or (in paediatrics,one third of patients total blood volume in pleural space)

39. a---The preferred access site for cardiac catheterization is(H) femoral artery and vein

40.b---Brockenbrough-Braunwald sign noted during cardiac catheterization is seen in(H) hypertrophic obstructive cardiomyopathy

41.a---Correct maching (H) mean right atrial pressure(0 to 5mmHg),mean pulmonary artery pressure(9 to 19 mmHg),mean pulmonary artery wedge pressure(4 to 12 mmHg),cardiac index(2.8 to 4.2 L-min/m^2)

42. b---Square root sign is noted in(H) constrictive pericarditis

43.d----Methods of cardiac output measurement are (H) Fick method,thermodilution method,use of left ventricular angiography

44.a---Gorlin formula is used to calculate(H) valve area

 5.b---The gold standard for assessing LV mass and volume(H) MRI

46.a---Investigation best suited for diagnosis of chronic thromboembolic disease is(H) V/Q SCAN

47.d--- The pathognomonic sign of the coarctation of aorta is(H) the '3' sign

48.a---The indentation of aorta at the site of coarctation and pre-and poststenotic dilation is known as(H) the '3' sign

49. c---- X ray features of the coarctation of aorta (H) are dilated left subclavian artery,dilated descending aorta,.inferior notching of ribs,the '3' sign

50. d---- rib notching noted in the coarctation of aorta is in inferior notching,third to ninth rib and due to development of collaterals

51.d--- Components of the tetralogy of Fallot are (H)malaligned VSD,obstruction to right RV outflow,aortic override of the VSD,RV hypertrophy

52.a---Boot shaped heart (Coeur en sabot) is feature of(H) TOF

53.c----Radiological finding notes in TOF are (H) normal sized heart,prominent right ventricle ,concavity in region of pulmonary conus,oligemia and right sided aortic arch and knob

54.d---Chest x ray finding in mitral stenosis are (H) straightening of upper left border of cardiac silhouette,promonence of main pulmonary arteries,dilataion of upper lobe pulmonary vein,posterior displacement of oesophagus

55.d---Feature of Kerley B lines in mitral stenosis are (H) horizontal lines,most prominent in lower and mid lung fields,due to distension of interlobular septae and lymphatics,resting mean LA pressure >20mmHg

56.b--- Calcification of the mitral annulus is particularly seen on which view of chest(H)lateral view

57.c---Systolic anterior motion of mitral valve is the classical finding on ECHO of(H) hypertrophic cardiomyopathy

58.a---normal amount of pericardial fluid is(H) 15-50 ml

59.a---Water bottle configuration of cardiac silhouette on chest x ray is noted in(H) pericardial effusion

60.a---On ECHO Small pericardial effusion appears as relatively echo free space between(H) posterior pericardium and left ventricular epicardium

61.a----The investigations that are key in distinguishing restrictive cardiomyopathy and chronic constrictive pericarditis(H) CE CT and MRI

62.a---Most common primary tumour in all age group(H) myxoma

63.a---Most common cause of myocardial ischemia is(H) atherosclerotic disease of coronary artery

64.c---Cold spot on myocardial perfusion scanning with[201] thallium indicate(H)acute infarct,chronic scar

65.b---Cardiac MRI imaging in STEMI (H) make use of Gadolinium,use of delayed enhacement technique and give bright signal in infarcted area and dark signal in normal myocardium

66.a--- Andreas Gruentzig first introduced PTCA as an alternative to CABG(H)

67.d---Second generation drug eluting stents use (H) everolimus,biolimus,zotarolimus

68.a---The gold standard for evaluation of renal artery stenosis is(H)contrast atreriography

69.c----The diameter of descending aorta in abdomen in adult is(H)1.8 to 2cm

70.d---Sensitive and specific tests for assessment of aneurysms of thoracic aorta are all except(H) CECT,MRI,conventional aortography

71.a---Tests used for screening of patients at risk for abdominal aortic aneurysm(H) is USG

72.d----USG screening is recommended for abdominal aortic aneurysm for (H) men ,65-75yrs of age with history of smoke,siblings or offspring of persons with abdominal aortic aneurysm,individuals with thoracic aortic aneurysm or peripheral arterial aneurysm

73.a---The investigation that provides most reliable view of mediastinal anatomy(H) CT

74.a---Lymphangioscintigraphy uses(SW) technetium 99m sulphur colloid

75.b---Heart is usually enlarged when cardiothoracic ratio (H)>50%

76.d---The Left border of cardiac shadow comprises all except(H) the aortic knob,the main and left pulmonary arteries,left ventricle

77.d---Structures contributing to the right border of cardiac silhouette are (H) superior vena cava,the ascending aorta,the right atrium

78.b---(H)the right sided aortic arch is found in TOF,pulmonary overcrculation is mainly associated with L-R shunt lesions,pulmonary undercirculation is associated with obstruction of outflow tract of right ventricle

79.a---Erlenmeyer flask type of cardiac contour is noted in(H) pericardial effusion

80.c---The most common pediatric cardiac tumour(H) rhabdomyoma

81.b---The most common cardiac tumour in adult(H) myxoma

82.b---Acynotic shunts are (GRAINGER) ASD/VSD,PDA,APW

83.a----Central cyanosis present within few hrs of birth may be due to(GRAINGER)UTGA

84.d---Increased pulmonary perfusion (plethora) is seen in (GRAINGER) ASD,VSD,PDA

85.c---Pulmonary plethro is recognized by (GRAINGER) enlarged central pulmonary and peripheral arteries and veins in all zones

86.d---In Eisenmenger reaction or syndrome shows(GRAINGER) enlarged central pulmonary and and smaller peripheral arteries in all zones

87.c---Increased bronchial circulation is noted in(GRAINGER) TOF

88.c---A vascular pedicle narrow in the frontal view and wide on lateral view is seen in(GRAINGER) uncorrected transposition

89.a---A very long convexity on the left upper mediastinal contour of ascending aorta is noted in(GRAINGER) congenitally corrected transposition

90.d--The feature that distinguish high cervical arch(pseudocoarctation) from coarctation of aorta is(GRAINGER) rib notching

91.d---rib notching in aortic coarctation (GRAINGER)involve lower margin of 3rd to 8th rib,usually bilaterally symmetrical,due to enlarged tortuous intercostals arteries,usually takes several years to develop seen

92.b---3D imaging investigation of choice of heart (GRAINGER) MRI

93.a---The most common cyanotic congenital heart disease(GRAINGER) TOF

94.c---The imaging modality of choice for initial diagnosis and assessment of TOF(GRAINGER) transthoracic usg

95.b----Boot-shaped heart, small hila and pulmonary oligemia are x ray features of(GRAINGER) isTOF

96.d--- Right-sided aortic arch is noted (GRAINGER) 30% of TOF

97.a----The 2nd most common cyanotic CHD in first year of life (GRAINGER) is transposition of great arteries

98.d---In cardiomegaly ,the cardiothoracic diameter in PA view exceed(GRAINGER) 50%

99.a----Double density through the heart on PA view is seen in (GRAINGER) left atrial enlargement

100.c---Appearance of mitral annulus calcification is(GRAINGER) C –shaped and J-shaped

101.b---In Ebstein anomaly,insertion of the septal cusp of the tricuspid valve is displaced towards the apex of right ventricle(GRAINGER)

102.a----Agatston calcium score is done for(GRAINGER) coronary artery calcification

103.d---ACC/AHA guideline for coronary angiography are (GRAINGER) severe resting left ventricular dysfunction(LVEF<35%),high risk treademill score(score=>11),severe execrcise left ventricular dysfunction(exercise LVEF<35%),stress induced large perfusion defect (particularly if anterior)

104.c---Kugel's anomaly is related to(GRAINGER) coronary artery circulation

105.a---The Kommerell diverticulum refers to(GRAINGER) nonresorbed element of the left fourth aortic arch

106.b---'3' sign in coarctation of aorta is due to(GRAINGER) enlargement of left subclavian artery above the coarctation

107.b---The imaging technique of choice for coarctation of aorta(GRAINGER)MRI

108.d--- Crawford,DeBakey,Stanford are all related to aortic dissection classification (GRAINGER).Todani classification is related to choledochal cyst.

109.a---Situs inversus is noted in(CHAPMAN) Kartagener's syndrome

110.d---Small heart is noted in (CHAPMAN) emphysema,addition disease,constrictive pericarditis

111.b---Uhl's disease involve (CHAPMAN) right ventricle

112.b---Radiological feature of enlarged left atrium are all except(CHAPMAN)prominent left atrial appendge, splying of carina,elevated left main bronchus.'Double' left heart border is feature of left atrial enlargement.

113.c---Right sided aortic arch is found in all except(CHAPMAN) TOF,truncus arteriosus,pulmonary atresia with VSD

114.d----Regarding thallium 201 scan (SW):initial uptake in myocardial cell is dependent on myocardial perfusion,delayed uptake myocardial cell is dependent on myocardial viability,fixed defect suggest nonviable myocardium

115.b---The best overall test to detect myocardial ischemia(SW)exercise thallium scan

116.a---drug used to provoke in thallium scan is(SW) dipyridamole

117.b---Calcium scoring is done using(SW) CT scan

118.c---Transmyocardial laser revascularistion is done by(SW) high powered co_2 laser,holmium:yttrium-aluminium-garnet laser

119.a---The straightening of left heart border is noted in (SW) mitral stenosis

120.a----The propenisity to atrial fibrillation is greatly increased when left atrial size(SW) is >4.5-5.0cm

121.b---'Coeur de stein' in which the entire visceral surface of heart is covered with an armour- like calcification is noted in(SW) constrictive pericarditis

122c---.Characteristic catheterization finding in constrictive pericarditis are(SW) square root sign,equalization of pressure

123.c---Chest x ray finding in ascending aortic aneurysm (SW) convex shadow to right of cardiac shilhouette,loss of retrosternal space

124.a---The most common imaging modality for evaluating thoracic aortic aneurysm(SW) isCECT

125.c--- CT and MRA should now be considered as gold standard for thoracic aortic disease(SW)

126.c----On CECT ,the double lumen aorta is classic diagnostic feature of(SW)aortic dissection,aortic an eurysm

127.a---The diagnostic modality of choice in hemodynamically unstable patients with suspected aortic dissection(SW) is TEE

128.c---Contrast used for MRI angiography(SW) is gadolinium

129.c---Gold standard in vascular imaging(SW) is catheter angiography

130.c---The most widely used screening tool to evaluate for atherosclerotic plaque and stenosis of extracranial carotid artery(SW) is USG

131.c--Regarding USG of carotid artery (SW) normal internal carotid artery(ICA) has low resistance flow,normal external carotid artery(ECA) has high resistance flow,flow pattern in CCA resemble that in ICA,the peak systolic velocity is increased at the site of vessel stenosis

132.a-- Normal parameter of carotid artery on Doppler study (SW) are ICA peak systolic velocity <125cm/s,ICA end diastolic velocity <40cm/s,ICA/CCA peak systiloic ratio<4

133.c---Doppler criteria to diagnose carotid artery stenosis>70% to less near occlusion ICA peak systolic velocity >230cm/s,ICA end diastolic velocity >100/s,ICA/CCA peak systiloic ratio >4,plaque estimate (diameter reduction)=>50%

134.d---Carotid stenting should be avoided in following carotid angiographic appearance (SW) extensive carotid calcification,polypoid or globular carotid lesions,severe tortuosity of common carotid artery,long segment stenoses(>2cm in length)

135.c--Carotid stenting should be avoided in following carotid angiographic appearance(SW): carotid artery occlusion,severe intraluminal thrombus,extensive middle cerebral artery thrombosis,exctensive carotid calcification

136.b---The most common location of abdominal aortic aneurysm is(SW) infrarenal aorta

137.d---Regarding abdominal aortic aneurysm (SW) normal size of aorta is 2-3 cm,the average aggregate :growth of aneurysm is 3-4mm/year,rupture risk is quite low for aneurysm< 5.5 cm,estimated annual risk of rupture is >50% for aneurysm size of 6-7cm

138.c---In abdominal aortic aneurysm size of aorta is(SW)>30mm and 1.5 times the adjacent diameter of the normal aorta

139.c---The screening modality of choice for abdominal aortic aneurysm(SW) is USG

140.a---The gold standard for determination of anatomic eligibility for endovascular repair is(SW) CECT

141.D---The inferior mesenteric artery provide collateral flow to the superior mesenteric artery through(SW) the marginal artery of Drummond ,arc of Riolan,maendering mesenteric arteries

142.c---Most common radiographic appearance of acute mesenteric ischemia (SW) is adynaic ileus and gasless abdomen

143.a---Investigation contraindicated in mesentric ischemia(SW) is Barium study

144.d---The defintive diagnosis of mesenteric vascular ischemia is(SW) biplanar arteriography

145.d---Dolichostenomelia is a feature of (SW) Marfan syndrome

146.b--- Scimitar sign on angiography is found in adventialial cystic disease of popliteal artery

147.a---The vein of Giacomini is related to(SW) small saphenous vein

148.d—Regarding perforators in lower legs(SW) the Cokett perforator veins drain the medial lower leg,the Cokett perforator connect the posterior arch vein (a tributary to great saphenous vein) and posterior tibial vein,the Boyd perforator veins connect the great saphenous vein to deep veins,the Boyd perforator lies approximately 10 cm below the knee

149.a---The most commonly performed test for detection of deep vein thrombosis(SW) is duplex USG

150.a--The primary method of detection of deep venous thrombosis is(SW) lack of coaptation

151.d--Duplex usg features of lower limb DVT(SW) are inability to compress the vein,lack of spontaneous flow,loss of respiratory flow variation,failure of filling of the lumen on color Doppler

152.a---Iodine 125 fibrinogen uptake investigation is meant for (SW) detection of DVT

153.d---The most definitive test for diagnosis of DVT in both symptomatic and asymptomatic patients (SW) is venography

154.c---The gold standard test for DVT(SW) is venography

155.c---Earliest sign of left atrial enlargement is posterior displacement of esophagus

156.c---Egg-on –side appearance is noted in TGA

GASTROINTESTINAL SYSTEM

1.Initial structural test performed in patients with suspected ulcer disease, esophagitis,neoplasm, malabsorption,and Barrett's esophagus is(H)
a.upper endoscopy
b.baruim study
c.USG
d.uclear scan

2.The procedure of choice for colon cancer screening and surveillance(H)
a.colonoscopy
b.occult blood test
c.USG
d.nuclear scan

3.The procedure of choice for diagnosis of colitis secondary to infection ,ischemia,radiation and inflammatory bowel disease is(H)
a.colonoscopy
b.occult blood test
c.USG
d.nuclear scan

4.Indications of endoscopic ultrasound are all except(H)
a.staging of GI malignancy
b.exclusion of choledocholithiasis
c.evaluation of chronic pancreatitis
d drainage of choledochal cyst

5.indications of ERCP are all except(H)
a.jaundice
b.pancreatic/ampullry /biliary mass
c.sphincter of Oddi manometry
d.staging of GI malignancy

6.Indications of capsule endoscopy are(H)
a.obscure GI bleeding
b.suspected Crohn's disease of small intestine
c.both
d.none

7.The initial procedure of evaluation of dysphagia(H)
a.barium swallow
b.upper GI endocopy
c.USG
d.nuclear scan

8.The procedure being evaluated as an alternative to colonoscopy for colon cancer screening(H)
a.USG
b.CT and MRI colonography
c.nuclear scan

d.barium enema

9.Investigation for intraabdominal abscess not visualized on CT is(H)

a.radiolabeled leucocyte scan

b.MRI

c.USG

d.barium study

10 Investigation that can be used for screen of mesenteric ischemia(H)

a.CTand MR technique

b.angiography

c.barium study

d.nuclear scan

11.Characteristic radiologic appearance of "bent inner tube"is noted in(H)

a.sigmoid volvulus

b.intestinal pseudo obstruction

c.intessusception

d. tumour of intestine

12.Esophageal stricture is better detected by(H)

a.barium study

b.endoscopy

c.PET

d.SPECT

13.Major application of Endoscopic ultrasound are all except(H)

a.to stage esophageal cancer

b.to evaluate dysplasia in Barret⋅s esophagus

c.to assess submucosal tumour

d.to diagnose achalasia

14.All are true about B ring except(H)

a.thin membranous narrowing

b.at the squamocolumnar mucasal junction in lower esophagus

c.also known as Schatzki rings when lumen diameter<13mm

d usually symptomatic

15.one of the most common causes of intermittent food impaction(steakhouse syndrome) (H)

a.Schatzki rings

b.webs

c.achalasia

d.none

16.Esophageal diverticula through Killian's triangle is known as(H)

a.epiphrenic diverticula

b.hypopharyngeal diverticula(Zenker's diverticula)

c.mid esophageal diverticula

d.none

17.The most sensitive diagnostic test for achalasia cardia is(H)

a.barium study

b.manometry

c.endoscopy

d.nuclear scan

18.Barium swallow x ray appearance of achalasia are all except(H)

a.tappering at LES(beak- like appearance)

b.dilatation of esophagus

c.air fluid level

d.stenotic cricopharyngeus muscle

19.Corkscrew esophagus is noted in(H)

a.achalasia

b.intramural diverticulosis

c.diffuse esophageal spasm

d.carcinoma esophagus

20 Sigmoid appearance of esophagus on barium is noted in (H)

a.achalasia

b.intramural diverticulosis

c.diffuse esophageal spasm

d.carcinoma esophagus

21.The test most sensitive in detecting mediastinal air(H)

a.CT

b.barium

c.x ray

d.nuclear scan

22.Esophageal perforation is confirmed by(H)

a.Contrast swallow

b.x ray

c.nuclear scan

d.MRI

23.First test used for documenting a gastric ulcer is(H)

a.barium study

b.endoscopy

c.CT scan

d.nuclear scan

24. Features of benign gastric ulcer on barium study are all except(H)

a.a discrete crater

b.radiating mucosal fold originating from ulcer margin

c.size <3cm

d.ulcer associated with mass

25.The most specific and sensitive approach for examining the upper GI tract(H)

a.endoscopy

b.barium study

c.EUS

d.CT

26.In Crohn's disease, early radiographic finding in the small bowel include(H)

a.the thickened fold and aphthous ulceration

b.strictures

c.fistula

d.abscesses

27.Cobblestoning is noted in(H)

a.Chrohn's disease

b.ulcerative colitis

c.typhoid

d.carcinoma

28.String sign is noted in(H)

a.Chrohn's disease

b.ulcerative colitis

c.typhoid

d.carcinoma

29.The earliest macroscopic findings of colonic Crohn's disease is(H)

a.apthous ulcer

b.stellate ulcer

c.sepiginous ulcer

d.linear ulcer

30.The first line test for the evaluation of suspected Crohn's disease and its complication(H)

a.CT /MR enterography

b.routine CT

c.barium study

d.USG

31.Radiographic finding which favour Crohn's disease are all except(H)

a.small bowel significantly abnormal

b.abnormal terminal ileum

c.segmental and asymmetric colitis

d.stricture rare

32.The gold standard for confirmation of mesenteric arterial occlusion(H)

a.mesentric angiography

b.MR angiography

c.CT angiography

d.none

33 .Radiographic finding pathognomonic of small bowel obstruction are all except(H)

a.fluid and gas filled distended small intestine

b.Step ladder pattern of intestine

c.air fluids level

d.abundant colonic gas

34.Strangulating closed loop obstruction may give rise to(H)

a.general haze in abdomen

b.coffee bean shaped mass

c.both

d.none

35.Bird's beak sign is seen in(H)

a.sigmoid volvulus

b.intessuception

c.gastric volvulus

d.none

36.All are true regarding radiography of small intestine except(H)

a.thick barium by mouth should be avoided in case of complete obstruction

b.CT is most commonly modality to evaluate intestinal obstruction

c.gastrograffin enema may help in demonstrating complete bowel obstruction

d.use oral barium in possible colonic obstruction

37.megaesophagus is produced by(N)

a.chagas disease

b.toxoplasmosis

c.malaria

d.parvo virus

38.The most commonly encountered foregut duplications(N)

a.esophageal duplication cysts

b.gastric duplication

c.ileal duplication

d.jejuna duplication

39.The most sensitive diagnostic test for achalasia(N)

a.barium study

b.manometry

c.chest x ray

d.none

40.Bird's beak appearance of esophagus on barium fluoroscopy is seen in(N)

a.achalasia

b.carcinoma esophagus

c.ring

d.scleroderma

41. on x ray , coin appears as(N)

a.flat in lateral view in esophagus

b.edge in AP view in esophagus

c.edge in AP view in trachea

d.edge in lateral view in trachea

42.USG Criteria for diagnosis of hypertrophic pyloric stenosis (N)

a.pyloric thickness-3 to 4 mm

b.an overall pyloric length—15 to 19 mm

c.pyloric diameter –10 to 14 mm

d.all

43. contrast study showing string sign,shoulder sign and double tract sign are all noted in(N)

a.duodenal atresia

b.jejunal atresia

c.pyloric atresia

d.none

44.Pyloric dimple in upper GI contrast series is noted in(N)

a.congenital gastric outlet obstruction

b.hypertrophic pyloric stenosis

c.duodenal atresia

d.none

45.All are features of mesenteroaxial volvulus on plain erect abdominal x ray except(N)

a.double fluid level

b.beak near the lower esophageal junction

c.stomach in vertical plane

d.single air fluid level

46.The most common congenital GI anomaly(N)

a.esophageal duplication cysts

b.Meckel's diverticulum

c.ileal duplication

d.jejuna duplication

47.The most sensitive study for Meckel' diverticulum is(N)

a.nuclear scan

b. barium study

c.USG

d. x ray

48.The most common cause of lower intestinal obstruction in neonate(N)

a.Hirschsprung disease

b.ileal atresia

c.functional

d.none

49.Currarino triad comprises all except(N)

a.anorectal malformations

b.sacral bone anomalies

c.pre-sacral anomaly

d.congenital cardiac anomaly

50.Barium enema study that suggest of Hirschsprung disease are all except(N)

a.abrupt narrow transition zone

b.the rectal diameter same or smaller than the sigmoid colon

c.retention of contrast in colon in delayed film(>24hrs film)

d.gradual transition zone

51.All are true regarding barium enema study in Hirschsprung disease except(N)

a. through bowel preparation needed

b.aid in diagnosis child older than one months

c. normal study in 10% noweborn with Hirschsprung disease

d.24hrs delayed film useful for diagnosis

52.Radiographic feature of

intussusceptions are all except(N)

a.longitudinal mass on USG

b.doughnut or target appearance on transverse image of USG

c.coiled ring appearance on barium enema

d.abrupt transition

53.Coiled ring appearance on barium enema is found in(N)

a.volvulus

b.intussusception

c.carcinoma of colon

d.superior masentric syndrome

54.In toxic megacolon , radiologically ,the diameter of colon(N)

a.>4cm

b.>5mm

c.>6mm

d.>7mm

55.Plain x ray finding in acute appendicitis may be all except(N)

a.sentinal loops and localized ileus

b.scoliosis

c.colonic air- fluid level above the right iliac fossa(colon cutoff sign)

d.fecolith in 40% cases

56.All are findings on CT scan of acute appendicitis except(N)

a.distentended thick walled appendix

b.normal surrounding mesenteric fat

c.pericecal phlegmon

d.abscess

57.Abdominal x ray findings in acute pancreatitis are all (N)

a.sentinel loop

b.dilataion of transverse colon(colon cutoff sign)

c.ileus

d.all

58.Investigation of first choice for detection of pseudocyst(N)

a.CT

b.USG

c. x ray

d.none

59.In infants with biliary atresia ,USG findings (N)

a.small or absent gall bladder

b.nonvisualisation of CBD

c.triangular cord sign

d.all

60.Increased echogenicity of liver on USG is noted in(N)

a.fatty change

b. abscess

c.cyst

d.all

61.Increase in liver density on CT scan is noted in(N)
a.diffuse iron deposition
b.glycogen storage
c.both
d.none

62.Radionuclide used in liver scan showing uptake by hepatocyte is(N)
a.^{99m}Tc sulphur colloid
b.^{99m}Tc iminodiacetic acid derivative
c.Gallium 67
d.none

63.Nuclear scan that can differentiate intrahepatic cholestasis from extrahepatic obstruction in neonates(N)
a.^{99m}Tc sulphur colloid
b.^{99m}Tc iminodiacetic acid derivative
c.Gallium 67
d.none

64.Bull's eye lesion on USG of liver is seen in(N)
a.liver candidiasis
b.hydatid cyst
c.tuberculosis
d.schistosomiasis

65.'Wheel within a wheel' and Bull's eye lesion in hepatic ultrasound is noted in(RUMACK)
a.liver abscess
b.hepatic candidiasis
c.hydatid disease
d.schistosomiasis

66.The modality of choice for the detection of gallstones,assessment of acute right upper quadrant pain and for evaluation of the patients with jaundice or elevated liver function tests(RUMACK)
a.USG
b.CT
c.MRI
d.none

67.All are sonographic criteria used to diagnose a simple cyst(RUMACK)
a.anechoic round or ovoid shape
b.acoustic enhancement
c.sharply defined,imperceptible ,smooth far wall
d.multiple septations

68.All are signs of retroperitoneal mass except(RUMACK)
a.phantom 's sign
b.embedded sign
c.claw sign or beak sign

d.corona sign

69.Whirlpol sign on color doppler of mesenteric vessel is seen in(RUMACK)

a.mid gut volvulus

b.duodenal atresia

c.sigmoid volvulus

d.Hirschsprung disease

70.For demonstarion free intra-abdiminal gas,which x ray is preffered(GRAINGER)

a.erect abdominal view

b.erect chest radiograph

c.supine abdominal

d.lateral decubitus abdomen

71.The investigation of choice for the uterus,ovaries and adnexa(GRAINGER)

a.USG

b.CT

c.MRI

d.PET

72.All are true regarding plain abdominal radiograph except(GRAINGER)

a.large amounts of gas normally present in stomach and colon

b.only small amount of gas is normally seen in the small bowel

c.fluid levels in colons is always abnormal

d.more than two fluid levels in dilated small levels(caliber>2.5cm) is said to be abnormal

73.Plain abdominal x ray showing gas filled ,slightly dilated bowel loop containing relatively little fluid,consequent upon excessive swallowing is noted in(GRAINGER)

a.meteorism

b.peritonism

c.bibliosim

d.urinism

74.Transeverse colon normally measures less than(GRAINGER)

a.5.5cm across

b.4.5cm across

c.3.5cm across

d.2.5cmm across

75.Critical diameter of caecum for perforation is(GRAINGER)

a.6cm

b.7cm

c.8cm

d.9cm

76.All are true except(GRAINGER)

a.small bowel is recognized by central position,multiple loops and valvulae conniventes b.presence of solid faeces is only reliable sign that the loop is large bowel

c.strangulated hernia account for three-fourths of small bowel obstruction in underdeveloped country

d.The string of beads appearance is virtually diagnostic of large bowel obstruction

77.CT sign of closed- loop obstruction are all except(GRAINGER)

a.dilated ,fluid-filled,V/U/radial shaped small bowel

b.tapering of loop (beak sign)

c.twisted mesentry (whorl sign)

d.normal orientation of mesenteric vessel

78.sigmoid volvulus shows all except(GRAINGER)

a.left flank overlap sign

b.liver overlap sign

c.pelvic overlap sign

d.apex under right hemidiaphragm

79.The bird of Prey sign on barium enema is noted in(GRAINGER)

a.caecal volvulus

b.gastric volvulus

c.sigmoid volvulus

d.paralytic ileus

80.As little as---ml of gas can be demonstrated radiographically in case of pneumoperitoneum(GRAINGER)

a.1ml

b.2ml

c.3ml

d.4ml

81.All are signs of pneumoperitoneum on x ray except(GRAINGER)

a.Rigler's(double) sign

b.football or air dome sign

c.'ghost-like' appearance of bowel

d.beak sign

82.All are signs of pneumoperitoneum on x ray except(GRAINGER)

a.inverted V sign

b.triangular sign

c.scrotal air in children

d.whorl sign

83.The most sensitive investigation of free peritoneal gas(GRAINGER)

a.x ray

b.CT

c.USG

d.none

84.The esophageal shiver is noted in(GRAINGER)

a.feline esophagus

b.corksrew esophagus

c.achalasia cardia

d.sclerodema involving esophagus

85.Hampton's line is noted in(GRAINGER)

a. base of rectal ulcer signifying its malignancy

b. base of oral mucosal ulcer signifying its malignancy

C base of esophageal ulcer signifying its benignancy

d.base of gastic ulcer signifying its benignancy

86.All are true regarding Giant ulcer in stomach except(GRAINGER)

a.size>3cm

b.almost always malignant

c.more chance of bleeding

d.more chance of perforation

87.Barium features suggesting benignancy of gastric ulcer are all except(GRAINGER)

a.irregularity of fold

b. normal areae gastricae extending to the ulcer crater

c.a pencil-thin line of lucency crossing the base of ulcer(Hampton's line)

d.2-4 mm smooth rim of lucency at the base of ulcer(ulcer collar)

88.Appearance of gastric ulcer on double contrast barium study (GRAINGER)

a.barium collection on dependent wall (en face)

b.ring shadow on non dependent surface(en face)

c. lesser curvature ulcer project beyond lumen of stomach (in profile)

d.all

89.Radiographically , upside-down stomach is noted in(GRAINGER)

a.eosophageal hernia

b.gastric volvulus

c.internal hernia

d.none

90.All are barium study features of malignant gasric ulcer except(GRAINGER)

a.irregular ulcer not extending beyond gastric wall

b.irregular,nodular,club shaped fold

c.Carman meniscus

d.Hampton's line

91.The most frequent site of GI lymphoma(GRAINGER)

a.stomach

b.small intestine

c.transverse colon

d.sigmoid colon

92.The size giant duodenal ulcer is (GRAINGER)

a.>1cm

b.>2cm

c.3cm

d.4cm

93.Which neoplasm of duodenum shows 'cauliflower' or 'soap-bubble' appearance on barium study(GRAINGER)

a.villous adenoma

b.benign lymphoid hyperplasia

c.GIST

d.Brunner's gland hyperplasia

94.Duodenal changes in carcinoma of head of pancreas on barium study (GRAINGER)

a.widening of duodenal loop

b.a double contour

c.irregularity of the inner border

d.all

95.Reversed '3' sign of Frostberg on barium study is characteristic of (GRAINGER)

a.carcinoma of duodenum

b.carcinoma head of pancreas

c.gastric carcinoma invading duodenum

d.gastric lymphoma invading duodenum

96.'Pseudo post-Billroth 1'(tubular narrowing of the antrum and proximal duodenum in continuity) appearance on barium study is found in(GRAINGER)

a.Crohn's disease

b.tuberculosis

c.progressive systemic sclerosis

d.carcinoma of duodenum

97.Bouveret's syndrome refers to(GRAINGER)

a.gallstone impacted in ileum

b.gallstone impacted in jejunum

c.gallstone impacted in the duodenal cap

d.gallstone impacted in 2rd part of duodenum

98.Sellink's methods and Nolan's tube is used for(GRAINGER)

a.esophageal dilatation in achalasia

b.for enteroclysis

d.for retrograde pyelography

e.for antegrade pyelography

99.Radiological signs of Crohn's disease are(GRAINGER)
a.aphthoid ulcer/fissure ulcer
b.longitudinal ulcer along mesentic border of ileum
c.Cobblestoning
d.all

100.A sandwitch like complex on CT /MRI of small intestine os noted in(GRAINGER)
a.carcinoid tumour
b.lymphoma
c.adenocarcinoma
d.Crohn's disease

101.Bull's eye/target appearance on barium study of small intestine is noted in(GRAINGER)
a.carcinoid tumour
b.lymphoma
c.adenocarcinoma
d.metastase of melanoma

102.All are true of ileocaecal tuberculosis of intestine (GRAINGER)
a.narowed and thickened terminal ileum
b.rigid, irregular ,gaping and incompetent ileocaecal valve
c.enlarged,mesentric nodes of low attenuation with enhancing peripheral ring
d.all

103.Pseudodiverticula,the 'wire spring/hidebound 'appearance on barium study of small intestine is noted in(GRAINGER)
a.progressive systemic sclerosis
b.nodular lymphoid hyperplasia
c.Whipple's disease
d.intestinal lymphangiectasia

104.Radiological feature suggesting ulcerative colitis over Crohn's disease is(GRAINGER)
a.ractum is always involved
b.granular mucosa
c.symmetrical disease
d.skip lesion

105.Accordion sign on CT scan of intestine is noted in(GRAINGER)
a.progressive systemic sclerosis
b.nodular lymphoid hyperplasia
c.Whipple's disease
d.pseudomembranous colitis

106.Bird's peak appearance on contrast enema and the swirl sign on CT is noted in(GRAINGER) a.sigmoid volvulus

b.intessusception

c.carcinoms of rectum

d.ischemic colitis

107.Free- fluid collection exceeding ---ml is considered to be ascites(GRAINGER)

a.100ml

b.150ml

c.200ml

d.250ml

108.CT appearance of prominent and wide –spaced recta traversing the proliferated mesenteric fat towards inflamed ileal loops (Comb sign) is noted in(GRAINGER)

a.diverticulitis

b.Crohn's disease

c.tuberculosis

d.carcinoid syndrome

109.Reidel's lobe is related to(GRAINGER)

a.thyroid gland

b.kidney

c.spleen

d.liver

110.Decrease of CT attenuation of liver in diffuse fatty liver is(GRAINGER)

a.1.6HU/per mg of triglyceride increase /gram of liver substance

b.0.6 HU/per mg of triglyceride increase /gram of liver substance

a.2.0HU/per mg of triglyceride increase /gram of liver substance

a.2.4HU/per mg of triglyceride increase /gram of liver substance

111.The most specific and sensitive technique for demonstrating hepatic fatty infiltration(GRAINGER)

a.USG

b.CT

c.MRI

d.PET

112.The 'corkscrew vessels' on hepatic arteriography is noted in(GRAINGER)

a.cirrhosis of liver

b.AVM

c.HCC

d.FNH

113.The most specific imaging technique for hemocromatosis is(GRAINGER)

a.USG

b.CT

c.MRI

d.PET

114.The most sensitive test for detection of portal vein gas(GRAINGER)

a.USG

b.CT

d.MRI

d.PET

115.Meyenburg's complexes is associated with(GRAINGER)

a.origin of true hepatic cysts

b.cystic metastases

c.hydatid cyst

d.biliary cystadenoma

116.Cyst with 'sand',daughter cysts,membrane sepration and wall calcification are all features of which hepatic cyst(GRAINGER)

a.simple cyst

b.biliary cystadenoma

c.hydatid cyst

d.cystic metastases

117.The commonest benign hepatic tumour(GRAINGER)

a.Haemangioma

b.FNH

c.adenoma

d.cystadenoma

118.The most specific and sensitive imaging examination for demonstrating hepatic haemangioma(GRAINGER)

a.USG

b.CT

d.MRI

d.PET

119.'Cotton wool' appearance on hepatic angiography is noted in(GRAINGER)

a.cirrhosis

b.haemangioma

c.AVM

d.none

120.'Chemical shift '/in-and-out-of-phase imaging of MRI is useful to demonstrate(GRAINGER)

a.protein

b.fat

c.calcification

d.all

121.'Spider web' appearance on hepatic angiography is characteristic of(GRAINGER)

a.cirrhosis

b.haemangioma

c.AVM

d.Budd-chiari syndrome

122.Magnetic resonance cholangio-pancreatography is based on(GRAINGER)

a.T1 weighted sequence

b.T2weighted sequence

c.Both

d.none

123.The most accurate modality for diagnosis of gall bladder stone(GRAINGER)
a.USG
b.CT
d.MRI
d.PET

124.Double arc sign on USG of gall bladder is noted in(GRAINGER)
a.gall bladder filled with stone
b.sludge
c.adenomyomatosis
d.emphysematous cholecystitis

125.The best initial imaging modality in patients with acute cholecystitis(GRAINGER)
a.PET
b.CT
d.MRI
d.USG

126.The most accurate modality for acute acalculous cholecystitis is(GRAINGER)
a.biliary scintigraphy
b.CT
d.MRI
d.USG

127.Comet- tail ring down artefact on USG of gall bladder is found in(GRAINGER)
a.gall stone
b.milk of calcium
c.adenomyomatuos hyperplasia
d.gall bladder polyp

128.A diameter of -- mm of common bile duct is commonly used as predictor of bile duct obstruction in jaundiced patients(GRAINGER)
a.>7mm
b.>10mm
c.>5mm
d.>11mm

129.Biliary cystic disease is best evaluated by(GRAINGER)
a.USG
b.cholangiography
c.both
d.none

130.ERCP showing adjacent strictures of both bile duct and the pancreatic duct(double duct sign) is highly suggestive of(GRAINGER)
a.pancreatic carcinoma
b.periampullary carcinoma
c.chronic pancreatitis
d.cholangiocarcinoma

131.The commonest congenital pancreatic anomaly(GRAINGER)
a.annular pancreas
b.pancreas divisum

209

c.ectopic panceas

d.pancreatic hypoplasia

132.The investigation of choice for assessment of pancreatic necrosis,peripancreatic inflammation and collection of fluid(GRAINGER)

a.NECT

b.CECT

c.MRI

d.USG

133.The most reliable imaging modality for the staging of acute pancreatitis (GRAINGER)

a.NECT

b.CECT

c.MRI

d.USG

134.Balthazar CT severity index is related to(GRAINGER)

a.acute pancreatitis

b.acute cholecystitis

c.acute appendicitis

d.acute diverticulitis

135.Intessusception is characterised by all except on USG(GRAINGER)

a.'traget 'appearance on transeverse image

b.'sandwitch 'appearance on longitudinal image

c.'crescent' on doughnut appearance on transverse image

d.'circle sign' on transverse image

136.USU finding of hypertrophic pyloric stenosis are all except(GRAINGER)

a.canal length>16mm

b.transeverse pyloric diameter>11mm

c.muscle wall thickness>4mm

d.pyloric canal does not open

137.Triangular cord sign and absent or small gall bladder on USG is predictive of(GRAINGER)

a.biliary atresia

b.cholangitis

c.choledochal cyst

d.duodenal atresia

138.The investigation used to differentiate severe cholestasis from biliary atresia (GRAINGER)

a.USG

b.MRI

c.$_{99m}$Tc DISIDA

d.PET

139.Linitis plastica is noted in all except(CHAPMAN)

a.gastric carcinoma

b.lymphoma

c.breast metastases

d.Menetrier's disease

140.All are radiological sign of infantile hypertrophic pyloric stenosis on barium study except(CHAPMAN)

a.string sign

b.shoulder sign

c.beak sign

d.sail sign

141.All are radiological sign of infantile hypertrophic pyloric stenosis

on barium study except(CHAPMAN)

a.string sign

b.shoulder sign

c.double track sign

d.notch

142.'Bull's eye'(target) lesions in the stomach is noted in all except(CHAPMAN)

a.submucosal metastases in melanoma

b.leimyoma

c.pancreatic rest

d.carcinoma of a stomach

143.All are radiological features of celiac disease except(CHAPMAN)

a.jejunal dilatation

b.Moulage sign

c.both

d.none

144.Thumbprinting in the colon is noted in(CHAPMAN)

a.ischemic colitis

b.coeliac disease

c.tuberculosis

d.none

145.Aphthoid ulcers are seen in all except(CHAPMAN)

a.Crohn's disease

b.Yersinia enterocolitis

c.amoebic colitis

d.lymphoma

146.Rokitansky-Ascoff sinuses is found in(CHAPMAN)

a.adenomyomatosis of Gall bladder

b. strawberry gallbladder

c. carcinoma gall bladder

d.none

147.Strawberry gall bladder refers to(CHAPMAN)

a.cholesterosis of gall bladder

b.adenomyomatosis of Gall bladder

c. carcinoma gall bladder

d.none

148.The commonest cause of neonatal abdominal calcification(CHAPMAN)

a.meconeum peritonitis

b.TORCH infection

c.hepatoblastoma

d.neuroblastoma

149.Alagille syndrome is characterized by all except(CHAPMAN)

a.hypolasia of intrahepatic ducts

b.butterfly vertebrae

c.perippheral pulmonary stenosis

d.normal facies

150.Pancreatic calcification is noted in all except(CHAPMAN)

a.alcoholic chronic pancreatitis

b.hyperparathyroidism

c.kwashiorkor

d.adenocarcinoma of pancreas

151 .All are true regarding oesophagus except(SW)

a.shows deviation to left in upper and lower portion of thorax

b.narrowest part of esophagus is at its entrance(1.5cm)

c. four normal areas of narrowing

d.Normal distance of lower esoplageal spincter from incisor teeth is 40cm in male

152.Hiatal hernia is best demonstrated in which position of barium study(SW)

a.supine

b.standing

c.prone

d.none

153.What is crucial in barium study to detect lower esophageal narrowing such as rings and strictures(SW)

a.fully distended view of esophagogastric region

b.fully collapsed view of esophagogastric region

c.both

d.none

154.Esophageal disorders clearly shown by a full column technique of barium study are all except(SW)

a.circumferential carcinoma

b.peptic strictures and lower esophageal ulcers

c.hiatal hernia

d.espophageal varices

155.Esophageal transit scintigraphy uses(SW)

a.^{99m}Tc sulphur colloid

b.^{99m}Tc DISIDA

 c.iodine

d.thallium

156.The best means available to evaluate complex functional abnormalities of esophagus is (SW)

a.manometry

b.videofluoroscopic imaging

c.manofluorography

d.scintigraphy

157.Common barium findings of neuromuscular disorders affecting pharyngoesophageal area are all except(SW)

a.misdirection of barium into trachea or nasopharynx

b.prominence of cricopharyngeal muscle

c.Zenker's diverticulum and narrow pharyngoesophageal segment

d.rapid transit of contrast in through vallecula or hypopharyngeal recesses

158.Reliable radiographic indicator of gastroesophageal reflux on barium study is(SW)

a.spontaneus regurgitation of barium into esophagus in the upright position

b.induced regurgitation of barium into esophagus in the upright position

c.spontaneus regurgitation of barium into esophagus in the supine position

d.induced regurgitation of barium into esophagus in the supine position

159.Cholescintigraphy uses(SW)

a.^{99m}Tc sulphur colloid

b.^{99m}Tc DISIDA

c.iodine

d.thallium

160.All are true regarding esophageal hiatal hernia except(SW)

a.sliding hernia(type I)--- upward dislocation of gastic fundus in posterior mediastinum

b.rolling hernia(type II)--- upward dislocation of gastric fundus,normally positioned cardia

c.mixed hernia(type III)--- upward dislocation of both the cardia and fundus

d.type IV esophageal hernia--- additional organ,like colon also herniated

161.Intrathoracic stomach is end result of (SW)

a.rolling hernia

b.sliding hernia

c.mixed hernia

d.rolling and siding hernia

162.Accuracy of barium study in diagnosis of gastroesophageal hernia is greater for(SW)

a.paraeophageal hernia

b.sliding hernia

c.equal accuracy

d.none

163.Schatzki's ring is located at(SW)

a.mid esophagus

b.upper esophagus

c.lower esophagus

d.none

164 Specific diagnostic indicator of scleroderma is noted in(SW)

a.manometry ---absent peristalsis in distal esophageal smooth muscle

b.barium study---dilated esophagus

c.CECT---dilated esophagus

d.scintigarphy---retained material in esophagus

165.Dilated esophagus with tapering or bird's beak- like narrowing of distal end of esophagus on barium esophagogram is noted in (SW)

a.achalasia

b.scleroderma

c.nutcracker's esophagus

d.carcinoma of esophagus

166.Corkscrew deformity on barium esophagogram is noted in(SW)

a.achalasia

b.diffuse esophageal spasm

c.nutcracker's esophagus

d.carcinoma of esophagus

167.The most common of primary esophageal motility disorder(SW)

a.achalasia

b.diffuse esophageal spasm

c.nutcracker's esophagus

d.hypertensive esophageal sphincter

168.The most reliable method of determining depth of cancer invasion in esophageal cancer is(SW)

a.EUS

b.CECT

c.MRI

d.PET

169.Smooth, intraluminal polypoid esophageal mass on barium study is suggestive of(SW)

a.sarcoma

b.carcinoma

c.leiomyoma

d.cyst

170.The most useful method to demonstrate a leimyoma of esophagus(SW)

a.CECT

b.MRI

c.PET

d.Barium swallow

171.Sharply demarcated,smooth,semilunar or crescent shaped filling defect that moves with swallowing on barium swallow in profile suggest of(SW)

a.sarcoma

b.carcinoma

c.leiomyoma

d.cyst

172.Which sign is often the earliest sign of esophageal perforation in chest /neck radiograph(SW)

a.air in the erector spinae muscle

b.mediastnal emphysema

c.pneumotharax

d.mediastinal widening

173.All are true of esophageal perforation in chest radiograph except(SW)

a.pleural effusion

b.mediastnal emphysema in 40% cases

c.pneumotharax in 77%cases

d.perfoarion on right side in 66% cases

174.Whih contrast is preffered to demonstrate esophageal perforation(SW)

a.gastrografin

b.barium

c.gadolinium

d.none

175.The diagnosis of esophageal perforation is confirmed by(SW)

a.contrast esophagoram

b. neck x ray

c.chest x ray

d.PET

176.Contrast esophagogram to demonstrate esophageal perforation is done in(SW)

a.erect position

b.supine position

c.lateral decubitus position

d.lordotic position

177.Preoperative imaging study of choice for gastrinoma is(SW)

a.somatostatin receptor scintigraphy

b.MRI

c.CECT

d.PET

178. Somatostatin receptor scintigraphy uses(SW)

a.indium labeled octreotide

b.technetium labeled sulphur colloid

c.technetium labeled DISIDA

d.technetuim labeled octreotide

179.The gold standard for the diagnosis of gastic malignancy is(SW)

a.double contrast barium study

b.endoscopy

c.CECT

d.MRI

180.Preoperative staging of gastric cancer is best accomplished with(SW)

a.NECT

b.CECT(IV and oral)

c.PET

d.EUS

181.The best way to stage gastic tumour locally is(SW)

a.NECT

b.CECT(IV and oral)

c.PET

d.EUS

182.The most accurate in distinguishing early gastric cancer from more advanced tumours(SW)

a.NECT

b.CECT(IV and oral)

c.USG

d.PET

183.Watermelon stomach refers to (SW)

a.gastric antral vascular ectasia

b.Menetrier 's disease(hypertrophic gastropathy)

c.gastric varices

d.lymphoma of stomach

184.Dieulafoy's lesion refers to(SW)

a.congenital AVM in brain

b.congenital AVM in liver

c.congenital AVM in spleen

d.congenital AVM in stomach

185.The most common cause of small bowel obstruction is(SW)

a.adhesion

b.hernias

c.malignant bowel obstruction

d.intestinal malrotation

186.Source of most of gas seen in small bowel obstruction is(SW)

a.swallowed air

b.gas produced within lumen

c.equal contribution

d.none

187.X ray finding most specific for small bowel obstruction are all except(SW)

a.dilated small bowel loops > 3cm

b.air –fluid seen on upright films

c.paucity of air in colon

d.Gas under diaphragm

188.All are true regarding abdominal radiograph in small bowel obstruction except(SW)

a.sensitivity -40 to 50%

b.ileus and colonic obstruction mimic small bowel obstruction

c.false negative finding in proximal small bowel obstruction

d.false negative finding in closed loop obstruction

189.CT finding of small bowel obstructions are all except(SW)

a.a discrete transition zone with dilation of bowel proximally

b.decompression of bowel distally

c.intraluminal contrast that does not pass beyond the transition zone

d.colon containing abundant fluid or gas

190.In which type of obstruction CT scan shows U or C –shaped dilated loop with radial distribution of mesenteric vessels converging towards a torsion point(SW)

a.Small bowel obstruction

b.large bowel obstruction

c.closed loop obstruction

d.superior artery mesenteric syndrome

191.CT features of intestinal strangulations are all except(SW)

a.thickening of bowel wall

b.air in the bowel wall(pneumatosis intestinalis)

c.portal venous gas

d.intense uptake of contrast in wll of affected part

192.All are true regarding CT in small bowel obstruction except(SW)

a.performed after oral water soluble contrast or diluted barium

b.low sensitivity(<50%) in detection of low grade or partial small bowel obstruction

c.sensitivity of 80 to 90% in detection of small bowel obstruction

d.<50% specificity in detection of small lowel obstruction

193.Substance used for enteroclysis is(SW)

a.mathylcellulose

b.gadolinium

c.metoclopramide

d.neostigmine

194.The earliest characteristic lesion of the Crohn's disease is(SW)
a.apthous ulcer
b.granuloma
c.abscess
d.stricture

195.All are true of Crohn's disease except(SW)
a.focal,transmural inflammation of intestine---pathological hallmark
b.the apthous ulcer----late appearance lesion
c.granulomas ----highly characteristic lesion
d.fat wrapping---vertually pathognomonic

196.The most useful initial test in Crohn's disease(SW)
a.CT scn with oral contrast
b.MRI
c.PET
d.barium study

197. All are true regarding hepatic tumour except
a.HCC and adenoma are hypervascular
b.adenoma enhance homogenously,especially in the portal venous phase in delayed image
c.HCC donot enhance in delayed image
d.CT is more sensitive than MRI in depicting the central scar of FNH

198.The test of choice for neoplasm of small intestine ,particularly for tumours located in distal small bowel(SW)
a.Small bowel follow through
b.enteroclysis
c.CT
d.MRI

199.The most accurate imaging test for diagnosing chronic radiation enteritis is(SW)
a.enteroclysis
b.CT
c.MRI
d.PET

200.The most prevalent congenital anomaly of the GI tract is(SW)
a.esophageal atresia
b.hypertrophic pyloric stenosis
c.Meckel's diverticulum
d.imperforate anus

201.All are true regarding 'rule of twos' in Meckel's diverticulum(SW) a.2%prevalence

b.2:I male predominance

c.location 2 feet proximal to ileocaecal valve in adults

d.1/2of symptomatic patients under two yrs of age

202.Which radionuclide scan can be helpful in diagnosis of Meckel's diverticulum(SW)

a.^{99m}Tc pertechnetate

b.^{99m}Tc DISIDA

c.^{99m}Tc octeotide

d.^{99m}Tc sulphur colloid

203.What percentage of Meckel's diverticulum contain heterotopic mucosa(SW)

a.20%

b.30%

c.40%

d.60%

204.The most sensitive test for diagnosing duodenal perforations is(SW)

a.MRI

b.x ray

c.CT scan

d.PET

205.CT findings of duodenal perforations (SW)

a.pneumoperitoneum/retroperitoneal fluid

b.contrast extravasation

c.paraduodenal fluids

d.all

206.Investigation of choice for intessusception(SW)

a.MRI

b.USG

c.CT

d.x ray

207. The imaging modality of choice for pancreatic cancer

a.Contrast MRI

b.double-phase,contrast – enhanced spiral CT

c.PET

d.USG

208.All are true regarding caecum except(SW)

a.widest part of colon(normal 7.5 to 8.5cm)

b.has thickest muscular wall

c.most vulnerable to perforation

d.least vulnerable to obstruction

209.The most common site of colonic diverticulosis(SW)

a.ascending colon

b.transverse colon

c.sigmoid colon

d.descending colon

210.The most accurate and most complete method for

examining the large bowel is(SW)

a.colonoscopy

b.CT scan

c.MRI

d.USG

211.Scimitar sign(sacrum with rounded border without any bony destruction) is pathognomonic radiographic appearance of(SW)

a.Anterior meningocele and myelomeningocele in sacrum region

b.sacral chordoma

c.sacral giant cell tumour

d.sacral tuberculosis

212.The most sensitive and most specific imaging study for retrorectal and presacral tumour(SW)

a.CECT

b.MRI

c.USG

d. PET

213.x ray showing 'bent inner tube or coffe baen appearance' with convexity of loop lying in right upper quadrant is characteristic of (SW)

a.caecal volvulus

b.transeverse colon volvulus

c.sigmoid volvulus

d.none

214.Bird's beak's appearance on gastrograffin enema is pathognomonic of(SW)

a.sigmoid volvulus

b.transeverse colon volvulus

c.caecal volvulus

d.intessuception

215.x ray of abdomen showing kidney shaped ,air filled structure in left upper quadrant is suggestive of(SW)

a.sigmoid volvulus

b.transeverse colon volvulus

c.caecal volvulus

d.intessuception

216.Thumbprinting on plain x ray is noted in(SW)

a.ischemic colitis

b.intestinal volvulus

c.intessusception

d.intestinal polyp

217.All are true regarding imaging in acute appendicitis(SW)

a.presence of fecolith on plan x ray is highly suggestive

b.if appendix is filled with barium ,appendicitis is excluded

c.rate of misdiagnosis has tremendously reduced.

d.graded compression sonography suggested as accurate way of diagnosis

218.Normal appendix on USG has following features except(SW)

a.blind-ending tubular structures

b.easily compressible

c.diameter=>6mm

d.tubular structure

219.All are USG features of acute appendicitis except(SW)

a.nonperistaltic bowel loop originating from caecum

b.blind- ending structure

c.compressible

d.anteroposterior diameter=>6mm

220.All are USG features of acute appendicitis except(SW)

a.appendicolith establish the diagnosis

b.thickening of appendiceal wall

c.presence of periappendiceal fluid

d.anteroposterior diameter =<5mm

221.False positive diagnosis of appendicitis on USG are due to all except(SW)

a.periappendicitis

b.dilated fallopian tube

c.inspissated stool

d.thin patients

222.false negative sonogram for acute appendicitis are due to all except(SW)

a.appendiceal tip appendicitis

b.retrocaecal appendix

c.markedly dilated/perforated appendix

d.periappendicitis

223.All are CT fatures of acute appendicitis except(SW)

a.appendix diameter<5cm and thickened wall

b.dirty fat ,thickened mesoappendix,phlegmon

c.fecolith

d.the arrowhead sign

224.The arrowhead sign on CT scan is suggestive of(SW)

a.caecal carcinoma

b.acute appendicitis

c.intussusception

d.volvulus

225.All are regarding anatomy of liver(SW)

a.Cantlie line divide left lobe of liver

b.caudate lobe correspond to segment 1

c.II,III and IV correspond to left lobe

d.V,VI,VII,VIII correspond to right lobe

226.Who divided liver into eight segment(SW)

a.Couinaud

b.Bismuth

c.Cantlie

d.Rex

227.Useful initial imaging test of liver(SW)

a.USG

b.CT

c.MRI

d.x ray

228.Contrast enhanced USG uses(SW)

a.iodine

b.barium

c.gadolinium

d.microbubbles

229.The gold standard for detecting liver lesions(SW)

a.preoperative USG

b.intraoperative USG

c.both

d.none

230.All are true regarding helical scanner(SW)

a.continuous patient –table motion

b.continuous CT gantary rotation

c.increased scan speed

d.more artifact due to respiration

231.All are true regarding CT evaluation of liver(SW)

a.tumours with arterial supply is well delineated in arterial phase

b.arterial phase—20 to 30s.after contrast delivery

c.venous/portal phase---60 to 70s. after contrast delivery

d.arterial phase provide optimal enhacement of liver parenchyma

232.Investigation producing images metabolic activity in tissues(SW)

a.CT

b.MRI

c.PET

d.USG

233. The accurate method of determining portal hypertension (SW)

a.USG

b.CECT

c.portal venography

d.PET

234.The initial investigation of choice for Budd-Chiari syndrome(SW)

a.USG

b.CECT

c.portal venography

d.PET

235.The definitive radiographic study to evalaute Budd-Chiari syndrome(SW)

a.USG

b.CECT

c.portal venography

d.PET

236.Biphasic CECT of liver reveals a lesion showing asymmetrical nodular enhancement and progressive centripetal enhancemet fill-in over time,the diagnosis is(SW)

a.adenoma

b.haemangioma

c.FNH

d.HCC

237. All are true regarding imaging features of liver lesions(SW)

a.adenoma appears 'cold'on nuclear imaging

b.FNH appears 'hot' on nuclear imaging

c.central scar noted in adenoma

d.centripetal enhancement in haemangioma

238.Imaging features of hepatocellular carcinoma are all except(SW)

a.hypervascular during arterial phase

b.relatively hypodense during delayed phase

c.presence of enhancing portal vein thrombus

d.late wash out of contrast

239. Correct pathological feature relevant to imaging are all except(SW)

a.HCC is predominantly supplied by hepatic artery

b.adenoma contain Kupffer's cells

c.FNH has central scar

d.HCC has tendency to invade portal vein

240.All may be used in treatment of HCC (SW)

a.radiofrequency ablation/chemoembolisation

b ethanol/cryosurgery/microwave ablation

c.yttrium 90 microshphere

d.all

241.All are true regarding common bile duct except(SW)

a.7-11cm in length

b.5-10mm in diameter

c.enters the first part of duodenum

d.opens at Ampulla of Vater

242.Initial investigation of any patients suspected of biliary tree(SW)

a.USG

b.CT

d.PET

d.MRI

243.USG will show gall stone with sensitivity and specificity of(SW)

a>60%

b>70%

c.>80%

d.>90%

244.All are features of gall stone except(SW)

a.acoustically dense

b.acoustic shadow

c. non-mobility

d.sediment/sludge formation

245.features of acute cholecystitis on USG are all except(SW)

a.contracted gall bladder

b.edematous gall bladder wall

c.edema between gall bladder and liver

d.lacal tenderness

246.A contracted, thick bladder wall on USG indicate of(SW)

a.acute cholecyctitis

b.chronic cholecystitis

c.hydrops

d.none

247.All are true regarding biliary radionuclide scanning except(SW)

a.use of i.v.^{99m}Tc HIDA

b.uptake by liver detected within 10 minutes

c.visualisation of the gall bladder,the CBD,the duodenum within 30 minutes in fasting states

d.HIDA cleared by Kuffer's cells of liver

248.All are indictions of biliary scintigraphy except(SW)

a.acute cholecystitis

b.biliary leaks

c.both

d.none

249.All are true regarding acute cholecystitis on biliary scintigraphy (SW)

a.Normal HIDA scan exclude acute cholecystitis

b.cystic duct obstruction(lack of filling of GB after 4hrs) highly sensitive and specific

c.both

d.none

250.The test of choice for suspected malignancy of gall bladder,the extrahepatic

biliary system,head of
pancreas(SW)

a.USG

b.CT

c.MRI

d.PET

251.Indication of
percutaneous transhepatic
cholangiography(SW)

a.management of
uncomplicated GB stone

b.management of bile duct
strictures and tumour

c.both

d.none

252.Which MRI technique
generate high resolution
images of biliary tree and
pancreatic duct(SW)

a.T1W images

b.T2W images

c.heavily T2W images

d.heavily T1W images

253.Advantages of endoscopic
retrograde
cholangiography(SW)

a.direct visualization of
ampullary region

b.direct access to distal
common bile duct

c.possibility of therapeutic
intervention/intraductal
endoscopy

d.All

254. Therapeutic procedure of
choice for CBD stone
associated with obstructive
jaundice,cholangitis or gall
stone pancreatitis(SW)

a.ERCP

b.Laproscopic surgery

c.open surgery

d.none

255.Definitive diagnostic test
of cholangitis is(SW)

a.Ultrasound

b.ERC(endoscopic retrograde
cholangiography)

c.CT scan

d.MRI

256. ERCP showing beading of
biliary tree suggests of(SW)

a.sclerosing cholangitis

b.bile duct cyst

c.cholangitis

d.none

257.Mirrizi's syndrome refers
to(SW)

a.biliary obstruction due to
cholecystolithiasis

b.biliary obstruction due to
calculus in CBD

c.biliary ostrction due to
cholangitis

d.biliary strictures

258.Diameter of dilated common bile duct on USG(SW)
a.>8mm
b.>6mm
c.>10mm
d.>12mm

259 The gold standard for diagnosing common bile duct stone(SW)
a.USG
b.CT
c.ERC
d.nuclear scan

260. Which investigation is as good as ERC for detecting common bile duct stone (SW)
a.transabdominal USG
b.endoscopic USG
c.CT
d.MRI

261.The diagnostic test of choice for acalculous cholecystitis(SW)
a.HIDA scan
b.USG
c.CT
d.MRI

262.Klatskin tumour refers to(SW)
a.perihilar cholangiocarcinoma
b.peripheral cholangiocarcinoma
c.ampullary carcinoma
d.none

263.The gold standard for detecting and assessing the severity of acute pancreatitis(SW)
a.CECT
b.NECT
c.USG
d.MRI

264. CECT finding in acute pancreatitis all except(SW)
a.uniform enhancement in interstitial pancreatitis
b.considerably decreased enhancement in necrotizing pancreatitis
c.air bubbles indicate of infected necrosis or pancreatic abscess
d.calcification in parenchyma

265.Parenchymal calcification in pancreas is noted in(SW)
a.chronic calcifying pancreatitis
b.hereditary pancreatitis
c.tropical (nutritional)pancreatitis
d.all

266.Size of pancreatic abnormalities that is picked up by endoscopic USG and laprascopic USG is(SW)
a.<1 cm

b.<2cm

c<3cm

d.<4cm

267.Cambridge classification of chronic pancreatitis is based on all except(SW)

a.ERCP finding

b.CT scan

c.USG

d.MRI

268.USG features of chronic pancreatitis are all except(SW)

a.pancreatic duct dilatation/calculi

b.cystic changes(<10mm)

c.homogenous echotexture

d.intrductal filling defect

269.Ductal changes seen on endoscopic ultrasound (EUS) in chronic pancreatitis are all except(SW)

a.ductal size <2mm

b.tortuous duct/side branch ectasia

c.echogenic intraductal foci

d.echogenic duct wall

270.All are true regarding imaging in case of chronic pancreatitis except(SW)

a.EUS is frequently used as a preliminary step in evaluation of pancreatic disease

b.EUS is superior to ERCP in detection of advanced changes in chronic pancreatitis

c.EUS may be more sensitive than ERCP in detection of mild changes of chronic pancreatitis

d.Small neoplasm seen in chronic pancreatitis may be invisible to all modalities except EUS

271.Earliest changes in chronic pancreatitis ,detected by EUS and ERCP are(SW)

a.dilatation of secondary ducts

b.heterogenous parenchymal changes

c.both

d.none

272.The gold standard for the diagnosis and staging of chronic pancreatitis (SW)

a.EUS

b.ERCP

c.MRI

d.CECT

273.The most sensitive radiological test for the diagnosis of chronic pancreatitis(SW)

a.EUS

b.ERCP

c.MRI

d.CECT

274.ERCP changes in moderate pancreatitis (SW)

a.normal main pancreatic duct,<3abnormal side branches

b.normal main pancreatic duct,=>3abnormal side branches

c.abnormal main pancreatic duct,>3abnormal side branches

d.abnormal main pancreatic duct and large cavity

275.Chain of lakes appearance is noted in(SW)

a.chronic pancreatitis

b.acute pancreatitis

c.pancreatic carcinoma

d.pancreatic divisum

276.The initial diagnostic imaging test of choice for pancreatic endocrine/exocrine tumour(SW)

a.Multi detector CT

b. USG

c.somatostatin scintigraphy

d.MRI

277. The most common endocrine neoplasm of pancrease(SW)

a.gastinoma

b.insulinoma

c.glucogonoma

d.VIPoma

278.The test of choice for gastrinoma(SW)

a.SSTR(octreotide) scintigraphy

b.EUS

c.CT

d.MRI

279.The most sensitive imaging method for VIPoma(SW)

a.SSTR(octreotide) scintigraphy

b.EUS

c.CT

d.MRI

280.The current diagnostic and staging test of choice for pancreatic cancer(SW)

a.multidetector ,dynamic CECT

b.EUS

c.MRI

d.none

281.The single most versatile and cost effective tool for diagnosis of pancreatic cancer(SW)

a CECT

b.EUS

c.MRI

d.none

282.Classic feature of chronic pancreatitis (SW)

a.calcification

b.beaded appearance of duct

c.both

d.none

283.Fish-eye lesion on ERCP is virtually diagnostic of(SW)

a.intraductal papillary mucinous neoplasm

b.solid pseudopapillary tumour

c.ductal adenocarcinoma

d.mucinos cystadenoma

284.The first imaging modality used to evaluate splenic trauma(SW)

a.USG

b.CECT

c.MRI

D.X RAY

285.Investigation especially helpful in locating accessory spleen after unsuccessful splenectomy for ITP(SW)

a.radioscintigrapgy with^{99m}Tc sulphur colloid

b.USG

c.CECT

d.MRI

286.Felty 's syndrome comprises all except(SW)

a.splenomegaly

b.hepatomegaly

c.rheumatoid arthritis

c.neutropenia

287.Feature of intestinal obstruction on x ray (H)

a.multiple air fluid level

b.intestinal dilation

c.both

d.none

288.All are criteria for grade III injury of liver and spleen (American association for surgery for trauma) except(SW)

a.subcapsular hematoma >50% of surface area

b.subcapsular hematoma >10cm in depth

c.laceration >3cm

d.hepatic avulsion/shattered spleen

289.The imaging technique of choice for evalution of soft tissue sarcomas of the extremities(SW)

a.CT supplanted with MRI

b.only MRI

c.USG

d.Nuclear scan

290.Golderhar complex comprises all except(SW)

a.branchial cleft anomalies

b.biliary atresia

c.congenital cardiac anomalies

d.renal anomalies

291.Criteria for ultrasonographic diagnosis of hypertrophic pyloric stenosis(SW)
a.pyloric channel length>16mm
b.pyloric thickness of>4mm
c.both
d.none

292.Double bubble sign on abdominal radiograph is seen in(SW)
a.duodenal atresia
b.jejunal atresia
c.biliary atresia
d.imperforate anus

293.Small intestinal atresia may appear on lapratomy as all except(SW)
a.orange-peel deformity
b.Christmas tree deformity
c.String of sausage deformity
d.strings of beads appearance

294.Pathognomonic radiographic finding in Necrotising enterocolitis(SW)
a.peumatosis intestinalis
b.presence of ileus
c.portal venous air
d.multiple fluid air level

295.Accurate and reliable imaging technique for biliary atresia(SW)
a.USG
b.Technetuim Tc ^{99m} disofenin using phenobarbital
c.cholangiogram
d.none

296.Alagille syndrome comprises(SW)
a.severe intrahepatic cholestasis
b.biliary hypoplasia
c.both
d.none

297.Initial evaluation of blunt abdominal trauma is done by(SW)
a.CT
b.x ray
c.FAST
d.MRI

298.FAST (focused abdominal ultrasonography for trauma) is use to identify free intraperitoneal fluid in all except(SW)
a.Morison's pouch
b.left upper quadrant
c.the pelvis
d.right upper quadrant

299. FAST (focused abdominal ultrasonography for trauma) is exquisitively sensitive for detecting intraperitoneal fluid(SW)

a.>100 ml
b.>200 ml
c.>250 ml
d.>300 ml

300.Malignant obstruction of intestine are suggested on CT by all except(H)
a.abrupt transition zone
b.irregular bowel thickening at obstruction site
c.mass at the site of obstruction
d.lack of adenopathy

301.'Double bubble' of stomach and duodenal cap is seen in(GRAINGER)
a.duodenal atresia
b.jejunal atresia
c.esophageal atresia
d.anal atresia

302. An ultrasound of abdomen can detect ascites as little as
a.100ml
b.200ml
c.50ml
d.150ml

303.Apple-core or napkin ring appearance on barium study of colon is noted in
a.carcinoma
b.adenoma
c.haemangioma
c.lymphoma

304.Excellent screening tool for hepatocellular carcinoma
a.CT
b.MRI
c.USG
d.PET

305.Characteristic vascular abnormalities of HCC
a.hypervascularity
b.portal vein thrombosis
c.both
d.none

306. All are true regarding ethiodol(lipiodol) except
a.ethiodised oil emulsion
b.retained by tumour cells
c.helpful for biopsy of small lesions
d.cotton seed oil

307.The most common benign tumour of liver
a.adenoma
b.focal nodular hyperplasia
c.haemangioma
d.lipoma

308.The most useful diagnostic differentiating tool for HCC,adenoma,FNH
a.triphasic CT scan
b.USG
c.MRI
d.neclear scan

309.The hepatic tumour wuth central scar which is hypovasclar on arterial phase and hypervascular on delayed phase CT is

a.adenoma

b.focal nodular hyperplasia

c.HCC

d.haemangioma

asked q

310.methods used for in situ ablation of liver secondaries are all except

a.alcohol

b.radiofrequency

c.utrasounds

d.cryotherapy

311.The investigation of choice for Hirschsprung disease

a.CT

b.MRI

c.contrast enema

d.USG

312.USG finding of adenomyomaosis are all except

a.tiny echogenic foci in the wall

b.thickening of wall due to presence of cystic spaces

c.commet-tail artefact

d.the presence of vascularity in the lesion

313.The USG features of cholesterolosis are all except

a.soft tissue lesion

b.attached to wall

c.no shadow

d.mobile

314.CT scan is least accurate for

a.gall stone

b.aneurysm of hepatic artery

c.lymph node in paraoartic organ

d.mass in tail of pancrease

315.All are true regarding Crohn's disease except(C)

a.most common site in small intestine---jejunum

b.asymetric involvement and skip lesions –characteristic

c.aphtoid ulcer—earliest sign

d.Cobblestone pattern

316. Accordian sign on CT of intestine is highly suggestive of

a.pseudomembranous colitis

b.colonic carcinoma

c.intestinal obstruction

d.none

317.Light bulb appearance on T2W image of liver is suggestive of

a.haemangioma

b.adenoma

c.FNH

d.HCC

318.The central dot sign on CT scan of liver is pathognomonic of

a.heamangioma

b.Caroli's disease

c.FNH

d.HCC

GASTROINTESTINAL SYSTEM
(ANSWERS)

1.a---Initial structural test performed in patients with suspected ulcer disease, esophagitis,neoplasm, malabsorption,and Barrett'sesophagus is(H) upper endoscopy

2.a---The procedure of choice for colon cancer screening and surveillance(H) colonoscopy

3.a---The procedure of choice for diagnosis of colitis secondary to infection ,ischemia,radiation and inflammatory bowel disease is(H) colonoscopy

4.d---Indications of endoscopic ultrasound are (H) staging of GI malignancy,exclusion of choledocholithiasis,evaluation of pancreatitis,drainage of pancreatic pseudocyst

5.d---indications of ERCP are (H)jaundice,pancreatic/ampullry /biliary mass,sphincter of Oddi manometry

6.c---Indications of capsule endoscopy are(H) obscure GI bleeding and suspected Crohn'sdisease of small intestine

7.a---The initial procedure of evaluation of dysphagia(H) barium swallow

8.b---The procedure being evaluated as an alternative to colonoscopy for colon cancer screening(H) is CT and MRI colonography

9.a---Investigation for intraabdominal abscess not visualized on CT is(H) radiolabeled leucocyte scan

10.a--- Investigation that can be used for screen of mesenteric ischemia(H) are CTand MR technique

11.a---Characteristic radiologic appearance of "bent inner tube"is noted in(H) sigmoid volvulus

12.a---Esophageal stricture is better detected by(H) barium study

13.d---Major application of Endoscopic ultrasound are (H) to stage esophageal cancer,to evaluate dysplasia in Barrett·ˢ esophagus,to assess submucosal tumour

14.d-- B ring (H) is a thin membranous narrowing ,at the squamocolumnar mucosal junction in lower esophagus,also known as Schatzki rings when lumen diameter<13mm,usually asymptomatic

15.a---one of the most common causes of intermittent food impaction(steakhouse syndrome) (H) Schatzki rings

16.b---Esophageal diverticula through Killian'ˢ triangle is known as(H)hypopharyngeal diverticula(Zenker'ˢ diverticula)

17.b---The most sensitive diagnostic test for achalasia cardia is(H) manometry

18.d---Barium swallow x ray appearance of achalasia are(H)tappering at LES(beak- like appearance),dilatation of esophagus,air fluid level

19.c---Corkscrew esophagus is noted in(H)diffuse esophageal spasm

20.a----Sigmoid appearance of esophagus on barium is noted in (H) achalasia

21.a---The test most sensitive in detecting mediastinal air(H) isCT

22.a----Esophageal perforation is confirmed by(H) Contrast swallow

23.a---First test used for documenting a gastric ulcer is(H) barium study

24.d--- Features of benign gastric ulcer on barium study are (H) a discrete crater,radiating mucosal fold originating from ulcer margin,size <3cm

25.a---The most specific and sensitive approach for examining the upper GI tract(H) endoscopy

26.a---In Crohn's disease, early radiographic finding in the small bowel include(H) the thickened fold and aphthous ulceration

27.a---Cobblestoning is noted in(H)Chrohn's disease

28.a---String sign is noted in(H) Chrohn's disease

29.a---The earliest macroscopic findings of colonic Crohn's disease is(H) apthous ulcer

30.a---The first line test for the evaluation of suspected Crohn's disease and its complication(H) is CT /MR enterography

31.d---Radigraphic finding which favour Crohn's disease are (H)small bowel significantly abnormal,abnormal terminal ileum,segmental and asymmetric colitis,common stricture

32.a---The gold standard for confirmation of mesenteric arterial occlusion(H) mesentric angiography

33 .d----Radiographic finding pathognomonic of small bowel obstruction are (H) fluid and gas filled distended small intestine,Step ladder pattern of intestine,air fluids level

34.c---Strangulating closed loop obstruction may give rise to(H)general haze in abdomen,coffee bean shaped mass

35.a---Bird's beak sign is seen in(H)sigmoid volvulus

36.d ---Regarding radiography of intestine (H) :thick barium by mouth should be avoided in case of complete obstruction,CT is most commonly modality to evaluate intestinal obstruction,gastrograffin enema may help in demonstrating complete bowel obstruction

37.a--Megaesophagus is produced by(N) chagas disease

38.a---The most commonly encountered foregut duplications is (N) esophageal duplication cysts

39.b---The most sensitive diagnostic test for achalasia(N) manometry

40.a---Bird's beak appearance of esophagus on barium fluoroscopy is seen in(N) achalasia

41.c--- on x ray , coin appears as(N)flat in AP view in esophagus,edge in LATERAL view in esophagus,edge in AP view in trachea,flat in lateral view in trachea

42.d---USG Criteria for diagnosis of hypertrophic pyloric stenosis (N) pyloric thickness-3 to 4 mm,an overall pyloric length—15 to 19 mm,pyloric diameter –10 to 14 mm

43. d--contrast study showing string sign,shoulder sign and double tract sign are all noted in(N) pyloric stenosis

44.a---Pyloric dimple in upper GI contrast series is noted in(N) congenital gastric outlet obstruction

45.d---Features of mesenteroaxial volvulus on plain erect abdominal x ray (N) are double fluid level,beak near the lower esophageal junction,stomach in vertical plane

46.a---The most common congenital GI anomaly(N) isMeckel's diverticulum

47.a---The most sensitive study for Meckel' diverticulum is(N) nuclear scan

48.a---The most common cause of lower intestinal obstruction in neonate(N) is Hirschsprung disease

49.d---Currarino triad comprises (N)anorectal malformations,sacral bone anomalies,pre-sacral anomaly

50.a---Barium enema study that suggest of Hirschsprung disease are (N) abrupt narrow transition zone,the rectal diameter same or smaller than the sigmoid colon,retention of contrast in colon in delayed film(>24hrs film),

51.a--- Regarding barium enema study in Hirschsprung disease(N):no bowel preparation needed,aid in diagnosis in child older than one months,normal study in 10% noweborn with Hirschsprung disease,24hrs delayed film useful for diagnosis

52.d---Radiographic feature of intussusceptions are (N) longitudinal mass on USG,doughnut or target appearance on transverse image of USG,coiled ring appearance on barium enema

53.b---Coiled ring appearance on barium enema is found in(N) intussusception

54.c---In toxic megacolon , radiologically ,the diameter of colon(N)>6mm

55.d---Plain x ray finding in acute appendicitis may be (N) sentinal loops and localized ileus,scoliosis,colonic air- fluid level above the right iliac fossa(colon cutoff sign) , fecolith in 5-to-10% cases

56.b--- CT scan finding of acute appendicitis are (N) distentended thick walled appendix,inflammatory stranding of mesenteric fat ,pericecal phlegmon,abscess

57.d---Abdominal x ray findings in acute pancreatitis are (N) sentinel loop,dilataion of transverse colon(colon cutoff sign),ileus

58.b---Investigation of first choice for detection of pseudocyst(N) is USG

59.d---In infants with biliary atresia ,USG findings (N) are small or absent gall bladder,nonvisualisation of CBD,triangular cord sign

60.a---Increased echogenicity of liver on USG is noted in(N) fatty change

61.c---Increase in liver density on CT scan is noted in(N) diffuse iron deposition and glycogen storage

62.c---Radionuclide used in liver scan showing uptake by hepatocyte is(N)^{99m}Tc iminodiacetic acid derivative

63.b---Nuclear scan that can differentiate intrahepatic cholestasis from extrahepatic obstruction in neonates(N) is ^{99m}Tc iminodiacetic acid derivative

64.a---Bull's eye lesion on USG of liver is seen in(N)liver candlasis

65.b---'Wheel -within -a wheel' and Bull's eye lesion in hepatic ultrasound is noted in(RUMACK) hepatic candidiasis

66.a---The modality of choice for the detection of gallstones,assessment of acute right upper quadrant pain and for evaluation of the patients with jaundice or elevated liver function tests(RUMACK) USG

67.d--- Sonographic criteria used to diagnose a simple cyst(RUMACK) are anechoic round or ovoid shape,acoustic enhancement,sharply defined,imperceptible ,smooth far wall

68.d---Signs of retroperitoneal mass are (RUMACK) phantom 's sign,embedded sign,claw sign or beak sign

69.a---Whirlpol sign on color doppler of mesenteric vessel is seen in(RUMACK) mid gut volvulus

70.b---For demonstarion free intra-abdiminal gas,which x ray is preffered(GRAINGER) erect chest radiograph

71.a---The investigation of choice for the uterus,ovaries and adnexa(GRAINGER) USG

72.c---Regarding plain abdominal radiograph(GRAINGER) large amounts of gas normally present in stomach and colon,only small amount of gas is normally seen in the small bowel,fluid levels are common in normal people and they usually lie   in colons is always abnormal,more than two fluid levels in dilated small levels(caliber>2.5cm) is said to be abnormal

73.a---Plain abdominal x ray showing gas filled ,slightly dilated bowel loop containing relatively little fluid,consequent upon excessive swallowing is known as(GRAINGER)meteorism

74.a---Transeverse colon normally measures less than(GRAINGER) 5.5cm across

75.d---Critical diameter of caecum for perforation is(GRAINGER) 9cm

76.d---(GRAINGER)Small bowel is recognized by central position,multiple loops and valvulae conniventes,presence of solid faeces is only reliable sign that the loop is large bowel,strangulated hernia account for three-fourths of small bowel obstruction in underdeveloped country,the string of beads appearance is virtually diagnostic of small bowel obstruction

77.d---CT sign of closed- loop obstruction are (GRAINGER) dilated ,fluid- filled,V/U/radial- shaped small bowel,tapering of loop (beak sign),twisted mesentry (whorl sign),radial distribution of mesenteric vessel

78.d--- Feature of sigmoid volvulus are (GRAINGER)left flank overlap sign,liver overlap sign,pelvic overlap sign,apex under left hemidiaphragm

79.c---The bird of Prey sign on barium enema is noted in(GRAINGER) sigmoid volvulus

80.a---As little as 1ml of gas can be demonstrated radiographically in case of pneumoperitoneum(GRAINGER)

81.d--- Signs of pneumoperitoneum on x ray are (GRAINGER) Rigler's(double) sign,football or air dome sign,'ghost-like' appearance of bowel

82.d---Signs of pneumoperitoneum on x ray are (GRAINGER) inverted V sign,triangular sign,scrotal air in children

83.b---The most sensitive investigation of free peritoneal gas(GRAINGER) CT

84.a---The esophageal shiver is noted in(GRAINGER)feline esophagus

85.d---Hampton's line is noted in(GRAINGER) base of gastic ulcer signifying its benignancy

86.b---Regarding Giant ulcer in stomach (GRAINGER) size>3cm,almost always benign,more chance of bleeding and perforation

87.a---Barium features suggesting benignancy of gastric ulcer arc (GRAINGER)normal areae gastricae extending to the ulcer crater,a pencil-thin line of lucency crossing the base of ulcer(Hampton's line),2-4 mm smooth rim of lucency at the base of ulcer(ulcer collar)

88.d---Appearance of gastric ulcer on double contrast barium study are (GRAINGER)barium collection on dependent wall (en face),ring shadow on non dependent surface(en face),lesser curvature ulcer project beyond lumen of stomach (in profile)

89.b---Radiographically , upside-down stomach is noted in(GRAINGER) gastric volvulus

90 .d---Features of malignant gasric ulcer are (GRAINGER)irregular ulcer not extending beyond gastric wall,irregular,nodular,club shaped fold,Carman meniscus

91.a---The most frequent site of GI lymphoma(GRAINGER) stomach

92.b---The size giant duodenal ulcer is (GRAINGER)>2cm

93.a---Which neoplasm of duodenum shows 'cauliflower' or 'soap-bubble' appearance on barium study(GRAINGER) villous adenoma

94.d---Duodenal changes in carcinoma of head of pancreas on barium study are (GRAINGER) widening of duodenal loop,a double contour,irregularity of the inner border

95.b---Reversed '3' sign of Frostberg on barium study is characteristic of (GRAINGER) carcinoma head of pancreas

 96.a---'Pseudo post-Billroth 1'(tubular narrowing of the antrum and proximal duodenum in continuity) appearance on barium study is found in(GRAINGER) Crohn's disease

97.c---Bouveret's syndrome refers to(GRAINGER) gallstone impacted in the duodenal cap

98.b---Sellink's methods and Nolan's tube is used for(GRAINGER) for enteroclysis

99.d---Radiological signs of Crohn's disease are(GRAINGER) aphthoid ulcer/fissure ulcer ,longitudinal ulcer along mesentic border of ileum,cobblestoning

100.b---A sandwitch like complex on CT /MRI of small intestine is noted in(GRAINGER) lymphoma

101.d---Bull's eye/target appearance on barium study of small intestine is noted in(GRAINGER) metastase of melanoma

102.d---Feature of ileocaecal tuberculosis of intestine are (GRAINGER) narowed and thickened terminal ileum, rigid, irregular ,gaping and incompetent ileocaecal valve,enlarged,mesentric nodes of low attenuation with enhancing peripheral ring

103.a---Pseudodiverticula,the 'wire spring/hidebound 'appearance on barium study of small intestine is noted in(GRAINGER) progressive systemic sclerosis

104.d---Radiological features suggesting ulcerative colitis over Crohn's disease are (GRAINGER) rectum is always involved rectum,granular mucosa and symmetrical disease

105.d---Accordion sign on CT scan of intestine is noted in(GRAINGER) pseudomembranous colitis

106.a---Bird's peak appearance on contrast enema and the swirl sign on CT is noted in(GRAINGER) sigmoid volvulus

107.a---Free- fluid collection exceeding 100 ml is considered to be ascites(GRAINGER)

108.CT appearance of prominent and wide –spaced recta traversing the proliferated mesenteric fat towards inflamed ileal loops (Comb sign) is noted in(GRAINGER) Crohn's disease

109.d---Reidel's lobe is related to(GRAINGER) liver

110.a---Decrease of CT attenuation of liver in diffuse fatty liver is(GRAINGER) 1.6HU/per mg of triglyceride increase /gram of liver substance

111.c---The most specific and sensitive technique for demonstrating hepatic fatty infiltration(GRAINGER) MRI

112.a---The 'corkscrew vessels' on hepatic arteriography is noted in(GRAINGER) cirrhosis of liver

113.c---The most specific imaging technique for hemocromatosis is(GRAINGER) MRI

114.a---The most sensitive test for detection of portal vein gas(GRAINGER) USG

115.a---Meyenburg's complexes is associated with(GRAINGER) origin of true hepatic cysts

116.c---Cyst with 'sand',daughter cysts,membrane sepration and wall calcification are all features of (GRAINGER)hydatid cyst

117.a---The commonest benign hepatic tumour(GRAINGER) is haemangioma

118.a---The most specific and sensitive imaging examination for demonstrating hepatic haemangioma(GRAINGER) USG

119.b---'Cotton wool' appearance on hepatic angiography is noted in(GRAINGER) haemangioma

120.b---'Chemical shift '/in-and-out-of-phase imaging of MRI is useful to demonstrate(GRAINGER) fat

121.d---'Spider web' appearance on hepatic angiography is characteristic of(GRAINGER) Budd-chiari syndrome

122.b---Magnetic resonance cholangio-pancreatography is based on(GRAINGER) T2weighted sequence

123.a---The most accurate modality for diagnosis of gall bladder stone(GRAINGER) is USG

124.a---Double arc sign on USG of gall bladder is noted in(GRAINGER) gall bladder filled with stone

125.d---The best initial imaging modality in patients with acute cholecystitis(GRAINGER) is USG

126.a----The most accurate modality for acute acalculous cholecystitis is(GRAINGER) biliary scintigraphy

127.c---Comet- tail ring down artefact on USG of gall bladder is found in(GRAINGER) adenomyomatuos hyperplasia

128.a---A diameter of -- mm of common bile duct is commonly used as predictor of bile duct obstruction in jaundiced patients(GRAINGER) 7mm

129.b---Biliary cystic disease is best evaluated by(GRAINGER) cholangiography

130.a---ERCP showing adjacent strictures of both bile duct and the pancreatic duct(double duct sign) is highly suggestive of(GRAINGER)pancreatic carcinoma

131.b---The commonest congenital pancreatic anomaly(GRAINGER)pancreas divisum

132.b---The investigation of choice for assessment of pancreatic necrosis,peripancreatic inflammation and collection of fluid(GRAINGER) CECT

133.b---The most reliable imaging modality for the staging of acute pancreatitis (GRAINGER) is CECT

134.a---Balthazar CT severity index is related to(GRAINGER) acute pancreatitis

135.d---Intessusception is characterised by USG(GRAINGER)'traget 'appearance on transeverse image,'sandwitch 'appearance on longitudinal image,'crescent' on doughnut appearance on transverse image

136.c---USU finding of hypertrophic pyloric stenosis are(GRAINGER)canal length>16mm,transeverse pyloric diameter>11mm,muscle wall thickness>2.5mm,pyloric canal does not open

137.a---Triangular cord sign and absent or small gall bladder on USG is predictive of(GRAINGER) biliary atresia

138.c---The investigation used to differentiate severe cholestasis from biliary atresia (GRAINGER) $_{99m}$Tc DISIDA

139.d---Linitis plastica is noted in(CHAPMAN)gastric carcinoma,lymphoma,breast metastases

140.d---Radiological sign of infantile hypertrophic pyloric stenosis on barium study are (CHAPMAN)string sign,shoulder sign,beak sign

141.d---Radiological sign of infantile hypertrophic pyloric stenosis on barium study are (CHAPMAN) string sign,shoulder sign,double track sign

142.d---'Bull's eye'(target) lesions in the stomach is noted in (CHAPMAN)submucosal metastases in melanoma,leimyoma,pancreatic rest

143.c---Radiological features of celiac disease are (CHAPMAN) jejunal dilatation andMoulage sign

144.a---Thumbprinting in the colon is noted in(CHAPMAN) ischemic colitis

145.d---Aphthoid ulcers are seen in (CHAPMAN)Crohn's diseaseYersinia enterocolitis,amoebic colitis

146.a---Rokitansky-Ascoff sinuses is found in(CHAPMAN) adenomyomatosis of Gall bladder

147.a---Strawberry gall bladder refers to(CHAPMAN) cholesterosis of gall bladder

148.a---The commonest cause of neonatal abdominal calcification(CHAPMAN) meconeum peritonitis

149.d---Alagille syndrome is characterized by (CHAPMAN) hypolasia of intrahepatic ducts,butterfly vertebrae,peripheral pulmonary stenosis

150.d---Pancreatic calcification is noted in (CHAPMAN) alcoholic chronic pancreatitis,hyperparathyroidism,kwashiorkor

151 .c---Regarding oesophagus :(SW)shows deviation to left in upper and lower portion of thorax,narrowest part of esophagus is at its entrance(1.5cm),three normal areas of narrowing,normal distance of lower esoplageal spincter from incisor teeth is 40cm in male

152.c---Hiatal hernia is best demonstrated in prone position of barium study(SW)

153.a---Fully distended view of esophagogastric region is crucial in barium study to detect lower esophageal narrowing such as rings and strictures(SW)

154.d---Esophageal disorders clearly shown by a full column technique of barium study are (SW)circumferential carcinoma,peptic strictures and lower esophageal ulcers,hiatal hernia

155.a---Esophageal transit scintigraphy uses(SW) ^{99m}Tc sulphur colloid

156.c---The best means available to evaluate complex functional abnormalities of esophagus is (SW) manofluorography

157.d---common barium findings of neuromuscular disorders affecting pharyngoesophageal area are (SW)misdirection of barium into trachea or nasopharynx,prominence of cricopharyngeal muscle,Zenker's diverticulum and narrow pharyngoesophageal segment,stasis contrast in through vallecula or hypopharyngeal recesses

158.a---Reliable radiographic indicator of gastroesophageal reflux on barium study is(SW) spontaneus regurgitation of barium into esophagus in the upright position

159.b---Cholescintigraphy uses(SW) ^{99m}Tc DISIDA

160.a---All are true regarding esophageal hiatal hernia (SW)sliding hernia(type I)---upward dislocation of cardia in posterior mediastinum,rolling hernia(type II)---upward dislocation of gastric fundus,normally positioned cardia,mixed hernia(type III)---upward dislocation of both the cardia and fundus,type IV esophageal hernia---additional organ,like colon also herniated

161.d---intrathoracic stomach is end result of(SW) rolling and siding hernia

162.a---Accurcy of barium study in diagnosis of gastroesophageal hernia is greater for(SW) paraeophageal hernia

163.c---Schatzki's ring is located at(SW) lower esophagus

164. Specific diagnostic indicator of scleroderma is noted in(SW) manometry ---absent peristalsis in distal esophageal smooth muscle

165.a---Dilated esophagus with tapering or bird's beak- like narrowing of distal end of esophagus on barium esophagogram is noted in (SW) achalasia

166.b---Corkscrew deformity on barium esophagogram is noted in(SW) diffuse esophageal spasm

167.c---The most common of primary esophageal motility disorder(SW) nutcracker's esophagus

168.a---The most reliable method of determining depth of cancer invasion in esophageal cancer is(SW) EUS

169.a---Smooth, intraluminal polypoid esophageal mass on barium study is suggestive of(SW) sarcoma

170.d---The most useful method to demonstrate a leimyoma of esophagus(SW) Barium swallow

171.c---Sharply demarcated,smooth,semilunar or crescent shaped filling defect that moves with swallowing on barium swallow in profile suggest of(SW) leiomyoma

172.a--- Air in the erector spinae muscle is often the earliest sign of esophageal perforation in chest /neck radiograph(SW)

173.d---Regarding esophageal perforation,chest radiograph shows (SW) pleural effusion,mediastnal emphysema in 40% cases,pneumotharax in 77%cases,perfoarion on left side in 66% cases

174.a--- Gastrophin contrast is preffered to demonstrate esophageal perforation(SW)

175.a---The diagnosis of esophageal perforation is confirmed by(SW) contrast esophagoram

176.c---Contrast esophagogram to demonstrate esophageal perforation is done in(SW) lateral decubitus position

177.a---Preoperative imaging study of choice for gastrinoma is(SW) somatostatin receptor scintigraphy

178. a---Somatostatin receptor scintigraphy uses(SW) indium labeled octreotide

179.b---The gold standard for the diagnosis of gastic malignancy is(SW) endoscopy

180.b---Preoperative staging of gastric cancer is best accomplished with(SW)CECT(IV and oral) .MRI is probably comprable

181.d---The best way to stage gastric tumour locally is(SW)EUS

182.c---The most accurate in distinguishing early gastric cancer from more advanced tumours(SW) is USG

183.a---Watermelon stomach refers to (SW)gastric antral vascular ectasia

184.d---Dieulafoy's lesion refers to(SW) congenital AVM in stomach

185.a---The most common cause of small bowel obstruction is(SW) adhesion

186.a---Source of most of gas seen in small bowel obstruction is(SW) swallowed air

187.d--X ray finding most specific for small bowel obstruction are (SW) dilated small bowel loops > 3cm,air –fluid seen on upright films,a paucity of air in colon

188.a----Regarding abdominal radiograph in small bowel obstruction:(SW)sensitivity -70 –to 80%,ileus and colonic obstruction mimic small bowel obstruction,false negative finding in proximal small bowel obstruction and in closed loop obstruction

189.d--CT finding of small bowel obstructions are(SW),a discrete transition zone with dilation of bowel proximally,decompression of bowel distally,intraluminal contrast that does not pass beyond the transition zone,colon containing little fluid or gas

190.c---In which type of obstruction CT scan shows U or C – shaped dilated loop with radial distribution of mesenteric vessels convering towards a torsion point(SW)closed loop obstruction

191.d---CT features of intestinal strangulations are (SW)thickening of bowel wall,air in the bowel wall(pneumatosis intestinalis),portal venous gas

192.d---Regarding CT in small bowel obstruction :(SW),performed after oral water soluble contrast or diluted barium,low sensitivity(<50%) in detection of low grade or partial small bowel obstruction,sensitivity of 80 to 90% in detection of small bowel obstruction,70—90%% specificity in detection of small lowel obstruction

193.a---Substance used for enteroclysis is(SW) mathylcellulose

194.a---The earliest characteristic lesion of the Crohn's disease is(SW)apthous ulcer

195.b—Regarding Crohn's disease (SW)focal,transmural inflammation of intestine---pathological hallmark,the apthous ulcer----early lesion,granulomas ----highly characteristic lesion,fat wrapping---vertually pathognomonic

196.a---The most useful initial test in Crohn's disease(SW) CT scn with oral contrast

197. d---Regarding hepatic tumour HCC and adenoma are hypervascular,adenoma enhance homogenously,especially in the portal venous phase in delayed image,HCC donot enhance in delayed image

198.b---The test of choice for neoplasm of small intestine ,particularly for tumours located in distal small bowel(SW)enteroclysis

199.a---The most accurate imaging test for diagnosing chronic radiation enteritis is(SW) enteroclysis

200.c---The most prevalent congenital anomaly of the GI tract is(SW) Meckel's diverticulum

201.b---Regarding 'rule of twos' in Meckel's diverticulum are (SW) 2%prevalence,2:I female predominance,location 2 feet proximal to ileocaecal valve in adults,1/2of symptomatic patients under two yrs of age

202.a--- Radionuclide scan helpful in diagnosis of Meckel's diverticulum(SW) ^{99m}Tc pertechnetate

203.d---Percentage of Meckel's diverticulum containing heterotopic mucosa(SW)60%

204.c---The most sensitive test for diagnosing duodenal perforations is(SW) CT scan

205.d--CT findings of duodenal perforations (SW) pneumoperitoneum/retroperitoneal fluid,contrast extravasation,paraduodenal fluids

206.c---Investigation of choice of intessusception(SW)CT

207.b--- The imaging modality of choice for pancreatic cancer double-phase,contrast –enhanced spiral CT

208.b---Regarding caecum :(SW)widest part of colon(normal 7.5 to 8.5cm),most vulnerable to perforation,least vulnerable to obstruction

209.c---The most common site of colonic diverticulosis(SW) is sigmoid colon

210.a---The most accurate and most complete method for examining the large bowel is(SW) colonoscopy

211.a---Scimitar sign(sacrum with rounded border without any bony destruction) is pathognomonic radiographic appearance of(SW) is anterior meningocele and myelomeningocele in sacrum region

212.b---The most sensitive and most specific imaging study for retrorectal and presacral tumour(SW) MRI

213.c---x ray showing 'bent inner tube or coffe baen appearance' with convexity of loop lying in right upper quadrant is characteristic of (SW) sigmoid volvulus

214.a---Bird's beak's appearance on gastrograffin enema is pathognomonic of(SW) sigmoid volvulus

215.c---x ray of abdomen showing kidney shaped ,air filled structure in left upper quadrant is suggestive of(SW) caecal volvulus

216.a---Thumbprinting on plain x ray is noted in(SW) ischemic colitis

217.c--Regarding imaging in acute appendicitis:(SW)presence of fecolith on plan x ray is highly suggestive,if appendix is filled with barium ,appendicitis is excluded,graded compression sonography suggested as accurate way of diagnosis

218.c---Normal appendix on USG has following features except(SW)blind-ending tubular structures,easily compressible,diameter<5mm,tubular structure

219.c---USG features of acute appendicitis are (SW) nonperistaltic bowel loop originating from caecum,blind-ending structure,non-compressible,anteroposterior diameter=>6mm

220.d---USG features of acute appendicitis are (SW) appendicolith establish the diagnosis,thickening of appendiceal wall,presence of periappendiceal fluid,anteroposterior diameter >6mm

221.d--False positive diagnosis of appendicitis on USG are due to (SW)periappendicitis,dilated fallopian tube,inspissated stool

222.d--false negative sonogram for acute appendicitis are due to (SW)appendiceal tip appendicitis,retrocaecal appendix.markedly dilated/perforated appendix

223.a--CT fatures of acute appendicitis are(SW)dirty fat ,thickened mesoappendix,phlegmon,fecolith,the arrowhead sign

224.b---The arrowhead sign on CT scan is suggestive of(SW) acute appendicitis

225.a---All are regarding anatomy of liver(SW)Cantlie line divide liver into right and left lobe,caudate lobe correspond to segment 1.II,III and IV correspond to left lobe.V,VI,VII,VIII correspond to right lobe

226.a--- Couinaud divided liver into eight segment(SW)

227.a---Useful initial imaging test of liver(SW) USG

228.d---Contrast enhanced USG uses(SW) microbubbles

229.b---The gold standard for detecting liver lesions(SW) intraoperative USG

230.d---Regarding helical scanner:(SW)continuous patient – table motion,continuous CT gantary rotation,increased scan speed

231.d---Regarding CT evaluation of liver(SW)tumours with arterial supply is well delineated in arterial phase,arterial phase—20 to 30s.after contrast delivery,venous/portal phase---60 to 70s. after contrast delivery,arterial phase doesnot provide optimal enhacement of liver parenchyma

232.c---Investigation producing images metabolic activity in tissues(SW) PET

233. c---The accurate method of determining portal hypertension (SW) portal venography

234.a---The initial investigation of choice for Budd-Chiari syndrome(SW) USG

235.a---The definitive radiographic study to evalaute Budd-Chiari syndrome(SW) USG

236.b---Biphasic CECT of liver reveals a lesion showing asymmetrical nodular enhancement and progressive centripetal enhancemet fill-in over time,the diagnosis is(SW) haemangioma

237. c- Imaging features of liver lesions:(SW) adenoma appears 'cold'on nuclear imaging,FNH appears 'hot' on nuclear imaging,centripetal enhancement in haemangioma

238.d---Imaging features of hepatocellular carcinoma are (SW)hypervascular during arterial phase,relatively hypodense during delayed phase ,presence of enhancing portal vein thrombus

239. b---Pathological feature relevant to imaging are (SW)HCC is predominantly supplied by hepatic artery,denoma doesnot contain Kupffer's cells,FNH has central scar,HCC has tendency to invade portal vein

240.d----Used in treatment of HCC: (SW)radiofrequency ablation/chemoembolisation,ethanol/cryosurgery/microwave ablation,yttrium 90 microshphere

241.c---Regarding common bile duct :(SW)7-11cm in length,5-10mm in diameter,enters the second part of duodenum ,opens at Ampulla of Vater

242.a----Initial investigation of any patients suspected of biliary tree(SW) USG

243.d---USG will show gall stone with sensitivity and specificity of(SW) >90%

244.c---Features of gall stone :(SW) acoustically dense,acoustic shadow,moves with change in position,sediment/sludge formation

245.a---features of acute cholecystitis on USG are (SW)edematous gall bladder wall,edema between gall bladder and liver,local tenderness

246.b---A contracted, thick bladder wall on USG indicate of(SW) chronic cholecystitis

247.c---Regarding biliary radionuclide scanning :(SW)use of i.v.^{99m}Tc HIDA,uptake by liver detected within 10 minutes,HIDA cleared by Kuffer's cells of liver

248.c--- indictions of biliary scintigraphy are (SW)acute cholecystitis,biliary leaks

249c--. Regarding acute cholecystitis on biliary scintigraphy :(SW) normal HIDA scan exclude acute cholecystitis,cystic duct obstruction(lack of filling of GB after 4hrs) highly sensitive and specific

250.b---The test of choice for suspected malignancy of gall bladder,the extrahepatic biliary system,head of pancreas(SW) CT

251.b---Indication of percutaneous transhepatic cholangiography(SW) management of bile duct strictures and tumour

252.c----Which MRI technique generate high resolution images of biliary tree and pancreatic duct(SW) heavily T2W images

253.d---Advantages of endoscopic retrograde cholangiography(SW) direct visualization of ampullary region,direct access to distal common bile duct,possibility of therapeutic intervention/intraductal endoscopy

254. a---Therapeutic procedure of choice for CBD stone associated with obstructive jaundice,cholangitis or gall stone pancreatitis(SW) ERCP

255.b---Definitive diagnostic test of cholangitis is(SW) ERC(endoscopic retrograde cholangiography)

256.a---- ERCP showing beading of biliary tree suggest of(SW) sclerosing cholangitis

257.a---Mirrizi's syndrome refers to(SW) biliary obstruction due to cholecystolithiasis

258.a----Diameter of dilated common bile duct on USG(SW) >8mm

259.c---- The gold standard for diagnosing common bile duct stone(SW)ERC

260. b---Which investigation is as good as ERC for detecting common bile duct stone (SW) endoscopic USG

261.b---The diagnostic test of choice for acalculous cholecystitis(SW) USG

262.a---Klatskin tumour refers to(SW) perihilar cholangiocarcinoma

263.a---The gold standard for detecting and assessing the severity of acute pancreatitis(SW) CECT

264.d--- CECT finding in acute pancreatitis are (SW)uniform enhancement in interstitial pancreatitis,considerably decreased enhancement in necrotizing pancreatitis,air bubbles indicate of infected necrosis or pancreatic abscess

265.d---Parenchymal calcification in pancreas is noted in(SW)chronic calcifying pancreatitis,hereditary pancreatitis,tropical (nutritional)pancreatitis

266.a---Size of pancreatic abnormalities that is picked up by endoscopic USG and laprascopic USG is(SW)<1 cm

267.d----Cambridge classification of chronic pancreatitis is based on (SW) ERCP finding,CT scan,USG

268.c---USG features of chronic pancreatitis are all except(SW) pancreatic duct dilatation/calculi,cystic changes(<10mm),intrductal filling defect

269.a---Ductal changes seen on endoscopic ultrasound (EUS) in chronic pancreatitis are (SW) ductal size <3mm,tortuous duct/side branch ectasia,echogenic intraductal foci,echogenic duct wall

270.b---Regarding imaging in case of chronic pancreatitis:(SW)EUS is frequently used as a preliminary step in evaluation of pancreatic disease,EUS is comparable to ERCP in detection of advanced changes in chronic pancreatitis,EUS may be more sensitive than ERCP in detection of mild changes of chronic pancreatitis,Small neoplasm seen in chronic pancreatitis may be invisible to all modalities except EUS

271.c---Earliest changes in chronic pancreatitis ,detected by EUS and ERCP are(SW) dilatation of secondary ducts,heterogenous parenchymal changes

272.b----The gold standard for the diagnosis and staging of chronic pancreatitis (SW) ERCP

273.b---The most sensitive radiological test for the diagnosis of chronic pancreatitis(SW) ERCP

274.c----ERCP changes in moderate pancreatitis (SW) abnormal main pancreatic duct,>3abnormal side branches

275.a---Chain of lakes appearance is noted in(SW) chronic pancreatitis

276.a---The initial diagnostic imaging test of choice for pancreatic endocrine/exocrine tumour(SW) Multi detector CT

277. b---The most common endocrine neoplasm of pancreas(SW) insulinoma

278.a---The test of choice for gastrinoma(SW)SSTR(octreotide) scintigraphy

279.b---The most sensitive imaging method for VIPoma(SW) EUS

280.a---The current diagnostic and staging test of choice for pancreatic cancer(SW) multidetector ,dynamic CECT

281.a---The single most versatile and cost effective tool for diagnosis of pancreatic cancer(SW) CECT

282.c---Classic feature of chronic pancreatitis are (SW) calcification,beaded appearance of duct

283.a---Fish-eye lesion on ERCP is virtually diagnostic of(SW) intraductal papillary mucinous neoplasm

284.a---The first imaging modality used to evaluate splenic trauma(SW) USG

285.a----Investigation especially helpful in locating accessory spleen after unsuccessful splenectomy for ITP(SW) radioscintigrapgy with[99m]Tc sulphur colloid

286.b---Felty 's syndrome comprises all except(SW) splenomegaly,rheumatoid arthritis,neutropenia

287. c---Feature of intestinal obstruction on x ray (H) multiple air fluid level,intestinal dilation

288.d---criteria for grade III injury of liver and spleen (American association for surgery for trauma) (SW) subcapsular hematoma >50% of surface area,subcapsular hematoma >10cm in depth,laceration >3cm

289.a---The imaging technique of choice for evalution of soft tissue sarcomas of the extremities(SW) CT supplanted with MRI

290.d---Golderhar complex comprises (SW)branchial cleft anomalies,biliary atresia,congenital cardiac anomalies

291.c---Criteria for ultrasonographic diagnosis of hypertrophic pyloric stenosis(SW) pyloric channel length>16mm,pyloric thickness of>4mm

292.a---Double bubble sign on abdominal radiograph is seen in(SW)duodenal atresia

293.Small intestinal atresia may appear on lapratomy as(SW) apple-peel deformity,Christmas tree deformity,String of sausage deformity,strings of beads appearance

294.a---Pathognomonic radiographic finding in Necrotising enterocolitis(SW) peumatosis intestinalis

295.b---Accurate and reliable imaging technique for biliary atresia(SW) Technetuim Tc ^{99m} disofenin using phenobarbital

296.c----Alagille syndrome comprises(SW) severe intrahepatic cholestasis,biliary hypoplasia

297.a---Initial evaluation of blunt abdominal trauma is done by(SW) FAST

298.d---FAST (focused abdominal ultrasonography for trauma) is use to identify free intraperitoneal fluid in (SW) Morison's pouch,left upper quadrant,the pelvis

299. c---FAST (focused abdominal ultrasonography for trauma) is exquisitively sensitive for detecting intraperitoneal fluid(SW)>250 ml

300.d---Malignant obstruction of intestine are suggested on CT by (H) abrupt transition zone,irregular bowel thickening at obstruction site,mass at the site of obstruction

301.a---'Double bubble' of stomach and duodenal cap is seen in(GRAINGER) duodenal atresia

302.a--- An ultrasound of abdomen can detect ascites as little as 100ml

303.a----Apple-core or napkin ring appearance on barium study of colon is noted in carcinoma

304.c---Excellent screening tool for hepatocellular carcinoma USG

305.c--Characteristic vascular abnormalities of HCC are hypervascularity,portal vein thrombosis

306.d--- True regarding ethiodol are (lipiodol)ethiodised oil emulsion,retained by tumour cells,helpful for biopsy of small lesions,poppy seed oil

307.c---The most common benign tumour of liver haemangioma

308.a---The most useful diagnostic differentiating tool for HCC,adenoma,FNH triphasic CT scan

309.b---The hepatic tumour wuth central scar which is hypovasclar on arterial phase and hypervascular on delayed phase CT is focal nodular hyperplasia

310.c----methods used for in situ ablation of liver secondaries are alcohol,radiofrequency,cryotherapy

311.c---The investigation of choice for Hirschsprung disease contrast enema

312.d---USG finding of adenomyomaosis are tiny echogenic foci in the wall,thickening of wall due to presence of cystic spaces,commet-tail artefact,no vascularity in the lesion

313.d---The USG features of cholesterolosis are soft tissue lesion ,attached to wall ,no shadow,non-mobile

314.a---CT scan is least accurate for gall stone

315.a---Regarding Crohn's disease :(C)most common site in small intestine---terminal ileum,asymetric involvement and skip lesions –characteristic,aphtoid ulcer—earliest sign,Cobblestone pattern

GENITOURINARY SYSTEM

1.Following conditions increases risk of iodinated contrast nephropathy(H)
a.Diabetes
b.Multiple myeloma
c.renal disease
d.all

2.True regarding contrast nephropathy (H)
a.iodinated contrast cause acute renal injury
b.resolve in a week
c.gadolinium cause nephrogenic systemic fibrosis
d.high risk even in normal renal function

3.The useful study for chronic renal diseases is(H)
a.x ray KUB
b.USG
c.CECT
d.MRI

4.USG finding of bilaterally small kidney(<8.5cm) indicate (H)
a.chronic renal disease
b.acut renal disease
c.polycystic renal disease
d.amyloidosis

5.Chronic renal disease with increased or normal renal size (H)
a.diabetic nephropathy
b.amyloidosis
c.HIV nephropathy
d.all

6.Enlarged kidney with multiple cysts are seen in(H)
a.polycystic kidneys
b.diabetic nephropathy
c.amyloidosis
d.HIV nephropathy

7.Suggested investigation for reflux nephropathy(H)
a.CECT
b.MRI
c.voiding cystogram
d.x ray

8.The procedure of choice for urinary obstruction in renal transplant rejection(H)
a.nuclear scan
b.USG
c.CECT
d.MRI

9.Criteria required to diagnose ADPKD are all except(H)
a.presence three or four cysts in one or both kidney (15-39yrs)
b.presence two or more cysts in each kidney(40-59yrs)

c.presence of four or more cysts in each kidney(>60yrs)

d.presence of two or more cysts in each kidney(15-39yrs)

10. Spider leg appearance on IVP is seen in

a.autosomal dominant polycystic kidney disease

b.autosomal recesssive polycystic kidney disease

c.sickle cell disease

d.pyelonephritis

11.All are true regarding ARPKD except(H)

a.large echogenic kidneys

b.cysts generally become visible only after birth

c.diagnosis can be made in utero after 24weeks of gestation in severe cases

d.presence of renal cysts in either parent

12.The kidney is small in all except(H)

a.nephronophthisis I

b.nephronophthisis II

c.nephronophthisis III

d.MCDK

13 Radiological features of medullary sponge kidney diseases are (H)

a.hyperdense papillae

b.cluster of small stones

c.paintbrush like features on IVP

d.all

14.The paintbrush like feature seen on IVP is best found in (H)

a.medullary sponge kidney

b.dysplastic kidney

c.ADPKD

d.tuberous sclerosis

15.In hemodynamically important renal artery lesion(above 60% lumen occlusion),velocity in renal artery is generally(H)

a.>200cm/sec

b.>300cm/sec

c.>100cm/sec

d.>400cm/sec

16. The investigation used to estimate fractional flow to each kidney (H)

a.nuclear scan

b.MRI

c.CECT

d.USG

17.Radionucleotide used to calculate single kidney glomerular filtration rate(H)

a.^{99}Tc mertiatide(^{99}Tc MAG 3)

b.Tc-labelled pentetic acid(DTPA)

c.both

d.none

18.The most common type of renal stone is(H)

a.calcium stone

b.uric acid stone

c.cystine stone

d.struvite stone

19.The standard radiological procedure for diagnosis of nephrolithiasis is(H)

a.helical CT with contrast

b.helical ct without contrast

c. x ray KUB

d.USG

20 .All renal stones are radiopaque except(H)

a.calcium stone

b.uric acid stone

c.cystine stone

d.struvite stone

21.Radiolucent renal stone is(H)

a.calcium stone

b.uric acid stone

c.cystine stone

d.struvite stone

22. Nature of staghorn calculi may be(H)

a.uric acid sone

b.struvite stone

c.cystine stone

d.all

23. Which stone does not form in absence of infection(H)

a.calcium stone

b.uric acid stone

c.cystine stone

d.struvite stone

24. What is the specificity and sensitivity of USG for diagnosis of hdyronephrosis(H)

a.90%

b.80%

c.70%

d.100%

25.False positive hydronephrosis on USG is noted in(H)

a.diuresis

b.renal cyst

c.extra renal pelvis

d.all

26.Hydronephrosis may be absent in USG in all except(H)

a.obstruction less than 48yrs old

b.staghorn calculi

c.retroperitoneal fibrosis

d.diuresis

27.The most common extracranial solid tumour in children and most commonly diagnosed malignancy in children(N)

a.neuroblatoma

b.lymphoma

c.wilm's tumour

d.mesoblatic nephroma

28.All are true regarding neuroblatoma except(N)

a.mass contain calcification and hemorrhage

b.^{123}I-MIBG is used to define extent of the disease

c.CT or MRI of abdomen to evaluate metastatic disease

d. CT or MRI of brain is routinely performed

29.The most common primary malignant renal tumour of childhood(N)

a.neuroblatoma

b.lymphoma

c.wilm's tumour

d.mesoblastic nephroma

30.A useful first study for suspected Wilm's tumour(N)

a.USG with Doppler imaging

b.CT scan

c.MRI

d.nuclear scan

31.Nutcracker syndrome refers to(N)

a.unilateral bleeding of varicose vein of the right ureter

b. unilateral bleeding of varicose vein of the left ureter

c.bilateral bleeding of varicose vein of the ureter

d.corkscrew esophagus with esophageal variceal bleed

32.Mottled nephrogram with brushlke medullary opacification on IVP is noted in(N)

a.ARPKD

b.ADPKD

c.cystic dysplastic kidneys

d.simple benign cyst

33.Bilateral renal agenesis is suspected in presence of all except(N)

a.absent kidneys

b.nonvisualistion of bladder

c.oligohydramnias

d.absent gastric bubble

34.Imaging useful in UTI are (N)

a.DMSA scan

b.USG

c.VCUG

d.all

35.For vesicoureteral reflux ,initial study is(N)

a.radionuclide cystogram

b.VCUG

c.USG

d.CT scan

36.'Spinning top' urethra(dilated urethra) in girls in VCUG is sign of(N)

a.voiding dysfunction

b.retention dysfunction

c.neurogenic bladder

d.flaccid bladder

37.All are features of grade 3 hydronephrosis (as per society for fetal urology) (N)

a.wide splitting pelvis dilated outside renal border

b.calices uniformly dilated

c.normal renal parenchymal thickness

d.convex calices

38.Renal parenchyma becomes thin in which grade of hydronephrosis(as per society for fetal urology) (N)

a.grade 1

b.grade 2

c.grade 3

d.grade 4

39.Voiding cystourethrogram is indicated in(N)

a.vesicoureteral reflux

b.posterior urethral valve

c.both

d.none

40.All are true regarding renal scintigraphy(N)

a.Mercaptoacetyl triglycine(MAG-3) is excreted by renal tubular secretion

b.Diethylene tetrapentaacetic acid(DTPA) is cleared by glomerular filtration

c.MAG-3 and DTPA are used to assess differential renal function

d.all

41.Renal cortical imaging agent used to assess renal differential function and renal cortical scar(N)

a.MAG-3

b.DTPA

c.DMSA

d.DISIDA

42.All are true regarding MAG-3 diuretic urogram except(N)

a.normal $t_{1/2}$ of clearance of radionuclide from pelvis 10-15 minutes

b. $t_{1/2}$ of clearance of radionuclide from pelvis in significant upper tract obstruction >20 minutes

c.after,20-30 minutes iv frusemide is given

d.MAG-3 is considered inferior to IVP in infants and children with respect to hydronephrosis

43.All are true regarding MR urography except(N)

a.permits assessment of differential renal function and drainage assessment

b.no radiation exposure

c.used when USG and nuclear scan fail to delineate complex pathology

d.no need of sedation in younger children

44.All are true regarding Whitaker test except(N)

a.antegrade pressure-perfusion flow study

b.pressure in bladder and renal pelvis is monitored

c.fluid is infused at measured rate ,usually 10ml/minute

d.pressure differences exceeding 40 cmH$_2$O suggest obstruction

45.The most common obstructive urinary tract obstructive lesion in childhood(N)

a.ureteropelvic junction obstruction

b.ureterovesical junction obstruction

c.ectopic ureter

d.mid ureter obstruction

46.The diagnosis of micropenis is made if the stretched penis is(N)

a.<1.9cm

b.<2.9cm

c.<3.9cm

d.<4.9cm

47.All types of calculi may be radiolucent except(N)

a.cystine stone

b.xanthine stone

c.uric acid stone

d.struvite stone

48.The most accurate study for suspected renal colic (N)

a.unenhanced spiral CT scan

b.contrast spiral CT scan

c.USG

d.x ray

49.The normal adult renal length in term of lumber vertebra is(GRAINGER)

a.height of two lumber vertebra

b.height of three lumber vertebra

c.height of fourlumber vertebra

d.height of five lumber vertebra

50.All are true regarding ureter except(GRAINGER)

a.25-30cm long,2-4mm in diameter

b.a ureter>2.5cm lateral to

transverse process is said to be laterally deviated

c.a ureter crossing over pedicle is suspected to be medially deviated

d.ureteral orifices in the bladder are approx. 2.5cm apart

51.The most accurate method of demonstrating vesicoureteric reflux(GRAINGER)

a.IVU

b.MCU

c.USG

d.CT

52.Knutsson's clamp is used in(GRAINGER)

a.cholecystectomy

b.intestinal resection

c.ascending urethrography

d.for limb amputation

53.Lymphotrophic supraparamagnetic nanoparticle(LSN) is useful in MRI imaging of(GRAINGER)

a.prostate

b.liver

c.spleen

d.pancreas

54.The first line treatment for uterine fibroids(GRAINGER)

a.myomectomy

b.hysterectomy

c.expectant management

d.uterine artery embolisation

55.All are true regarding renal pathology except(GRAINGER)

a.chronic glomerulonephritis cause bilateral diffuse parenchymal loss with no papillary /caliceal abnormality

b.Obstructive nephropathy cause bilateral diffuse parenchymal loss with papillary /caliceal abnormality

c. renal artery stenosis cause unilateral diffuse parenchymal loss with no papillary /caliceal abnormality

d.papillary necrosis cause bilateral parenchymal loss with papillary /caliceal abnormality

56.The principal radiographic sign of acute cortical necrosis is(GRAINGER)

a.calcification

b.air

c.both

d.none

57.Characteristic of papillary necrosis are all except(GRAINGER)

a.tracks and horns from the calices

b.The 'egg-in-cup' appearance

c.ring shadows

d.truncated calices

58.All are features of renal tuberculosis except(GRAINGER)

a.coudy appearance of calcification

b.autonephrectomy

c.beaded calcification of ureter and vas

d.large bladder

59.The most useful technique for investigating and characterizing solid renal masses(GRAINGER)

a.CT

b.MRI

c.USG

d.PET

60.Which phase of renal CT is best for detection of renal masses(GRAINGER)

a.corticomedullay phase

b.nephrographic phase

c.both

d.none

61.Simple renal cyst is charecterised by all except(GRAINGER)

a.well defined mass with CT value 0-20HU

b.imperceptible wall

c.hyperintense on T1W and hyporintense on T2W

d.no enhancement after contrast

62.The best technique for diagnosis and staging of renal and perinephric abscess(GRAINGER)

a.CT

b.USG

c.MRI

d.PET

63.All are true of renal angiomyolipoma except(GRAINGER)

a.seen in case of tuberous sclerosis

b.malignant lesions composed of fat,mescles and abnormal blood vessels

c.presence of fat within the lesion(HU 15) is diagnostic

d.multiple aneurysm and 'onion' layer appearance on angiography

64.Renal cell carcinoma is characetrised by all except(GRAINGER)

a.mostly solid

b.enhncament more than 20HU

c.may be associated with VHL

d.calcification in 50% cases

65.The most characteristic abnormalities of acute obstruction on IVU(GRAINGER)
a.asymmetric nephrographic abnormality and excretion of contrast material
b.modest kidney enlargement
c.spontaneou pyelosinus extravasation
d.none

66. The imaging technique most frequently used to assess the primar tumor of prostate
a.TRUS
b CT
c.MRI
d.PET

67.The characteristic radiological feature of retoperitoneal fibrosis is(GRAINGER)
a.medial displacement of ureter
b.ureter narrowed at the L4-5
c.both
d.none

68.Which renal calculus escape detection of even non contrast helical CT(GRAINGER)
a.pure matrix stone
b.stone made of indinavir
c.both
d.none

69.Normal bladder wall thickness ,when distended is(GRAINGER)
a.1mm
b.2mm
c.3mm
d.5mm

70.Bow-tie appearance on on transverse view of USG is noted of(GRAINGER)
a.prostate
b.seminal vesicle
c.bladder
d.none

71.Colapinto and McCllum classification and Goldman and Sandler classification are related to(GRAINGER)
a.renal injury
b.ureteral injury
c.urethral injury
d.seminal vesicle injury

72.The method of choice for imaging scrotal contents(GRAINGER)
a.USG
b.CT
c.MRI
d.PET

73.Yo-Yo reflux is noted in(GRAINGER)
a.incomplete duplication of pelvis

b.hydronephrosis

c.ectopic insertion of ureter

d.crossed fused ectopia

74.All are causes of adrenal calcification except(CHAPMAN)

a.addition disease

b.neuroblastoma

c.adenoma

d.carcinoma

75.All are causes of adrenal calcification except(CHAPMAN)

a.cystic disease

b.wolman's disease

c.tuberculosis

d.all

76.Wolman's disease is characterized by all except(CHAPMAN)

a.hepatomegaly

b.splenomegaly

c.adrenomegaly with punctate calcification

d.cardiomegaly

77.All are true regarding adrenal gland except(CHAPMAN)

a.width of limb is normally less than 1 cm

b.the right adrenal lies above the right kidney

c.the left adrenal lies above of left kidney

d.the right adrenal lies behind the IVC

78.Causes of nephrocalcinosis are all except(CHAPMAN)

a.hyperparathyroidism

b.renal tubular acidosis

c.medullary sponge kidney

d.diabetes mellitus

79. Causes of nephrocalcinosis are all except(CHAPMAN)

a.renal papillary necrosis

b.primary hyperoxaluria

c.acute cortical necrosis

d.all

80.The commonest cause of medullary nephrocalciosis is(CHAPMAN)

a.hyperparathyroidism

b.renal tubular acidosis

c.medullary sponge kidney

d.primary hyperoxaluria

81.Bunch of grapes appearance of calculi in kidney is seen in(CHAPMAN)

a.hyperparathyroidism

b.renal tubular acidosis

c.medullary sponge kidney

d.primary hyperoxaluria

82.Tramline calcification in kidney is noted in(CHAPMAN)

a.hyperparathyroidism

b.renal tubular acidosis

c.acute cortical necrosis

d.primary hyperoxaluria

83.Dromedary hump is found in(CHAPMAN)

a.right kidney

b.left kidney

c.right dome of diaphragm

d.left dome of diaphragm

84.Drooping flower appearance of kidney on IVP is noted in(CHAPMAN)

a.duplex kidney with hydronephrotic upper moiety

b.multiple renal cysts

c.renal tumour

d.none

85.The most common solid renal tumour in the newborn(CHAPMAN)

a.Wilms'tumour

b.rabdoid tumour of kidney

c.congenital mesoblastic nephroma

d.nephroblastomatosis

86.Scalloped nephrogram with negative pyelogram is noted in(CHAPMAN)

a.severe hydronephrosis

b.acute tubular necrosis

c.medullary sponge kidney

d.acute pyelonephritis

87.Most frequent cause of renal papillary necrosis(CHAPMAN)

a.analgesics

b.sickle-cell anaemia

c.diabetes

d.pyelonephritis

88.Strings of beads appearance is noted in(CHAPMAN)

a.atherosclerosis of renal artery

b.fibromuscular dysplasia

c.aneurysm of renal artery

d.none

89.Dilatation of single calyx due to compression by an intrarenal artery is noted in(CHAPMAN)

a.Fanconi's syndrome

b.Fraley syndrome

c.Apert 's syndrome

d.poland 's syndrome

90.The most common cause bladder wall calcification worldwide is(CHAPMAN)

a.tuberculosis

b.schistosomiasis

c.TCC

d.cyclophosphamide intake

91.The commonest cause of bladder outflow obstructuin in male child is(CHAPMAN)

a.vesical diverticulum
b.urethral stricture
c.posterior urethral valve
d.meatal stenosis
92.The commonest cause of bladder outflow obstructuin in female child is(CHAPMAN)
a.vesical diverticulum
b.ectopic ureterocoele
c.calculus
d.none
93.Prune- belly syndrome is characterized by(CHAPMAN)
a.bilateral hydronephrosis and hydroureter
b.distended bladder
c.undescended testes
d.normal anterior abdominal wall
94.Oval calcification with lucent centre ,often arranged in the direction of muscle fibres is found in(CHAPMAN)
a.cysticerci
b.guinea worm
c.loa-loa
d.armillifer
95.Strings of beads appearance in renal artery is seen in(SW)
a.atheroclerosis
b.fibromuscular dysplasia
c.renal artery dissection
d.takayasu arteritis
96.The initial sceening test for patients with suspected renal artery occlusive disease(SW)
a.CECT
c.MRI
d.Duplex USG
d.captopril renal scan
97.drug used in nuclear renal scan in suspected renal artery occlusive disease(SW)
a.dipyridamole
b.captopril
c.indomethacin
d.amlodipine
98.The presence of severe artery stenosis(>60%) is suggested on dulplex USG by(SW)
a.peak systolic velocity(PSV) >180cm/s
b.PSV of renal artery/PSV of aorta>3.5
c.both
d.all
99.The gold standard to assess renal artery occlusive disease(SW)
a.DSA
b.CECT
c.MRA
d.renal scan

100.All are true regarding renal artery occlusive vascular disease except(SW)
a.renal vein rennin ratio >1.5 is indicative of functionally important renovascular hypertention
b.renal:systemic rennin index(RSRI) of affected kidneys in suspected renovascular hypertention is>0.24
c.Captopril increases time to peak activity to more than 11minutes in positive renal scan
d.PSV in normal renal artery >180cm/s

101.Angiographic criteria of renal artery revascularization are all except(SW)
a.fibromuscular dysplasia
b.pressure gradient>20mmHg
c.affected/unaffected kidney ratio>1.5:1
d.all

102.All are true regarding Bosniak classification system of renal cyst except(SW)
a.used to assess likelihood of malignancy
b.based on septations ,calcification and enhancement pattern
c.thin walled cyst with water density with no septations and calcification belong to category 1
d.cyst with solid enhancing component belongs to category III

103.Hyperdense cyst < 3cm on CT scan belong to which Bosniak category of renal cyst(SW)
a.category i
b.category ii
c.category iii
d.category iv

104.Bosniak classification system is used for(SW)
a.renal cyst
b.hapatic cyst
c.adrenal cyst
d.ovarian cyst

105.The most sensitive test for ureteral injury(SW)
a.retrograde pyelogram
b.IVP
c.CT urogram
d.none

106.The study of choice to evaluate for urolithiasis(SW)
a.Contrast CT
b.Noncontrast CT
c.USG
c.x ray

107.The diagnostic modality of choice for diagnosis of ureteropelvic junction obstruction(SW)
a.IVP
b.nuclear scan(mercaptoacetyltriglycine or ^{99m}tc DTPA)
c.CT
d.MRI

108.The most common cause of hydronephrosis on prenatal ultrasound(SW)
a. ureteropelvic junction obstruction
b.vesicoureteral reflux
c.posterior urethal valve
d.horse-shoe kidney

109.Vesicoureteral reflux is evaluated by(SW)
a.IVP
b.VCUG
c.USG
d.MRI

110.Posterior urethral valves is established with (SW)
a.IVP
b.VCUG
c.USG
d.MRI

111.The most sensitive investigation to diagnose renal tuberculosis in early stage
a.CT
b.MRI
c.USG
d.IVP

112.which feature is most important in case of significant of renal artery stenosis
a.collaterals presence
b.post stenotic dilatation of artery
c.diameter reduction>70%
d.systolic pressure gradient >20mmHg across the lesion

113.Agent used to measure GFR is
a.iodohippurate
b.Tc99m-DTPA
c.Tc99m-MAG3
d.Tc99m-DMSA

114.Dense nephrogram is obtained by all except
a.dehydrating the patients
b.increasing dose of contrast
c.rapid injection of dye
d.use of non ionic contrast

115.Cobra head appearance on IVU is noted in(SUTTON)
a.hydronephrosis
b.ureterocoles
c.ureteric diverticulum
d.duplication of ureter

116.Drooping lily sign on IVU is seen in(SUTTON)

a.Duplex kidney
b.hydatid cyst of kidney
c.APKD
d.multicystic kidney

GENITOURINARY SYSTEM (ANSWERS)

1.d---Following conditions increases risk of iodinated contrast nephropathy(H) Diabetes.Multiple myeloma,renal disease

2.d--Regarding contrast nephropathy (H).iodinated contrast cause acute renal injury,resolve in a week,gadolinium cause nephrogenic system fibrosis,not high risk even in normal renal function

3.b---The useful study for chronic renal diseases is(H) USG

4.a----USG finding of bilaterally small kidney(<8.5cm) indicate (H) chronic renal disease

5.d---Chronic renal disease with increased or normal renal size (H) diabetic nephropathy,amyloidosis,HIV nephropathy

6.a---Enlarged kidney with multiple cysts are seen in(H) polycystic kidneys

7.c---Suggested investigation for reflux nephropathy(H) voiding cystogram

8.b---The procedure of choice for urinary obstruction in renal transplant rejection(H) USG

9.d---Criteria required to diagnose ADPKD are (H) presence three or four cysts in one or both kidney (15-39yrs),presence two or more cysts in each kidney(40-59yrs),presence of four or more cysts in each kidney(>60yrs)

10.a---Spider leg appearance on IVP is seen in autosomal dominant polycystic kidney disease

11.d---Regarding ARPKD :(H)large echogenic kidneys,cysts generally become visible only after birth,diagnosis can be made in utero after 24weeks of gestation in severe cases

12.b---The kidney is small in (H) nephronophthisis I,nephronophthisis III,MCDK

13 d---Radiological features of medullary sponge kidney diseases are (H) hyperdense papillae,cluster of small stones,paintbrush like features on IVP

14.a---The paintbrush like feature best seen on IVP is found in (H) medullary sponge kidney

15.a---In hemodynamically important renal artery lesion(above 60% lumen occlusion),velocity in renal artery is generally(H)>200cm/sec

16.a--- The investigation used to estimate fractional flow to each kidney (H)nuclear scan

17.b---Radionucleotide used to calculate single kidney glomerular filtration rate(H) ^{99}Tc mertiatide(^{99}Tc MAG 3),Tc-labelled pentetic acid(DTPA)

18.a---The most common type of renal stone is(H) calcium stone

19.b---The standard radiological procedure for diagnosis of nephrolithiasis is(H) helical ct without contrast

20.b---All renal stones are radiopaque (H)calcium stone,cystine stone,struvite stone

21.b---radiolucent renal stone is(H)uric acid stone

22. d---Nature of staghorn calculi may be(H) uric acid sone,struvite stone,cystine stone

23.d--- Which stone doesnot form in absence of infection(H) struvite stone

24.a---the specificity and sensitivity of USG for diagnosis of hdyronephrosis is (H) 90%

25.d---False positive hydronephrosis on USG is noted in(H) diuresis,renal cyst,extra renal pelvis

26.d---Hydronephrosis may be absent in USG in (H)obstruction less than 48yrs old,staghorn calculi,retroperitoneal fibrosis

27.a---The most common extracranial solid tumour in children and most commonly diagnosed malignancy in children(N) neuroblatoma

28.d---Regarding neuroblatoma (N)mass contain calcification and hemorrhage,^{123}I-MIBG is used to define extent of the disease,CT or MRI of abdomen to evaluate metastatic disease

29.c---the most common primary malignant renal tumour of childhood(N) wilm's tumour

30.a---A useful first study for suspected Wilm's tumour(N) USG with Doppler imaging

31.b---Nutcracker syndrome refers to(N)unilateral bleeding of varicose vein of the left ureter

32.a----Mottled nephrogram with brushlke medullary opacification on IVP is noted in(N) ARPKD

33.d---Bilateral renal agenesis is suspected in presence of (N) absent kidneys,nonvisualistion of bladder,oligohydramnias

34.d----Imaging useful in UTI are (N)DMSA scan,USG,VCUG

35.b---For vesicoureteral reflux ,initial study is(N) VCUG

36.a---'Spinning top' urethra(dilated urethra) in girls in VCUG is sign of(N) voiding dysfunction

37.d---Features of grade 3 hydronephrosis (as per society for fetal urology) (N)wide splitting pelvis dilated outside renal border,calices uniformly dilated,normal renal parenchymal thickness

38.d---Renal parenchyma becomes thin in which grade of hydronephrosis(as per society for fetal urology) (N) grade 4

39.c---Voiding cystourethrogram is indicated in(N) vesicoureteral reflux,posterior urethral valve

40.d--Regarding renal scintigraphy(N) Mercaptoacetyl triglycine(MAG-3) is excreted by renal tubular secretion,Diethylene tetrapentaacetic acid(DTPA) is cleared by glomerular filtration,MAG-3 and DTPA are used to assess differential renal function

41.c---Renal cortical imaging agent used to assess renal differential function and renal cortical scar(N) DMSA

42.d---Regarding MAG-3 diuretic urogram :(N)normal $t_{1/2}$ of clearance of radionuclide from pelvis 10-15 minutes,$t_{1/2}$ of clearance of radionuclide from pelvis in significant upper tract obstruction >20 minutes,after,20-30 minutes iv frusemide is given

d.MAG-3 is considered inferior to IVP in infants and children with respect to hydronephrosis

43.d---Regarding MR urography (N)permits assessment of differential renal function and drainage assessment,no radiation exposure,used when USG and nuclear scan fail to delineate complex pathology,need of sedation in younger children

44.d---Regarding Whitaker test:(N)antegrade pressure-perfusion flow study,pressure in bladder and renal pelvis is monitored,fluid is infused at measured rate ,usually 10ml/minute,pressure differences exceeding 20cmH$_2$O suggest obstruction

45.a---The most common obstructive urinary tract obstructive lesion in childhood(N) ureteropelvic junction obstruction

46.a---The diagnosis of micropenis is made if the stretched penis is(N) <1.9cm

47.d---Types of   radiolucent calculi :(N) cystine stone,xanthine stone,uric acid stone

48.a---The most accurate study for suspected renal colic (N) unenhanced spiral CT scan

49.a--The normal adult renal length in term of lumber vertebra is(GRAINGER) height of three lumber vertebra

50.b---Regarding ureter(GRAINGER) 25-30cm long,2-4mm in diameter,a ureter crossing over pedicle is suspected to be medially deviated,ureteral orifices in the bladder are approx. 2.5cm apart

51.b---The most accurate method of demonstrating vesicoureteric reflux(GRAINGER) MCU

52.c---Knutsson's clamp is used in(GRAINGER) ascending urethrography

53.a---Lymphotrophic supraparamagnetic nanoparticle(LSN) is useful in MRI imaging of(GRAINGER) prostate

54.d---The first line treatment for uterine fibroids(GRAINGER) uterine artery embolisation

55.d---Regarding renal pathology (GRAINGER)chronic glomerulonephritis cause bilateral diffuse parenchymal loss with no papillary /caliceal abnormality,Obstructive nephropathy cause bilateral diffuse parenchymal loss with papillary /caliceal abnormality,renal artery stenosis cause unilateral diffuse parenchymal loss with no papillary /caliceal abnormality,papillary necrosis cause no parenchymal loss with papillary /caliceal abnormality

56.a---The principal radiographic sign of acute cortical necrosis is(GRAINGER) calcification

57.d---Characteristic of papillary necrosis are (GRAINGER) tracks and horns from the calices,The 'egg-in-cup' appearance,ring shadows

58.d---Features of renal tuberculosis :(GRAINGER) coudy appearance of calcification,autonephrectomy,beaded calcification of ureter and vas,smallbladder

59.a---The most useful technique for investigating and characterizing solid renal masses(GRAINGER) CT

60.b---Phase of renal CT is best for detection of renal masses(GRAINGER) nephrographic phase

61.c---Simple renal cyst is charecterised by (GRAINGER) well defined mass with CT value 0-20HU,imperceptible wall,hypointense on T1W and hyperintense on T2W,no enhancement after contrast

62.a---The best technique for diagnosis and staging of renal and perinephric abscess(GRAINGER) CT

63.b--True about renal angiomyolipoma :(GRAINGER)seen in case of tuberous sclerosis,benign lesions composed of fat,mescles and abnormal blood vessels,presence of fat within the lesion(HU 15) is diagnostic ,multiple aneurysm and 'onion' layer appearance on angiography

64.d---Renal cell carcinoma is characetrised by (GRAINGER) mostly solid,enhncament more than 20HU,may be associated with VHL

65.a---The most characteristic abnormalities of acute obstruction on IVU(GRAINGER) asymmetric nephrographic abnormality and excretion of contrast material

66.a--- The imaging technique most frequently used to assess the primar tumor of prostate TRUS

67.c--The characteristic radiological feature of retoperitoneal fibrosis is(GRAINGER) medial displacement of ureter,ureter narrowed at the L4-5

68.c---Renal calculus escape detection of even non contrast helical CT(GRAINGER) pure matrix stone,stone made of indinavir

69.b---Normal bladder wall thickness ,when distended is(GRAINGER) 2mm

70.b---Bow-tie appearance on on transverse view of USG is noted of(GRAINGER) seminal vesicle

71.c---Colapinto and McCllum classification and Goldman and Sandler classification are related to(GRAINGER) urethral injury

72.a---The method of choice for imaging scrotal contents(GRAINGER) USG

73.a---Yo-Yo reflux is noted in(GRAINGER) incomplete duplication of pelvis

74.c---Causes of adrenal calcification except(CHAPMAN) addition disease,neuroblastoma,carcinoma

75.d---Causes of adrenal calcification :(CHAPMAN)cystic disease,wolman's disease,tuberculosis

76.d---Wolman's disease is characterized by (CHAPMAN)hepatomegaly ,splenomegaly,adrenomegaly with punctate calcification

77.c---Regarding adrenal gland :(CHAPMAN) width of limb is normally less than 1 cm,the right adrenal lies above the right kidney,the left adrenal on medial side of left kidney,the right adrenal lies behind the IVC

78.d---Causes of nephrocalcinosis are(CHAPMAN)hyperparathyroidism,renal tubular acidosis,medullary sponge kidney

79. a---Causes of nephrocalcinosis are (CHAPMAN) renal papillary necrosis,primary hyperoxaluria,acute cortical necrosis

80.c---The commonest cause of medullary nephrocalciosis is(CHAPMAN)medullary sponge kidney

81.c---Bunch of grapes appearance of calculi in kidney is seen in(CHAPMAN)medullary sponge kidney

82.c---Tramline calcification in kidney is noted in(CHAPMAN)acute cortical necrosis

83.b---Dromedary hump is found in(CHAPMAN)left kidney84.a---Drooping flower appearance of kidney on IVP is noted in(CHAPMAN)duplex kidney with hydronephrotic upper moiety

85.c----The most common solid renal tumour in the newborn(CHAPMAN)congenital mesoblastic nephroma

86.a----Scalloped nephrogram with negative pyelogram is noted in(CHAPMAN)severe hydronephrosis

87.d---Most frequent cause of renal papillary necrosis(CHAPMAN)diabetes

88.b---Strings of beads appearance is noted in(CHAPMAN) fibromuscular dysplasia

89.b---Dilatation of single calyx due to compression by an intrarenal artery is noted in(CHAPMAN) Fraley syndrome

90.b---The most common cause bladder wall calcification worldwide is(CHAPMAN) schistosomiasis

91.c---The commonest cause of bladder outflow obstructuin in male child is(CHAPMAN)posterior urethral valve

92.b---The commonest cause of bladder outflow obstructuin in female child is(CHAPMAN) ectopic ureterocoele

93.d---Prune- belly syndrome is characterized by(CHAPMAN) bilateral hydronephrosis and hydroureter,distended bladder,undescended testes,abnormal anterior abdominal wall

94.a---Oval calcification with lucent centre ,often arranged in the direction of muscle fibres is found in(CHAPMAN) cysticerci

95.b---Strings of beads appearance in renal artery is seen in(SW) fibromuscular dysplasia

96.d---The initial sceening test for patients with suspected renal artery occlusive disease(SW) Duplex USG

97.b---drug used in nuclear renal scan in suspected renal artery occlusive disease(SW) captopril

98.c---The presence of severe artery stenosis(>60%) is suggested on dulplex USG by(SW) peak systolic velocity(PSV) >180cm/s,.PSV of renal artery/PSV of aorta>3.5

99.a---The gold standard to assess renal artery occlusive disease(SW) DSA

100.d---Regarding renal artery occlusive vascular disease (SW) renal vein rennin ratio >1.5 is indicative of functionally important renovascular hypertention,renal:systemic rennin index(RSRI) of affected kidneys in suspected renovascular hypertention is>0.24,Captopril increases time to peak activity to more than 11minutes in positive renal scan,PSV in normal renal artery <180cm/s

101.d---Angiographic criteria for renal artery revascularization (SW) fibromuscular dysplasia lesion,pressure gradient>20mmHg,affected/unaffected kidney ratio>1.5:1

102.Regarding Bosniak classification system of renal cyst :(SW)used to assess likelihood of malignancy,based on septations ,calcification and enhancement pattern,thin walled cyst with water density with no septations and calcification belong to category 1

103.b---Hyperdense cyst < 3cm on CT scan belong to which Bosniak category of renal cyst(SW)category ii

104.a---Bosniak classification system is used for(SW) renal cyst

105.a---The most sensitive test for ureteral injury(SW)retrograde pyelogram

106.b---The study of choice to evaluate for urolithiasis(SW) Noncontrast CT

107.b---The diagnostic modality of choice for diagnosis of ureteropelvic junction obstruction(SW) nuclear scan(mercaptoacetyltriglycine or ^{99m}tc DTPA)

108.a----The most common cause of hydronephrosis on prenatal ultrasound(SW) ureteropelvic junction obstruction

109.b---Vesicoureteral reflux is evaluated by(SW)VCUG

110.b---Posterior urethral valves is established with (SW)VCUG

111.d---The most sensitive investigation to diagnose renal tuberculosis in early stage IVP

112.a---feature that is most important in case of significant of renal artery stenosis is collaterals presence

113.b---Agent used to measure GFR is Tc99m-DTPA

114.d---Dense nephrogram is obtained by dehydrating the patients,increasing dose of contrast,rapid injection of dye

115.B---Cobra head appearance on IVU is noted in(SUTTON) ureterocoles

116.a---Drooping lily sign on IVU is seen in(SUTTON) Duplex kidney

ENDOCRINOLOGY

1. All are true regarding ^{123}I except (SW)
a.emits low dose radiation
b.$t_{1/2}$ =12-14hrs
c.used to image lingual thyroids or goiters
d.used to treat lingual thyroids

2. All are true regarding ^{131}I except (SW)
a.emits higher- dose radiation
b.$t_{1/2}$ =8-10 days
c.used treat differentiated thyroid cancers
d.used to image goitre

3.All are true regarding thyroid radionuclide imaging except(SW)
a.cold lesions refers to areas that trap less radioactivity than surrounding tissue
b.risk of malignancy is higher in cold lesions (20%) compared to hot/warm lesions(<5%)
c.^{99m}Tc pertechnetate is taken up by the thyroid gland,and is sensitive for nodal metastase
d.FDG PET is routinely used in evaluation of thyroid nodules

4.Subperiosteal resoption in hyperparathyroidism is most apparent on (SW)
a.the radial aspect of the middle phalanx of the second and third fingers
b.the ulnar aspect of the middle phalanx of the second and third fingers
c.the radial aspect of the distal phalanx of the second and third fingers
d.the ulnar aspect of the distal phalanx of the second and third fingers

5.All are true regarding radiological featrures of hyperparathyroidism except (SW)
a.subperiosteal resorption
b.bone cysts/brown tumour
c.tufting of distal phalanges
d.high metacarpal index

6.The most widely used and accurate modality for detection of parathyroid adenoma(SW)
a.^{99m}Tc sestamibi
b.USG
c.^{131}I scan
d.MRI

7.Radionuclide used for localization of adrenal adenoma(SW)
a.^{99m}Tc sestamibi
b.^{131}I NP-59

c.^{123}I scan

d.^{99m}Tc pertechnetate

8.All are true regarding adrenal imaging except (SW)

a.CT and MRI are useful in distinguishing adrenal adenoma from carcinoma

b.adrenal adenoma appear brighter than liver on T2W imaging

c.NP-59 can be used to distinguish adenoma from hyperplasia

d.petrosal/peripheral vein ACTH level of >2 in basal state and >3 after CRH stimulation is diagnostic of pituitary tumour

9.The Single most important criterion to diagnose adrenocortical malignancy (SW)

a.size

b.tumour heterogeneity

c.hemorrhage

d.margin irregularity

10.MRI features suggesting adrenocortical malignancy are all except(SW)

a.moderately bright signal intensity on T2W

b.significant lesion enhancement

c.fast washout of contrast

d.invasion of IVC

11.All are true regarding imaging in phaechromocytomas(SW)

a.CT imaging with Contrast is must

b.MRI almost 100% specific

c.MRI is study of choice in pregnant women

d.^{131}I MIBG is especially useful in localisation of ectopic position

12.All are imaging characteristics of adrenal adenoma except(SW)

a.homogenous

b.well encapsulated

c.smooth and regular margin

d.hyperattenuating >19HU

13.All are true regarding imaging of adrenal lesions except(SW)

a.adrenal cancer tend to be hypoattenuating<10HU

b.adenoma show low signal intensity compared to liver(adrenal mass to liver ratio<1.4) on T2W image

c.carcinoma and metastases have moderate intensity(adrenal mass to liver ratio 1.2:2.8) on T2W image d.phaecromocytoma have extremly bright (adrenal mass to liver ratio>3) on T2W image

14.For RAIU study ,which agent is used
a.I 132
b.I 131
c.I 123
d.I 125

15.CT features of adrenal adenoma are all except
a.low attenuation (<10HU)
b.sharpy marginated ,homogenous mass
c.calcification rare
d.relatively rapid uptake and delayed washout of contrast(ans rapid washout)

16.Following USG features of thyroid nodule suggest of malignancy except
a.hypoechogenicity
b.hyperechogenicity
c.nonhomogenous
d.microcalcification

17.All are features of spine in acromegaly except(H)
a.reduced intervertabral disc
b.hypertrophic anterior osteophyte
c.ligamental calcification
d.simulate DISH

18.All are features of acromegaly except(H)
a.barrell shaped chest
b.spadelike distal tuft
c.thin heel pad
d.chondrocalcinosis

19.Rotting fence –post appearance of the proximal femur, basketwork appearance of cortex and pepper-pot skull are features of (C)
a.acromegaly
b.Cushing's syndrome
c.hyperprarathyroidism
d.hyperthyroidism

20. features of hyperparathyroidism are all except(C)
a.rotting fence-post appearance of proximal femur
b.basketwork appearance of cortex
c.triradiate pelvis
d.buffalo's hump

21.Subperiosteal resorption seen in hyperparathyroidism particularly affects
a. the radial side of distal phalanx of the middle finger
b. the ulnar side of distal phalanx of the middle finger

c.the radial side of middle
phalanx of the middle finger
d.the ulnar side of middle
phalanx of the middle finger
22.The investigation of choice
for detection of

microadenoma of pituitary
gland(GRAINGER)
a.CT
b.MRI
c.PET
d.USG

ENDOCRINOLOGY(ANSWERS)

1.d--- true regarding ^{123}I:(SW) emits low dose radiation,$t_{1/2}$ =12-14hrs,used to image lingual thyroids or goiters

2. d---true regarding ^{131}I: (SW) emits higher- dose radiation,$t_{1/2}$ =8-10 days,used to screen and treat patients with differentiated thyroid cancers for metastatic disease

3.d--Regarding thyroid radionuclide imaging:(SW) Cold lesions refers to areas that trap less radioactivity than surrounding tissue,risk of malignancy is higher in cold lesions (20%) compared to hot/warm lesions(<5%),.^{99m}Tc pertechnetate is taken up by the thyroid gland,and is sensitive for nodal metastase.FDG is not routinely used in evaluation of thyroid nodule.

4.a---Subperiosteal resoption in hyperparathyroidism is most apparent on(SW) the radial aspect of the middle phalanx of the second and third fingers

5.d---Radiological featrure of hyperparathyroidism are (SW) subperiosteal resorption,bone cysts/brown tumour,tufting of distal phalanges .Osteitis fibrosa cytica occurs in less than 5% cases.

6.a---The most widely used and accurate modality for detection of parathyroid adenoma(SW)^{99m}Tc sestamibi

7.c---Radionuclide used for localization of adrenal adenoma(SW) ^{131}I NP-59

8.b--Regarding adrenal imaging(SW) CT and MRI are useful in distinguishing adrenal adenoma from carcinoma,adrenal adenoma appear darker than liver on T2W imaging,NP-59 can be used to distinguish adenoma from hyperplasia,petrosal/peripheral vein ACTH level of >2 in basal state and >3 after CRH stimulation is diagnostic of pituitary tumour

9.a---The Single most important criterion to diagnose adrenocortical malignancy (SW) size

10.c---MRI features suggesting adrenocortical malignancy are (SW) .moderately bright signal intensity on T2W,significant lesion enhancement,slow washout of contrast,invasion of IVC

11.a---Regarding imaging in phaechromocytomas(SW).MRI almost 100% specific,MRI is study of choice in pregnant women,^{131}I MIBG is especially useful in localisation of ectopic position,CT without contrast is done to minimize the hypertensive crisis

12.d---Imaging characteristics of adrenal adenoma :(SW)homogenous ,well encapsulated,smooth and regular margin,hypoattenuating <10HU on CT scan

13.a---Regarding imaging of adrenal lesions :(SW)adrenal cancer tend to be hyperattenuating>19HU,adenoma show low signal intensity compared to liver(adrenal mass to liver ratio<1.4) on T2W image,carcinoma and metastases have moderate intensity(adrenal mass to liver ratio 1.2:2.8) on T2W image,phaecromocytoma have extremly bright (adrenal mass to liver ratio>3) on T2W image

14.c---For RAIU study ,I 123 is used

15.d---CT features of adrenal adenoma are low attenuation (<10HU),sharpy marginated ,homogenous mass,calcification rare,relatively rapid uptake and rapid washout of contrast

16.b--- USG features of thyroid nodule that suggest of malignancy hypoechogenicity,nonhomogenous,microcalcification

17.a---Features of spine in acromegaly(H) thickened intervertabral disc,hypertrophic anterior osteophyte,ligamental calcification,simulate DISH

18.c---Features of acromegaly :(H) barrell shaped chest,spadelike distal tuft,thick heel pad,chondrocalcinosis

19.c---Rotting fence –post appearance of the proximal femur, basketwork appearance of cortex and pepper-pot skull are features of (C) hyperprarathyroidism

20. d---features of hyperparathyroidism are (C) rotting fence-post appearance of proximal femur,basketwork appearance of cortex,triradiate pelvis

21.c---Subpriosteal resorption seen in hyperparathyroidism particularly affect(C)the radial side of middle phalanx of the middle finger

22.b---The investigation of choice for detection of microadenoma of pituitary gland(GRAINGER) MRI

OBSTETRICS AND GYNAECOLOGY

1.Transvaginal ultrasound shows gestational sac and yolk sac by(DUTTA)

a.5 menstrual weeks

b.5.5 menstrual weeks

c.6 menstrual weeks

d.6.5menstrual weeks

2.Transvaginal ultrasound shows fetal pole and cardiac activity by(DUTTA)

a.5 menstrual weeks

b.5.5 menstrual weeks

c.6 menstrual weeks

d.6.5menstrual weeks

3.Between 7-12 weeks ,the fetal gestational age is best determined by(DUTTA)

a.fetal sac diameter

b.CRL

c.BPD

d.all

4. Transvaginal ultrasound shows embryonic movement by(DUTTA)

a.7 menstrual weeks

b.5 menstrual weeks

c.6 menstrual weeks

d.6.5menstrual weeks

5.BPD is measured at the level of(DUTTA)

a.thalami and cavum septum pellucidum

b.at level of cerebellum

c.at the level of shortest diameter

d.at the level of longest diameter

6.AFI in oligohydramnios is(DUTTA)

a.<5

b.<7

c.<3

d.<8

7.AFI in polyhydramnios is(DUTTA)

a.>15

b.>35

c.>25

d.>30

8.Ossification centres in lower end of femur appear at(DUTTA)

a.36-37week

b.34-35week

c.38-40week

d.41-42 week

9.Formula used to calculate fetal weight in sonography is(DUTTA)

a.Shepherd 's

b.Hadlock's

c.both

d.none

10.Radiological evidence of fetal skeletal shadow may be visible as early as (DUTTA)
a.12 week
b.14 week
c.16 week
d.18week

11.Biophysical profile parameters are all exept(DUTTA)
a.nonstress test
b.fetal breathing movement and gross body movement
c.fetal muscle tone and amniotic fluid
d.heart rate

12.The single ultrasonographic fetal parameter that best reflects the nutrion is(DUTTA)
a.biparietal diameter
b.abdominal circumference
c.femur length
D.head circumference

13.IUGR is suspected when the HC/AC ratio is ---after 34 weeks(DUTTA)
a.<1
b.>1
c.>2
d.>3

14.All are true regarding Doppler in pregnancy(DUTTA)

a.uterine artery Doppler is helpful to assess the downstream vascular resistance
b.umblical vein Doppler provide cardiac forward function.
c.in normal pregnancy,the S/D ratio,pulsatility index and resistance index decreases as the gestational age advnces.
d.normal uterine vein flow is diphasic.

15.Pulsatility index refers to(DUTTA)
a.S—D/M
b.S/D
c.S—D/S
d.D—S/M

16.Resistive index refers to(DUTTA)
a.S—D/M
b.S/D
c.S—D/S
d.D—S/M

17.All are abnormal umbilical artery flow velocity waveform except(DUTTA)
a.reduced end diastolic flow
b.absent end diastolic flow
c.reversed end diastolic flow
d.increased systolic flow

18.Brain sparing effect in response to fetal hypoxemia is reflected in Doppler study as(DUTTA)

a.increased diastolic flow

b.decreased S/D ratio

c.decreased PI

d.all

19.Amniotic fluid index refers to(DUTTA)

a.the sum of vertical pockets from two quadrant of uterine cavity

b.the sum of vertical pockets from four quadrant of uterine cavity

c.the sum of vertical pockets from three quadrant of uterine cavity

d.the depth of maximally vertical pocket of amniotic fluid

20.A vertical pocket of amniotic fluid -----cm is considered normal(DUTTA)

a.=>2cm

b=>3cm

c.=>4cm

d.=>5cm

21.All are assigned score of two in BPS(during observation period of 30 minutes) except(DUTTA)

a.fetal breathing movement =>1episode lasting >30sec.

b.=>3 discrete body/ limb movements

c.=>episode of extention (limb or trunk)with return of flexion

d.=>2pockets (measuring 2cm)of amniotic fluid in two perpendicular planes(2x2cm pocket)

22.Suspect chronic asphyxia if BPS is(DUTTA)

a.10

b.8

c.6

d.4

23.USG finding favouring ectopic pregnancy are (DUTTA)

a.absence of intrauterine pregnancy with positive pregnancy test

b.echogenic fluid in Pouch of Douglas

c.adnexal mass seprate from ovary

d.all

24.'Ring of fire' pattern of blood flow on color doppler outside the uterine cavity is noted in(DUTTA)

a.ovarian cyst

b.ectopic pregnancy

c.dermod cyst of ovary

d.all

25.Snow storm appearance on USG of uterus is characteristic of(DUTTA)

a.hydatidiform mole

b.intrauterine haemorrhage

c.intrauterine collection

d.all

26.Lambda/Twin peak sign in USG of pregnancy is noted in(DUTTA)

a.dichorionic-diamniotic twin

b.monochorionic-diamniotic twin

c.monochorionic-monomniotic twin

d.all

27.The maximum vertical diameter of amniotic fluid in oligohydramnios is(DUTTA)

a.<2cm

b<4cm

c<3cm

d.<5cm

28.The investigation of choice for placenta previa(DUTTA)

a.transabdominal USG

b.MRI

c.transvaginal USG

d.all

29.The anterior landmark for diagnosing placenta previa (DUTTA)

a.uterovesicle angle

b.head of fetus

c.both

d.none

30.The earliest diagnosis of fetal death is possible with(DUTTA)

a.x ray

b.USG

c.clinical

d.none

31.The irregular overlapping of the cranial bones on one another noted in intrauterine death is known as(DUTTA)

a.Spalding sign

b.Robert's sign

c.lemon sign

d.banana sign

32.Appearance of gas shadow in the chambers of the heart and great vessels in intrauterine death is known as(DUTTA)

a.Spalding sign

b.Robert's sign

c.lemon sign

d.banana sign

33.The earliest sign noted in x ray after intrauterine death is(DUTTA)

a.Spalding sign(usually 7days)

b.Robert's sign as early as 12hrs)

c.hyperflexion of the spine

d.crowding of ribs

34.All are features of IUD except(DUTTA)

a.Spalding sign(usually 7days)

b.Robert's sign (as early as 12hrs)

c.hyperflexion of the spine and crowding of rib

d.all

35.'Buddha position' of fetus with halo around the head in x ray is noted in(DUTTA)

a.hydrops fetalis

b.IUD

c.both

d.none

36.The most common type of pelvis is(DUTTA)

a.anthropoid

b.android

c.gynaecoid

d.platypelloid

37.Rachitic pelvis is characterized by all except(DUTTA)

a.'reniform' shape of the inlet

b.widening of transverse diameter of the outlet and the pubic arch

c.backward tilting of sacrum

d.increased anteroposterior diameter of inlet

38.Triradiate shaped inlet of pelvis is noted in(DUTTA)

a.ricket

b.osteomalacia

c.Robert's pelvis

d.Naegele 's pelvis

39.Pelvis resulting from arrested development of one ala of the sacrum (DUTTA)

a.ricketic pelvis

b.osteomalacic

c.Robert's pelvis

d.Naegele 's pelvis

40.Pelvis resulting from absent ala of both sides and sacrum fused with the innominate bone(DUTTA)

a.ricketic pelvis

b.osteomalacic

c.Robert's pelvis

d.Naegele 's pelvis

41.With conventional x ray pelvimetry,radiation exposure to gonads is(DUTTA)

a.885millirad

b.380millird

c.275millirad

d.105millirad

42.USG features of placenta accrete (DUTTA)

a.loss of normal hypoechoic retroplacental myometrial zone

b.thinning and disruption of the uterine serosa –bladder interface

c.focal exophytic mass within the placenta

d.all

43.All are true regarding HC/AC ratio(DUTTA)

a.>1 before 32weeks

b.approx.1 at 32-34weeks

c.<1 after 34weeks

d.remain elevated (>1) in symmetric IUGR

44.The single most sensitive parameter to detect IUGR(DUTTA)

a.AC

b.FL

c.HC

d.BPD

45.All are true regarding IUGR except(DUTTA)

a.HC/AC remain elevated in asymmetric IUGR

b.FL/AC ratio greater than 23.5suggest IUGR

c.FL is not affected in asymmetric IUGR

d.A vertical pocket of <5cm suggests IUGR

46.All are true regarding IUGR except(DUTTA)

a.S/D ratio elevated

b.presence of diastolic notch in uterine artery

c.Ponderal index below the 10th percentile

d.no diastolic flow as brain sparing effect

47.Invertogram is taken to diagnose(DUTTA)

a.imperforate anus

b.duodenal atresia

c.tracheo-esophgeal fistula

d.jejunal atresia

48.Commonly used frequency in TVS is(DUTTA)

a.1-3MHz

b. 3-5MHz

c.5-7MHz

d.7-10MHz

49.Ultrasound travels through tissues of body at(DUTTA)

a.1540m/sec

b.1240m/sec

c.1040m/sec

d.840m/sec

50.The mode used to study moving structures such as fetal heart(DUTTA)

a.B-mode

b.M-mode

c.both

d.none

51.All are true regarding 3D except(DUTTA)

a.view of complex structure in a single image

b.later review without patient

c.No improved diagnosis of prenatal anomaly

d.increased parental bonding due to life like images

52.Effects of ultrasound on tissues are all except(DUTTA)

a.temperature elevation

b.micobubbles

c.cavitation

d.all

53.All are true regarding gestational sac on usg in first trimester except(DUTTA)

a.eccentric in position in the endometrium

b.double decidua sign

c.presence of yolk sac and fetal pole confirm pregnancy

d.true gestational sac increases at rate of 3 mm/day

54.All are true finding on TVS except(DUTTA)

a.mean sac diameter 5-8mm, yolk sac

b.mean sac diameter 12mm, embryo

c.mean sac diameter 15-18mm , cardiac activity

d.embryo CRL=>7mm,cardiac activity

55.Cardiac activity is noted on TVS at(DUTTA)

a.4week

b.6week

c.7week

d.8week

56.Which is an accurate predictor of gestational age when measured between14-28weeks(DUTTA)

a.transcerebellar diameter

b.pons diameter

c.thalamus diameter

d.frontal diameter

57.All are true except(DUTTA)

a.gestational sac grows at rate of 1.1mm/day

b.CRL in mm+42=approx.gestational age in days

c.MSD in mm+50 =approx gestational age in days

d.failure to visualize an embryo when MSD is 6 mm indicate pregnancy loss

58.Nuchal thickness ---mm is strong marker of chromosomal anomalies(DUTTA)

a.>2mm

b.>3mm

c.>4mm

d.>5mm

59.Banana sign refers to(DUTTA)

a.flattening of cerebellar hemisphere

b.scalloping of frontal bones

c.flattening of cerebrum

d.none

60.Lemon sign and banana sign are found in(DUTTA)

a.open spina bifida

b.Arnold-Chiari malformation

c.both

d.none

61.Ventriculomagaly is diagnosed when width of lateral ventricle is(DUTTA

a.>10mm

b.>12mm

c.>14mm

d.>16mm

62.Which anomaly is characterized by absence of cranium and telencephalon(DUTTA)

a.anencephaly

b.Arnold-Chiari malformation

c.both

d.none

63.Diagnosis of anencephaly is possible at about (DUTTA)

a.10week

b.13week

c.15week

d.16week

64.Gastoschisis is characterized by all except(DUTTA)

a.praraumblical defect

b.herniated loops float freely in amniotic fluid

c.not covered with membrane

d.associated with chromosomal anomaly

65.All are true regarding omphalocele except(DUTTA)

a.usually midline defect

b.cord insertion on the herniated mass

c.not covered by membrane

d.associated with chromosomal anomaly

66.Placental thickness more than-- --mm is abnormal at any period of gestation (DUTTA)

a.30mm

b.25mm

c.40mm

d.45mm

67.Placental thickness at term is about (DUTTA)

a.20mm

b.25mm

c.30mm

d.35mm

68.Placenta previa is excluded from diagnosis when the distance between the internal OS and placental edge is more than(DUTTA)

a.20mm

b.25mm

c.30mm

d.35mm

69.Ultrasound marker of chromosomal anomalies (DUTTA)

a.choroid plexus cyst

b.strawberry skull

c.holoprosencephaly

d.all

70.All are marker of trisomy 21 except(DUTTA)

a.wide gap between 1st and 2nd toes

b.short femur

c.omphalocele

d.Rockerbottom foot

71.Absorbed radiation by the fetus in abdominal x ray(DUTTA)

a.0.263 rad

b.0.5 rad

c.0.001 rad

d.1.0 rad

72.Exposure to DES produce (DUTTA)

a.T –shaped uterus

b.unicornuate uterus

c.bicornuate uterus

d.none

73.Who first introduced ultrasound in the field of medicine(DUTTA)

a.Ian Donald

b.Felix Bloch

c.Jeffcoat

d.Williams John

74.Transabdominal USG requires full bladder in order to(DUTTA)

a.displace bowel out of pelvis

b.acts as an acoustic window

c.both

d.none

75.Tissue resolution of---mm can be obtained by ultrasound(DUTTA)

a.<0.2mm

b.>0.4mm

c.<0.1mm

d.<0.3mm

76.Higher is the frequency of ultrasound wave (DUTTA)

a.better is the resolution

b.lesser is the depth of tissue penetration

c.both

d.none

77.All are true regarding TVS except(DUTTA)

a.no need of full bladder

b.operates at frequeny of 5-8MHz

c.detailed examination of pelvis possible

d.easy in vergins and postmenopausal women

78.Sonohysterography involves (DUTTA)

a. infusion of saline in uterine cavity

b.infusion of saline in pelvis

c.infusion of saline in vagina

d.infusion of saline in rectum

79.Endometrial thickness of ----mm is considered as atrophic(DUTTA)

a.<2mm

b.<3mm

c.<4mm

d.<5mm

80.Who first described phenomenon of MRI(DUTTA)

a.Ian Donald

b.Felix Bloch and Edward Purcell

c.Jeffcoat

d.Williams John

81.Which is safe in pregnancy(DUTTA)

a.CT

b.MRI

c.PET

d.none

82. Hysterosalpingographic finding in female genital tuberculosis (DUTTA)

a.lead-pipe tube with nodulations

b.'Tobacco pouch' appearance with blocked fimbrial end

c.beaded appearance of tubes with variable filling density

d.all

83.Hysterosalpingographic finding in female genital tuberculosis (DUTTA)

a.distal tube obstruction/bilateral cornual block

b.coiling of the tubes/calcified shodow at places

c.tubal diverticula and /or fluffiness of tubal outline

d.all

84.Hysterosalpingographic finding in uterus in female genital tuberculosis (DUTTA)

a.irregular outline

b.honeycomb appearance

c.presence of uterine synechae

d.all

85.Saline infusion sonography is useful in all except(DUTTA) a.endometrial polyps

b.submucous fibroid

c.septate/subseptate uterus

d.ovarian cyst

86.Ultrasonographic finding of malignant ovarian tumour (DUTTA)

a.cystic areas with irregular heterogenous solid part more than 50% of total tumour volume

b.neovascularisation

c.low resistance flow with pulsatility index <1.

d.all

87.Presence of an adnexal mass with mixed attenuation due to the presence of large amount of fat,calcification and teeth suggest of(DUTTA)

a.dermoid cyst

b.mucinous cyst adenoma

c.serous cyst adenoma

d.none

88.Ultrasound showing enlarged uterus with honeycomb/swiss cheese pattern and increased vascularity suggest of(DUTTA)

a.fibroid

b.adenomyosis/endometriosis interna

c.secretory stage of menstrual cycle

d.post menopausal uterus

89.All are true of polycystic ovarian syndrome except(DUTTA)

a.enlarged ovary

b.>12 peripherally arranged cyst

c.increased ovarian stroma

d.all

90.All are specific features of cystic dermoid of ovary except(RUMACK)

a.cystic mass with echogenic mural nodule(plug)

b.'tip-of-the-iceberg' sign

c.multiple linear hyperechogenic interfaces floating within the cystic mass(mesh)

d.multiple cystic lesions in periphery

91.Which sign is noted in ultrasound of acute PID(RUMACK)

a.cogwheel sign

b.beads on string sign

c.tip-of-iceberg sign

d.none

92.'Trouser sign' on usg of heart is noted in (RUMACK)

a.RVOT

b.LVOT

c.TOF

d.VSD

93.The diagnosis of anencephaly can be made with 100% accuracy after(RUMACK)

a.14weeks of menstrual age

b.10weeks of menstrual age

c.11weeks of menstrual age

d.12weeks of menstrual age

94.T sign at two amnion junctions suggests of(RUMACK)

a.DC/DA

b.MC/DA

c.MC/MA

d.none

95.Wolfe classification is related to(GRAINGER)

a.to describe density of breast on mammography

b.to describe density of breast on CT

c.to describe density of breast on MRI

d.all

96.Bicornis bicollis refers to(GRAINGER)

a.two vagina,two cervices,two seprate uterine horn

b.single vagina,sngle cervix,two seprate uterine horn

c.single vagina,two cervices,single uterine horn

d.single vagina,two cervices,two seprate uterine horn

97.first structure to be visualized on TVS within chorionic sac (GRAINGER)

a.yolk sac

b.embryo

c.amniotic sac

d.all

98.Lemon shaped skull on antenatal usg is noted in(GRAINGER)

a.neural tube defect

b.down syndrome

c.achondroplasia

d.osteogenesis imperfect

99.Rain shower appearance of uterus on USG is noted in(GRAINGER)

a.adenomyosis

b.myoma

c.polyp

d.endometriosis

100.The most reliable predictor of cervical incompetence is(GRAINGER)

a.length of cervix

b.width of cervical canal

c.both

d.none

101.A normal gestational sac grows at the rate of (from 5 weeks to11 weeks)(CHAPMAN)

a.0.7—1.75mm/day

b.>2mm/day

c.>3mm/day

d.>4mm/day

102.ultrasounnd signs of an empty sac(blighted ovum)(CHAPMAN)

a.no fetal parts with sac diameter>30mm

b.no yolk sca with sac diameter >20mm

c.both

d.none

103.Lemon sign(abnormally pointed frontotemporal region) in head on USG is seen in(CHAPMAN)

a.anencephaly

b.spina bifida

c.hydroephalus

d.all

104.Banana sign(abnormally shaped cerebellum) on USG ia seen in(CHAPMAN)

a.anencephaly

b.spina bifida

c.hydroephalus

d.all

105.Causes of thickened placenta are all except(CHAPMAN)

a.Diabetes

b.Rhesus isoimmunisation

c.fetal hydrops and triploidy

d.hypertension

106.Routine use of screening mammography in woman>50yrs reduces cancer mortality by(SW)

a.33%

b.20%

c10%

d50%

107.The disease of thrombophlebitis of superficial veins of anterior chest wall and breast is known as(SW)

a.mondor's disease

b.Teitz disease

c.poland's syndrome

d.none

108.Conventional mammography delivers a radiation dose of (SW)

a.o.1cGy/study

b.o.2cGy/study

a.o.3cGy/study

a.o.4cGy/study

109.All are true regarding mammography except(SW)

a.increased cancer risk with screening mammography

b.screening mammography is done in asymptomatic women

c.diagnostic mammography is done in symptomatic women

d.MLO view images greatest volume of breast

110.Which view is used to evaluate upper outer quadrant and axillary tail of Spence(SW)

a.the craniocaudal view

b.the mediolateral view

c. 90 degree lateral view

d.none

111.All are true regarding compression view of breast are except(SW)

a.minimizes motion artefact

b.improves definition

c.seprates overlying tissue

d.increases radition dose

112.Mammographic finding that suggest a diagnosis of breast cancer are all except(SW)

a.solid mass with or without stellate features

b.asymmetric thickening of breast tissues

c. clustered microcalcifications

d.popcorn calcification

113.All are true regarding mammography except(SW)

a.screen film mammography requires lower dose than xeromammography

b. xeromammography provides positive image

c.digital provide better diagnostic accuracy than sceen film mammography

d.screen film mammography and xeromammographyprovide similar image quality

114.Digital mammography is more accurate than screen mammography in(SW)

a.< 50yrs of women

b.mammographically dense breast

c.premenopausal women/perimenopausal women

d.all

115.Yearly screening mammogram should be taken starting at age of(SW)

a.50yrs

b.45yrs

c.35yrs

d.40yrs

116.Breast USG does not reliably detect lesions (SW)

a.=<4cm

b.=<2cm

c.=<3cm

d.=<1cm

117.Chorionic villous sampling is performed between(SW)

a.10-12 weeks

b.12-14 weeks

c.08-10 weeks

d.14-16 weeks

118.Amniocentesis is performed after about(SW)

a.10 weeks

b.13 weeks

c.15 weeks

d.17 weeks

119.All are true regarding calcification in breast(CHAPMAN)

a.microcalcificatio size <0.5mm

b.microcalcification seen in 30-40% of carcinoma of breast

c.popcorn calcification in fibroadenoma

d.cluster microcalcifiation favor benign pathology

120.No of ovarian cysts as per the Rotterdam criteria for diagnosis of polycystic ovarian syndrome should be(H)

a.=>10 immature follicles

b.=>12 immature follicles

c.=>14 immature follicles

d.=>16 immature follicles

121.Heryln-Werner-Wunderlich syndrome comprises all except(H)

a.uterine – didelphysb.obstructed hemivagina

c.ipsilateral renal agenesis

d.arcuate uterus

122.Meyer-Rokitansky-Kuster-Hauser Syndrome comprises all except(H)

a.aplasia or agenesis of uterus

b.vaginal agenesis

c. ovarian agenesis

d.attenuated fallopian tube

123.Largest vertical pocket of amniotic fluid in polyhydramnios is(DUTTA)

a.>6cm

b.>8cm

c.>10cm

d.>11cm

124.Lemon sign refers to(DUTTA)

a.flattening of cerebellar hemisphere

b.scalloping of frontal bones

c.flattening of cerebrum

d.none

125.Shape of cervix which indicate imminent labour in preterm on TVS is

a.T

b.U

c.Y

d.O

126.Doppler umbilical artery finding in IUGR ,associated with worst prognosis is

a.absent diastolic flow

b.reversal of diastolic flow

c.absent systolic flow

d.dicrotic notch

GYNAECOLOGY AND OBSTETRICS(ANSWERS)

1.a---Transvaginal ultrasound shows gestational sac and yolk sac by(DUTTA) 5 menstrual weeks

2.a---Transvaginal ultrasound shows fetal pole and cardiac activity by(DUTTA) 6 menstrual weeks

3.b---Between 7-12 weeks ,the fetal gestational age is best determined by(DUTTA) CRL

4. a---Transvaginal ultrasound shows embryonic movement by(DUTTA) 7 menstrual weeks

5.a---BPD is measured at the level of(DUTTA) thalami and cavum septum pellucidum

6.a---AFI in oligohydramnios is(DUTTA) <5

7c---.AFI in polyhydramnios is(DUTTA) >25

8.a---Ossification centres in lower end of femur appear at(DUTTA) 36-37week

9.c---Formula used to calculate fetal weight in sonography is(DUTTA) Shepherd 's and Hadlock's

10.c---Radiological evidence of fetal skeletal shadow may be visible as early as (DUTTA) 16 week

11.d---Biophysical profile parameters are all exept(DUTTA) heart rate

12.b---The single ultrasonographic fetal parameter that best reflects the nutrion is(DUTTA) abdominal circumference

13.b---IUGR is suspected when the HC/AC ratio is >1after 34 weeks(DUTTA)

14.d---Regarding Doppler in pregnancy(DUTTA) uterine artery Doppler is helpful to assess the downstream vascular resistance,umblical vein Doppler provide cardiac forward function,in normal pregnancy,the S/D ratio,pulsatility index and resistance index decreases as the gestational age advnces,normal uterine vein flow is monophasic.

15.a---Pulsatility index refers to(DUTTA) S—D/M

16.c---Resistive index refers to(DUTTA) S—D/S

17.d---Abnormal umbilical artery flow velocity waveform :(DUTTA) reduced end diastolic flow,absent end diastolic flow,reversed end diastolic flow

18.d---Brain sparing effect in response to fetal hypoxemia is reflected in Doppler study as(DUTTA) increased diastolic flow,decreased S/D ratio,decreased PI

19.b---Amniotic fluid index refers to(DUTTA) the sum of vertical pockets from four quadrant of uterine cavity

20.a---A vertical pocket of amniotic fluid =>2cm is considered normal(DUTTA)

21.d---Score of two in BPS(during observation period of 30 minutes) :(DUTTA)fetal breathing movement =>1episode lasting >30sec.,.=>3 discrete body/ limb movements,=>episode of ex tention (limb or trunk)with return of flexion,=>1pockets (measuring 2cm)of amniotic fluid in two perpendicular planes(2x2cm pocket)

22.c---Suspect chronic asphyxia if BPS is(DUTTA) 6

23.d---USG finding favouring ectopic pregnancy are (DUTTA) absence of intrauterine pregnancy with positive pregnancy test,echogenic fluid in Pouch of Douglas,adnexal mass seprate from ovary

24.b---'Ring of fire' pattern of blood flow on color doppler outside the uterine cavity is noted in(DUTTA) ectopic pregnancy

25.a---Snow storm appearance on USG of uterus is characteristic of(DUTTA) hydatidiform mole

26.a---Lambda/Twin peak sign in USG of pregnancy is noted in(DUTTA) dichorionic-diamniotic twin

27.a---The maximum vertical diameter of amniotic fluid in oligohydramnios is(DUTTA) <2cm

28.a----the investigation of choice for placenta previa(DUTTA) transabdominal USG

29.a---The anterior landmark for diagnosing placenta previa (DUTTA) uterovesicle angle

30.b---The earliest diagnosis of fetal death is possible with(DUTTA) USG

31.a---The irregular overlapping of the cranial bones on one another noted in intrauterine death is known as(DUTTA) Spalding sign

32.b---Appearance of gas shadow in the chambers of the heart and great vessels in intrauterine death is known as(DUTTA) Robert's sign

33.b---The earliest sign noted in x ray after intrauterine death is(DUTTA) Robert's sign as early as 12hrs)

34.d---All are features of IUD except(DUTTA)Spalding sign(usually 7days),Robert's sign (as early as 12hrs),hyperflexion of the spine and crowding of rib

35.a---'Buddha position' of fetus with halo around the head in x ray is noted in(DUTTA) hydrops fetalis

36.c---The most common type of pelvis is(DUTTA)gynaecoid

37.d---Rachitic pelvis is characterized by (DUTTA) 'reniform' shape of the inlet,widening of transverse diameter of the outlet and the pubic arch,backward tilting of sacrum

38.b---Triradiate shaped inlet of pelvis is noted in(DUTTA)osteomalacia

39.d---Pelvis resulting from arrested development of one ala of the sacrum (DUTTA)Naegele 's pelvis

40.c---Pelvis resulting from absent ala of both sides and sacrum fused with the innominate bone(DUTTA)Robert's pelvis

41.a----With conventional x ray pelvimetry,radiation exposure to gonads is(DUTTA) 885millirad

42.d---USG features of placenta accreta (DUTTA) loss of normal hypoechoic retroplacental myometrial zone,thinning and disruption of the uterine serosa –bladder interface,focal exophytic mass within the placenta

43.d---Regarding HC/AC ratio(DUTTA)>1 before 32weeks,approx.1 at 32-34weeks,<1 after 34weeks

44.a---The single most sensitive parameter to detect IUGR(DUTTA)AC

45.d---Regarding IUGR (DUTTA)HC/AC remain elevated in asymmetric IUGR,FL/AC ratio greater than 23.5suggest IUGR,FL is not affected in asymmetric IUGR

46.d---Regarding IUGR :(DUTTA) S/D ratio elevated,presence of diastolic notch in uterine artery,Ponderal index below the 10th percentile ,increase in diastolic flow as brain sparing effect

47.a---Invertogram is taken to diagnose(DUTTA) imperforate anus

48.c---Commonly used frequency in TVS is(DUTTA) 5-7MHz

49.a---Ultrasound travels through tissues of body at(DUTTA) 1540m/sec

50.b---The mode used to study moving structures such as fetal heart(DUTTA) M-mode

51.c---Regarding 3D (DUTTA) view of complex structure in a single image,later review without patient , improved diagnosis of prenatal anomaly,increased parental bonding due to life like images

52.d---Effects of ultrasound on tissues are all except(DUTTA) temperature elevation ,micobubbles,cavitation

53.d---Regarding gestational sac on usg in first trimester (DUTTA) eccentric in position in the endometrium,double decidua sign,presence of yolk sac and fetal pole confirm pregnancy

54.d---Finding on TVS: (DUTTA) mean sac diameter 5-8mm, yolk sac,mean sac diameter 12mm, embryo,mean sac diameter 15-18mm , cardiac activity

55.b---Cardiac activity is noted on TVS at(DUTTA)6week

56.a---transcerebellar diameter is an accurate predictor of gestational age when measured between14-28weeks(DUTTA)

57.c---Regarding first trimester usg (DUTTA) gestational sac grows at rate of 1.1mm/day,CRL in mm+42=approx.gestational age in days,MSD in mm+30 =approx gestational age in days,failure to visualize an embryo when MSD is 6 mm indicate pregnancy loss

58.b---Nuchal thickness ---mm is strong marker of chromosomal anomalies(DUTTA)>3mm

59.a----Banana sign refers to(DUTTA) flattening of cerebellar hemisphere

60.c---Lemon sign and banana sign are found in(DUTTA) open spina bifida and Arnold-Chiari malformation

61.a---Ventriculomagaly is diagnosed when width of lateral ventricle is(DUTTA >10mm

62.a—anomaly characterized by absence of cranium and telencephalon(DUTTA)anencephaly

63.b---Diagnosis of anencephaly is possible at about (DUTTA) 13week

64.d---Gastoschisis is characterized by (DUTTA)praraumblical defect,herniated loops float freely in amniotic fluid,not covered with membrane,not associated with chromosomal anomaly

65.c---Regarding omphalocele :(DUTTA) usually midline defect,cord insertion on the herniated mass,covered by membrane,associated with chromosomal anomaly

66.d--Placental thickness more than 45–mm is abnormal at any period of gestation (DUTTA)

67.c---Placental thickness at term is about (DUTTA) 30mm

68.a---Placenta previa is excluded from diagnosis when the distance between the internal OS and placental edge is more than(DUTTA) 20mm

69.d---Ultrasound marker of chromosomal anomalies (DUTTA) choroid plexus cyst,strawberry skull,holoprosencephaly

70.d---marker of trisomy 21 :(DUTTA) wide gap between 1st and 2nd toes,short femur,omphalocele

71.a---Absorbed radiation by the fetus in abdominal x ray(DUTTA) 0.263 rad

72.a---Exposure to DES produce (DUTTA) T –shaped uterus

73.a---Who first introduced ultrasound in the field of medicine(DUTTA) Ian Donald

74.b---Transabdominal USG requires full bladder in order to(DUTTA) displace bowel out of pelvis,acts as an acoustic window

75.a--- resolution of<0.2mm can be obtained by ultrasound(DUTTA)

76.c---Higher is the frequency of ultrasound wave (DUTTA)better is the resolution,lesser is the depth of tissue penetration

77.d---Regarding TVS :(DUTTA)no need of full bladder,operates at frequeny of 5-8MHz,detailed examination of pelvis possible,difficult in vergins and postmenopausal women

78.a---Sonohysterography involves (DUTTA) infusion of saline in uterine cavity

79.d----Endometrial thickness of <5mm is considered as atrophic(DUTTA)

80.b---Felix Bloch and Edward Purcell first described phenomenon of MRI(DUTTA)

 81.b---MRI is safe in pregnancy(DUTTA)

82.d--- Hysterosalpingographic finding in female genital tuberculosis: (DUTTA) lead-pipe tube with nodulations,'Tobacco pouch' appearance with blocked fimbrial end,beaded appearance of tubes with variable filling density

83.d---Hysterosalpingographic finding in female genital tuberculosis (DUTTA) distal tube obstruction/bilateral cornual block,coiling of the tubes/calcified shodow at places,tubal diverticula and /or fluffiness of tubal outline

84.d---Hysterosalpingographic finding in uterus female genital tuberculosis (DUTTA) irregular outline,honeycomb appearance,presence of uterine synechae

85.d---Saline infusion sonography is useful in (DUTTA)endometrial polyps,submucous fibroid,septate/subseptate uterus

86.d---Ultrasonographic finding of malignant ovarian tumour (DUTTA) cystic areas with irregular heterogenous solid part more than 50% of total tumour volume,neovascularisation,low resistance flow with pulsatility index <1.

87.a---Presence of an adnexal mass with mixed attenuation due to the presence of large amount of fat,calcification and teeth suggest of(DUTTA dermoid cyst

88.b---Ultrasound showing enlarged uterus with honeycomb/swiss cheese pattern and increased vascularity suggest of(DUTTA) adenomyosis/endometriosis interna

89.d---True of polycystic ovarian syndrome :(DUTTA) enlarged ovary,>12 peripherally arranged cyst,increased ovarian stroma

90.d---Specific features of cystic dermoid of ovary :(RUMACK) cystic mass with echogenic mural nodule(plug),'tip-of-the-iceberg' sign,multiple linear hyperechogenic interfaces floating within the cystic mass(mesh)

91.a--- cogwheel sign is noted in ultrasound of acute PID(RUMACK)

92.a---'Trouser sign' on usg of heart is noted in (RUMACK)RVOT

93.a---The diagnosis of anencephaly can be made with 100% accuracy after(RUMACK) 14weeks of menstrual age

94.b---T sign at two amnion junctions suggests of(RUMACK) MC/DA

95.a----Wolfe classification is related to(GRAINGER) to describe density of breast on mammography

96.d---Bicornis bicollis refers to(GRAINGER) single vagina,two cervices,two seprate uterine horn

97.a----first structure to be visualized on TVS within chorionic sac (GRAINGER) yolk sac

98.a---Lemon shaped skull on antenatal usg is noted in(GRAINGER) neural tube defect

99.a----Rain shower appearance of uterus on USG is noted in(GRAINGER) adenomyosis

100.b---The most reliable predictor of cervical incompetence is(GRAINGER) width of cervical canal

101.a---A normal gestational sac grows at the rate of (from 5 weeks to11 weeks) (CHAPMAN) 0.7—1.75mm/day

102.c---ultrasounnd signs of an empty sac(blighted ovum) (CHAPMAN) no fetal parts with sac diameter>30mm,no yolk sac with sac diameter >20mm

103.b---Lemon sign(abnormally pointed frontotemporal region) in head on USG is seen in(CHAPMAN) spina bifida

104.b---Banana sign(abnormally shaped cerebellum) on USG ia seen in(CHAPMAN) spina bifida

105.d---Causes of thickened placenta are (CHAPMAN) Diabetes,Rhesus isoimmunisation,fetal hydrops and triploidy

106.a---Routine use of screening mammography in woman>50yrs reduces cancer mortality by(SW) 33%

107.a---The disease of thrombophlebitis of superficial veins of anterior chest wall and breast is known as(SW) mondor's disease

108.a---Conventional mammography delivers a radiation dose of (SW) o.1cGy/study

109.a---Regarding mammography (SW)screening mammography is done in asymptomatic women,diagnostic mammography is done in symptomatic women,MLO view images greatest volume of breast

110.b---The mediolateral view is used to evaluate upper outer quadrant and axillary tail of Spence(SW)

111.d---Regarding compression view of breast are (SW) minimizes motion artefact,improves definition,seprates overlying tissue,decrease radition dose

112.d----Mammographic finding that suggest a diagnosis of breast cancer are (SW) solid mass with or without stellate features,asymmetric thickening of breast tissues, clustered microcalcifications

113.c---Regarding mammography (SW)screen film mammography requires lower dose than xeromammograph,xeromammography provides positive image,digital doesnot provide better diagnostic accuracy than sceen film mammography,screen film mammography and xeromammographyprovide similar image quality

114.d---digital mammography is more accurate than screen mammography in(SW)< 50yrs of women,mammographically dense breast,premenopausal women/perimenopausal women

115.d---Yearly screening mammogram should be taken starting at age of(SW) 40yrs

116.d---Breast USG does not reliably detect lesions (SW) =<1cm

117.a---Chorionic villous sampling is performed between(SW) 10-12 weeks

118.b--Amniocentesis is performed after about(SW) 13 weeks

119.d---Regarding calcification in breast(CHAPMAN) segmental and cluster microcalcifiation favor malignant pathology

120.b---No of ovarian cysts as per the Rotterdam criteria for diagnosis of polycystic ovarian syndrome should be(H).=>12 immature follicles

121.d----Heryln-Werner-Wunderlich syndrome comprises all except(H)uterine –didelphys.,obstructed hemivagina,ipsilateral renal agenesis

122.c---Meyer-Rokitansky-Kuster-Hauser Syndrome comprises (H) aplasia or agenesis of uterus,vaginal agenesis,attenuated fallopian tube

123.b---Largest vertical pocket of amniotic fluid in polyhydramnios is(DUTTA)>8cm

124.b---Lemon sign refers to(DUTTA).scalloping of frontal bones

125.b---Shape of cervix which indicate imminent labour in preterm on TVS is U

126.b---Doppler umbilical artery finding in IUGR ,associated with worst prognosis is reversal of diastolic flow

BONE AND JOINTS DISORDER

1.The most common form of chronic inflammatory polyarthritis(H)
a.rheumatoid arthritis
b.osteoarthritis
c.anklylosing spondylitis
d.gout

2.The symmetric polyarthritis is seen in(H)
a.rheumatoid arthritis
b.osteoarthritis
c.anklylosing spondylitis
d.gout

3.Cartilge hair hypolasia involve(H)
a.metaphyseal ends
b.epiphysis
c.diaphysis
d.none

4.Cartilge hair hypoplasia is characterized by(H)
a.short –limb dwarfism
b.metaphyseal dysostosis
c.sparse hair
d. all

5.Musculoskeletal manifestations of SLE are all except(H)
a.intermittent polyarthritis
b.erosive arthropathy
c.may be ischemic necrosis of bone
d. hands, wrists and joints most commonly affected

6.The frequently involved joints in rheumatoid arthritis are all except(H)
a.wrist joint
b.metecarpophalangeal joint(MCP)
c.proximal interphalangeal joint(PCP)
d.shoulder joints

7.The deformities seen in rheumatoid arthritis are(H)
a.Swan neck deformity
b.Boutonniere deformity
c.Z-line deformity
d.all

8.The deformity showing hyperextension of the PIP joint with flexion of DIP joint is known as(H)
a.Swan neck deformity
b.Boutonniere deformity
c.Z-line deformity
d.piano-key movement

9.The deformity showing flexion of the PIP joint with hyperextension of DIP joint is known as(H)
a.Swan neck deformity
b.Boutonniere deformity

c.Z-line deformity

d.piano-key movement

10.The rheumatoid arthritis involve all except(H)

a.atlantoaxial involvement of cervical spine

b.metatarsophalangeal joint(MTP)

c.temporomandibular joint

d.thoracic and lumbar spine

11.The initial radiographic finding in rheumatoid arthritis is(H)

a.juxta articular osteopenia

b.symmetric joint space loss

c.subchondral erosion

d.soft tissue swelling

12.Which MTP joint of foot is targeted first in rheumatoid arthritis(H)

a.fifth MTP

b.fourth MTP

c.third MTP

d.second MTP

13.All are features of joint involvement in acute rheumatic fever except(H)

a.polyarthritis

b.migratory

c.almost always large joint

d.asymmetric

14.Acro-osteolysis in noted in(H)

a.systemic sclerosis

b.rheumatoid arthritis

c.acute rheumatic fever

d.osteoarthritis

15.HRCT feature of systemic sclerosis are all except(H)

a.subpleural reticular linear opacities,predominantly in lower lobe

b.ground glass opacification predict rapid progression of disease

c.gound glass opacification indicate fibrosis,not alveolitis

d.extent of disease is predictive of mortality

16.Which feature is often the earliest manifestations of ankylosing spondylitis(H)

a.peripheral arthritis

b. symmetrical sacroiliitis

c.enthesitis

d.none

17.Syndesmophyte is found in(H)

a.rheumatoid arthritis

b.systemic sclerosis

c.ankylosing spodylitis

d.acute rheumatic fever

18.Bamboo spine is found in(H)

a.rheumatoid arthritis

b.systemic sclerosis

c.ankylosing spodylitis

d.acute rheumatic fever

19.All are true regarding ankylosing spondylitis except(H)

a.squaring/barreling of vertabra

b.descending progression of disease

c.enthesitis –a characteristic lesion

d.calcification of outer annulus fibres

20.The earliest change in sacroiliac joint in ankylosing spondylitis in x ray is(H)

a.blurring of the subcotical margin of the subchondral bone

b.erosions and sclerosis

c.pseudowidening of joint

d.fibrous and bony ankylosis

21.Which modality is being increasingly used for diagnosis of ankylosing spondylitis(H)

a.x ray

b .MRI

c.CT

d.nuclear scan

22.Periostitis with reactive bone formation is characteristic of(H)

a.Spondyloarthropathy

b.rheumatoid arthritis

c.acute rheumatic fever

d.gout

23.Characteristic of peripheral psoriatic arthritis are all except(H)

a.DIP involvement

b.whiskering

c.small joint ankylosis

d.PIP involvement

24.Characteristic of peripheral psoriatic arthritis are all except(H)

a.pencil- in- cup deformity

b.osteolysis of phalangeal and metacarpal bones

c.telescoping of digits

d.Z-deformity

25.Characteristic of peripheral psoriatic arthritis are all except(H)

a.pencil- in- cup deformity

b.osteolysis of phalangeal and metacarpal bones

c.periostitis and proliferative new bone formation at sites of enthesitis

d.Boutonniere deformity

26. Characteristic of axial psoriatic arthritis which differentiate it from ankylosing spondylitis are all except(H)

a.asymmetric sacroiliitis

b.less zygapophyseal joint arthritis

c.fewer and less symmetric and delicate syndesmophyte

d.involvement of thoracolumbar spine

27. Characteristic of axial psoriatic arthritis which differentiate it from ankylosing spondylitis are all except(H)

a.fluffy hyperostosis on anterior vertebral bodies

b.atlantoaxial subluxation

c.paravertebral ossification

d.symmetric scaroiliitis

28.Pencil in cup deformity is seen in(H)

a.psoriatic arthritis

b.rheumatoid arthritis

c.ankylosing arthritis

d.gout

29.Telescoping of digit is seen in(H)

a.psoriatic arthritis

b.rheumatoid arthritis

c.ankylosing arthritis

d.gout

30.The most commonly used method to diagnose pulmonary involovement in sarcoidosis(H)

a.chest x ray

b.CT

c.MRI

d.nuclear scan

31.Stage 2 of pulmonary involvement in sarcoidosis refers to(H)

a.hilar adenopathy,particularly right paratracheal

b.hilar adenopathy +pulmonary infiltrates

c.pulmonary infiltrates only

d.pulmonary fibrosis

32.Upper lobe chest non infectious disease are all except(H)

a.sarcoidosis and silicosis

b.hypersensitivity pneumonitis

c.Langerhans cell histiocytosis

d.CWP

33. Upper lobe chest disease are all except(H)

a.sarcoidosis

b.tuberculosis

c.pneumocystitis pneumonia

d.idiopathic pulmonary fibrosis

34.Radiological features of sarcoidosis include all except(H)

a.bilateral hilar adenopathy

b.peribronchial thickening

c.reticular nodular

opacity,predominantly subpleural

d.lower lobe predominance of pathology

35.Features which favors sarcoidosis rather than multiple sclerosis are all except(H)

a.meningeal enhancement

b.hypothalmic involvement

c.pulmonary involvement

d.optic neuritis

36.Heberdon's node is noted in(H)

a.osteoarthritis

b.acute rheumatic fever

c.rheumatoid arthritis

d.sarcoidosis

37.Bouchard's node is noted in(H)

a.osteoarthritis

b.acute rheumatic fever

c.rheumatoid arthritis

d.sarcoidosis

38.Location of Heberdon'S node is(H)

a.PIP

b.DIP

c.MCP

d.CMC

39.Location of Bouchard'S node is(H)

a.PIP

b.DIP

c.MCP

d.CMC

40.The preferred method for evaluation of Baker's cyst,rotator cuff tears,tendinitis and tendon injury and suspected early synovitis(H)

a.USG

b.x ray

c.CT

d.MRI

41.Which radionuclide is used for metastatic bone survey and evaluation of Paget's disease(H)

a.^{99m}Tc

b.^{111}In-WBC

c.^{67}Ga

d.all

42.Which radionuclide is used for prosthetic infection(H)

a.^{99m}Tc

b.^{111}In-WBC

c.^{67}Ga

d.all

43.The most common type of arthritis is(H)

a.osteoarthritis

b.rheumatoid arthritis

c.ankylosing arthritis

d.gout

44.Joints commonly affected in osteoarthritis are all except(H)
a.Cervical and lumbosacral spine
b.wrist joint
c.knee joint
d.first metatarsophalangeal joint

45.Joints usually spared in osteoarthritis are all except(H)
a.wrist joint
b.ankle joint
c.elbow joint
d.hip joint

46.Joints of hand often involved in osteoarthritis are all except(H)
a.PIP
b.DIP
c. the base of thumb
d.wrist joint

47.Characteristic features of advanced chronic tophaceous gout are(H)
a.cystic changes
b.well defined erosion with sclerotic margins
c.overhanging bony edges
d.all

48.Chondrocalcinosis is noted in(H)
a.CPPD deposition disease
b.rheumatic arthritis
c.osteoarthritis
d.gout

49. All are true regarding infectious arthritis except(H)
a.Staph aureus causes acute monoarticular arthritis
b.subacute or chronic monoarthritis suggests mycobacterial or fungal infection
c.N. Meningitidis causes polyarticular arthritis
d.N.neisseria causes acute monoarticular arthritis

50.Episodic inflammation of joint is seen in (H)
a.Syphilis
b.lyme diseases
c.reactive arthritis following chlymdial urethritis
d.all

51.A reactive symmetric form of polyarthritis that affect a person with visceral or disseminated tuberculosis is known as(H)
a.charcot's joint
b.Poncet's disease
c.still's disease
d.Reiter's syndrome

52.True regarding arthritis (H)
a.tuberculous osteomyelitis

typically involves thoracic and
lumbar spine

b.tuberculous arthritis
particularly involves the
hip,knee and ankle joint

c.reactiv arthritis may follow
HIV urethritis

d.all

53.All are features of spine in
acromegaly except(H)

a.reduced intervertabral disc

b.hypertrophic anterior
osteophyte

c.ligamental calcification

d.simulate DISH

54.All are features of
acromegaly except(H)

a.barrell shaped chest

b.spadelike distal tuft

c.thin heel pad

d.chondrocalcinosis

55.Which joint is often the first
and prominent joints affected
in arthropathy of
hemochromatosis(H)

a.second MCP

b.third MCP

c.both

d.none

56.The joint first affected in
hemophilic arthropathy(H)

a.knee joint

b.ankle joint

c.elbow joint

d.shoulder joint

57.All are true regarding sickle
cell disease except(H)

a.Hand foot syndrome
commonly seen after five yrs
of age

b.osteomyelitis commonly in
long bones

c.infarction of bone and bone
marrow

d.avascular necrosis in
humeral head

58.Osteomyelitis in sickle cell
disease is particularly caused
by(H)

a.staph aureus

b.N.meningitidis

c.mycobacterial infection

d.salmonella

59.All are true about
arthropathy except(H)

a.symmetric ankle arthropathy
in thallassemia

b.avascular necrosis in
thallasemia

c.protrusio acetabuli in sickle
cell anemia

d.bone infarction in sickle cell
anemia

60.The most frequent cause of
neuropathic joint disease is(H)

a.diabetes mellitus

b.leprosy

c.syringomelia

d.amyloidosis

61.Disorders associated with neuropathic joint disease are all except(H)

a.diabetes mellitus

b.leprosy

c.syringomelia

d.tuberculosis

62.Disorders associated with neuropathic joint disease are all except(H)

a.Tabes dorsalis

b.meningomyelocele

c.peroneal muscular atrophy

d.congenita myotonica

63.The most commonly affected joints in tabes dorsalis are all except(H)

a.knees

b.hips

c.ankles

d.elbow

64.The most commonly affected joints in syringomyelia are all except(H)

a.knees

b.glenohumeral joint

c.wrist joint

d.elbow

65.The most commonly affected joint in diabetes mellitus is(H)

a.tarsal joints and tarsometatarsal joints

b.metatarsophalangeal joint

c.talotibial joints

d.elbow

66.The Rocker foot is noted in(H)

a.diabetes mellitus

b.leprosy

c.syringomelia

d.tuberculosis

67.The resorption and tapering of distal metatarsal bones is noted in(H)

a.diabetes mellitus

b.leprosy

c.syringomelia

d.tuberculosis

68.The destructive changes at tarsometatarsal joints is known as(H)

a.Lisfranc fracture dislocation

b.pott's fracture

c.jones fracture

d.none

69.The most common rheumatic disease in children(N)

a.Juvenile rheumatic disease

b.ankylosing spodylitis

c.reactive arthritis

d.SLE

70.Criteria for classification of JRA are all except(N)

a.age of onset <16yrs

b.arthritis=>1 joints

c.duration of disease =>6 weeks

d.polyarthritis variety =>6 joints in first six month after onset

71.An 'exoskeleton' of calcium deposition may be seen in(N)

a.juvenile dermatoyositis

b.SLE

c.JRA

d.ankylosing spodylitis

72.Acro-osteolysis may be seen in(N)

a.SLE

b.JRA

c.ankylosing spodylitis

d.systemic scleroderma

73.The most common chest finding in sarcoidosis(N)

a.isolated bilateral hilar lymphadenopathy

b.parenchymal infiltrates

c.miliary lesions

d.pleural effusion

74.Coronary artery aneurysm may be seen in(N)

a.Kawasaki's disease

b.SLE

c.scleroderma

d.sarcoidosis

75.Which is predominantly large vessel vasculitis(N)

a.Kawasaki's disease

b.Takayasu arteritis

c.Wegener's granulomatosis

d.Churg-Straus syndrome

76.Classic beads on string appearance may be noted in(N)

a.PAN

b.SLE

c.Takayasu 's arteritis

d.Wegener 's granulomatosis

77.Late manifestation of congenital syphilis are all except (N)

a.Olympian brow

b.saber shins

c.mulberry molars

d.saber trachea

78.Late manifestations of congenital syphilis are all except (N)

a.Hutchinson teeth

b.saddle nose/clutton joint

c.hutchinson's triad

d.craniotabes

79.Highoum Naki's sign(unilateral/bilateral thickening of sternoclavicular third of the clavicle)is feature of(N)

a.congenital syphilis
b.congenital leprosy
c.congenital toxoplasmosis
d.congenital harpes

80.Olympian brow is seen in(N)

a.congenital leprosy
b.congenital syphilis
c.congenital toxoplasmosis
d.congenital herpes

81.Radiographic abnormalities of congenital syphilis are all except(N)

a.Wimberger's line
b.osteochondritis
c.periostitis of long bones
d.dense metaphyseal line

82.Wimberger's line is noted in(N)

a.congenital leprosy
b.congenital syphilis
c.congenital toxoplasmosis
d.congenital herpes

83.Metaphyseal demineralistion of medial aspect of the proximal tibia in congenital syphilis is known as(N)

a.Wimberger's sign
b.Wimbeger 's line
c.shaber shin
d.ant eater sign

84.Presence of Scoliosis is defined by(N)

a.Cobb's angle > 10degrees
b.Cobb's angle > 20degrees
c.Cobb's angle > 05degrees
d.Cobb's angle > 15degrees

85.The most common primary malignant bone tumour in children and adolescent(N)

a.Ewing's sarcoma
b.osteosarcoma
c.chondrosarcoma
d.fibrosarcoma

86.Characetristics of osteochondroma are all except(N)

a.stalks from the surface of bone
b.diection usually towards the adjacent joint
c.a cap of cartilage
d.cortex and marrow space of bone continuous with the lesion

87.All are true regarding osteoid osteoma except(N)

a.oval metaphyseal/diaphyseal lucency(central lucency or nidus)
b.surrounding sclerotic bone
c.intense uptake on bone scan

d.MRI better than CT to detect the lesion

88.Ant eater sign on lateral view of foot is noted in(N)

a.calcaneal spur

b.calcaneonavicular coalition

c.talocalcaneal coalition

d.fracture of calcaneum

90.Harish view of the heel refers to(N)

a.lateralview

b.AP view

c.axial view

d.oblique view

91. Continuous C-sign on lateral view of foot is noted in(N)

a.calcaneal spur

b.calcaneonavicular coalition

c.talocalcaneal coalition

d.fracture of calcaneum

92.Blount's disease is characterized by all except(N)

a.metaphyseal –diaphyseal angle <11 degrees

b.medial sloping of the epiphyses

c.widening of epiphyses

d.fragmentation of the metaphyses

93.Notch view of knee refers to(N)

a.tunnel view of knee

b.AP view of knee

c.lateral view of knee

d.oblique view of knee

94.The diagnostic modality of choice for development dysplasia of hip(DDH) before 4-6months(N)

a.x ray

b.USG

c.CT

d.MRI

95.All are true regarding USG exam of suspected DDH except(N)

a.a normal alpha angle is <60 degrees

b.a normal beta angle is <55degrees

c.alpha angle represents depth of acetabulum

d.beta angle represents the cartilaginous roof of acetabulun

96.Graf technique of USG is used for (N)

a.hip joint

b.knee joint

c.shoulder joint

d.elbow joint

97.True regarding DDH (N)

a.alpha angle < 60 degree imply acetabular dysplasia

b.beta angle increases as femoral head subluxates

c.both

d.none

98.Lines used for assessment of DDH are all except(N)

a.Hilgrenreiner's line

b.Perkin's line

c.Shenton's line

d.Klein's line

99.Ossific nucleus of femoral head is normally located in(N)

a.medial lower quadrant of intersection of Hilgrenreiner's and Perkin's line

b.medial upper quadrant of intersection of Hilgrenreiner's and Perkin's line

c.lateral lower quadrant of intersection of Hilgrenreiner's and Perkin's line

d.lateral upper quadrant of intersection of Hilgrenreiner's and Perkin's line

100.All are true regarding lines except(N)

a.The Higrenreiner's line is drawn through the triradiate cartilage

b.The perkin's line is drawn perpendicular to the Hilgrenreiner's line at the lateral edge of acetabulum

c.The Shenton's line curves along the femoral metaphyses to lower border of superior pubic ramus

d.The acetabular index is angle between line drawn along the margin of the acetabulum and the Perkin's line

101.All are true except(N)

a.Ossific nucleus of femoral head is outside of medial lower quadrant in DDH

b.continuous shenton's line in DDH

c.Normal acetabular angle should be no more than 30 degrees

d.the center-edge angle is a useful measure of femoal head coverage

102.The primary diagnostic tool for Legg-Calve-Perthes disease is(N)

a.MRI

b.CT

c.USG

d.X ray

103. Lauenstein(frog –leg) view of hip is used to diagnose(N)

a. Legg-Calve-Perthes disease

b.slipped capital femora epiphysis

c.both

d.none

104.Cage 's sign (a radiolucent horizontal V in the lateral aspect of the femoral physis) is feature of(N)

a.DDH

b. Legg-Calve-Perthes disease

c.septic arthritis

d.Paget's disease

105.Lateral pillar classification of Legg-Calve-Perthes disease has been given by(N)

a.Herring

b.Catterall

c.Paget

d.Lucas

106.'Blanch sign of Steel'on x ray of hip is noted in (N)

a. DDH

b. Legg-Calve-Perthes disease

c.Slipped capital femoral epiphysis

d.septic arthritis

107.Which line is used to diagnose Sliped capital femoral epiphysis(N)

a.Hilgrenreiner's line

b.Perkin's line

c.Shenton's line

d.Klein's line

108.The pars on spine is best visualized on view(N)

a.AP

b.lateral

c.oblique

d.all

109.Pars defect on oblique view of spine is known as(N)

a.Blanch sign of Steel

b.Cage sign

c.Scotty dog sign

d.ant eater sign

110.For the diagnosis of atlantoaxial instability,atlantodens interval(ADI) should be(N)

a.<5mm

b.<4mm

c.<3mm

d.<2mm

111.A normal atlantodens interval in patients with Down 's syndrome is(N)

a.<4 mm

b.<4.5mm

c.<3.5mm

d.<2.5mm

112.Sprengel's deformity refers to(N)

a.congenital elevation of scapula

b.acquired elevation of scapula

c.congenital fusion of cervical vertebra

d.aquired fusion of cervical vertebra

113.Madelung deformity is related to(N)

a.knee

b.elbow

c.wrist

d.foot

114.Wassal classification is related to (N)

a.thumb duplication

b.little finger duplication

c.radial bone duplication

d.ulnar bone duplication

115.All are true regarding torus(buckle fracture) fracture except(N)

a.a compression fracture

b.usually at junction of metaphysis and diaphysis

c.especially in distal radius

d.inherently unstable

116.A fracture where bone is bent and fracture line does not propagate to concave side of bone is called(N)

a.torus fracture(buckle fracture)

b.greenstick fracture

c.spiral fracture

d.none

117.The most sensitive and specific test for osteomyelitis is(N)

a.Nuclear scan

b.x ray

c.MRI

d.CT

118.All are true regarding role of x ray in osteomyelitis except(N)

a.displacement of deep muscle plane from adjacent affected metaphysis within 72 yrs of onset

b.lytic bone changes seen after 30-50% bone matrix is destroyed

c.no lytic changes in tubular bones for 7-14 days after onset of infection

d.lytic changes in flat bone appear earlier than long bones

119.Which investigation is ideal for detecting gas in soft tissue(N)

a.MRI

b.USG

c.CT

d.x ray

120.All are true regarding role of MRI in osteomyelitis(N)

a.more sensitive than CT or nuclear scan

b.best imaging technique for identifying abscesses

c.best imaging technique for differentiating bone and soft tissue infection

d.purulent pus appear hyperintense on T1W and hypointense on T2W

121.All are true regarding role of radionuclide study in a case of osteomyelitis(N)

a.ability to image entire skeleton to detect multiple foci

b.uptake of radionuclide in third phase(4-6hrs)

c.can detect infection within 24-48 hrs of onset

d.sensitivity in neonates is much higher than adult

122.Which radionuclide is used for imaging in osteomyelitis(N)

a.^{99m}Tc metylene diphosphonate

b. ^{99m}T DMSA

c.^{99m}Tc MAG-3

d.^{99m}Tc MIBG

123.Obturator sign (medial displacement of obturator muscle in pelvis) is noted in(N)

a.perthes disease

b.septic arthritis of hip

c.DDH

d.rheumatoid arthritis of hip

124.All are true regarding skeletal dysplasis except(N)

a.radiological hallmark of spondyloepiphyseal dysplasia is abnormal development of vertebral bodies and of epiphyses

b.normal metaphyses in pyknodysostosis

c.severe platyspondyly in metatrophic dysplasia

d.telephone handle like femur in achondroplasia

125.Femur ,curved –like telephone receiver is noted in(N)

a.thanatophoric dysplasia

b.achondroplasia

c.spondyloepiphyseal dysplasia

d.Jansen dysplasia

126.Hitchhiker appearance (proximal displacement of thumb)is noted in(N)

a.thanatophoric dysplasia

b.achondroplasia

c.diastrophic dysplasia

d.Jansen dysplasia

127.Absent clavicle with multiple wormian bone is noted in(N)

a.thanatophoric dysplasia

b.achondroplasia

c.diastrophic dysplasia

d.cleidocranial dysplasia

128.Iliac horn is seen in(N)

a.nail-patella syndrome

b.achondroplasia

c.diastrophic dysplasia

d.cleidocranial dysplasia

129.Bone –in-bone appearance is seen in(N)

a.diastrophic dysplasia

b.cleidocranial dysplasia

c.osteopetrosis

d.pyknodysostosis

130.Metatrophic dysplasia is charecterised by all except(N)

a.severe platyspondyly

b.dumbbell-shaped long bones

c.halbred appearance of pelvis

d.absent clavicle

131.Dumbbell-shaped long bones and halbred appearance of pelvis is noted in(N)

a.diastrophic dysplasia

b.cleidocranial dysplasia

c.osteopetrosis

d.metatrophic dysplasia

132.Caffey disease is characterized by all except(N)

a.bone fusion like radius and ulna or ribs

b.calcification

d.cortical hyperostosis

d.involve phalanges and vertebral bodies

133.The most common genetic cause of osteoporosis(N)

a.osteogenesis impefecta

b.homocystinuria

c.Turner syndrome

d.Ehler-Danlos syndrome

134.The popcorn appearance of metaphyses is seen in(N)

a. Turner syndrome

b.homocystinuria

c.osteogenesis imperfecta

d.Ehler-Danlos syndrome

135.Silence classification is related to(N)

a. Turner syndrome

b.homocystinuria

c.osteogenesis imperfecta

d.Ehler-Danlos syndrome

136.Walker-Murdoch or wrist sign is noted in(N)

a. Turner syndrome

b.homocystinuria

c.Marfan syndrome

d.Ehler-Danlos syndrome

137.The Steinberg or thumb sign is noted in(N)

a.Marfan syndrome

b.homocystinuria

c.Turner syndrome

d.Ehler-Danlos syndrome

138.All are features of Marfan syndrome except(N)

a.pectus excavatum/pectus carnatum

b.arachnodactly

c.camptodactyly

d.brachycephaly

139.Hypophosphatasia radiologically resemble(N)

a.scurvy

b.ricket

d.thalessemia

d.sickle cell anemia

140. Hyperphosphatasia is characterized by all except(N)

a.bowing and thickening of diaphyses

b. large and thickened cranium

c.bony texture mix of teased cotton –wool appearance,lucent areas and pseudocysts

d.diffuse sclerosis

141.Pellegrini-Steida lesion lesion is noted in(G)

a.knee

b.elbow

c.shoulder

d.ankle

142.All are true regarding magic angle phenomenon in MRI imaging except(G)

a.artefactual increased signal from tendons on short TE imaging sequence

b.angle of alignment of tendon to static magnetic field is apprex.55 degree

c.magic angle effect is not seen in ligament ,cartilage or menisci`

d.magic angle effect is not persistent on long TE sequence

143.Black synovium on MRI is noted in all except(G)

a.pigmented villonodular synovitis

b.amyloid deposition

c.hemophiliac arthropathy

d.rheomatoid arthritis

144.Appearance of water/edema in mri imaging(G)

a.dark on T1W

b.bright on T2W

C.both

d.none

145.The most common underlying process for pathological fracture is(G)

a.paget's disease

b.renal osteodystrophy

c.osteogenesis imperfect

d.metastatic disease

146.Orientation of pathological fracture in long bones(G)

a.transverse

b.oblique

c.spiral

d.variable

147.Transverse fracture noted in pathological fracture in long bones is known as(G)

a.banana fracture

b.stress fracture

c.mango fracture

d.aale fracture fracture

148.All are true regarding stress fracture except(G)

a.due to chronic repetitive trauma

b.skeletal scintigraphy and MRI very sensitive for detection

c.March fracture noted in metatarsal shafts in military recruits

d.fracture line is easily identified

149.Radiographic 'five Ds'of diabetic neuropathic foot are all except (G)

a.destruction and dislocation

b.disorganisation and debris

c.density(heterotopic new bone and sclerosis)

d.delayed healing

150.Judet view is done to assesss(G)

a.iliac crest

b.acetabula

c.pubic rami

d.sacro-iliac joint

151.'Open book' appearance of x ray of pelvis shows(G)

a.disruption of both SI joint and pubic symphysis

b.disruption of single SI joint and pubic symphysis

c.disruption of both SI joint only

d.disruption of pubic symphysis only

152.Malgaigne complex ,a pattern of injury is noted in(G)

a.chest

b.shoulder

c.vertebra

d.pelvis

153.Which pelvic injury is commonly seen in a bicycle accident(G)

a.straddle injury

b.open book injury

c.Malgaigne complex

d.none of above

154.Honda sign on scintigraphy of pelvis is noted in(G)

a.ilaic fracture

b.pubic bone ftracture

c.sacral insufficiency fracture

d.ischial spine fracture

155.Grashey view of x ray is done for(G)

a.glenohumeral joint

b.hip joint

c.elbow joint

d.knee joint

156.Hill-Sachs deformity refers to(G)

a.notch in the posterolateral head of humerous

b fracture the antero-inferior glenoid rim

c.notch in the posteromedial head of humerous

d.notch in the coracoids process

157.Bankart's lesion refers to(G)

a.fracture of the antero-inferior glenoid rim

b.notch in the posterolateral head of humerous

c.notch in the coracoids process

d.notch in the posteromedial head of humerous

158.Light bulb sign on x ray of shoulder joint is seen in(G)

a.anterior dislocation

b.posterior dislocation

c.both

d.none

159.X ray showing humeral head located inferomedial to the glenoid beneath the coracoid process suggest of (G)

a.anterior dislocation

b.posterior dislocation

c.coarcoid fracture

d.scapular fracture

160.Positive fat pad sign and sail sign are indirect sign of(G)

a.shoulder joint effusion

b.knee joint effusion

c.elbow joint effusion

d.knee joint effusion

161.All are correctly matched except(G)

a.Colles's fracture –impacted fracture of distal radius with dorsal displacement of distal fragment fracture

b.Smith's fracture--- fracture of distal radius with volarly displaced distal fragment fracture

c.Barton's fracture----displaced fracture of the volar lip of the distal radius without involvement of dorsal lip

d.Hutchinson's(Chauffeur's crank handle fracture)--- an

isolated fracture of the ulnar styloid process

162.For suspected scaphoid fracture ,X ray may be taken to show fracture line(G)

a.immediately

b.3 days after the original trauma

c.7-10 days after original trauma

d.3weaks after original trauma

163.Terry Thomas sign/David Letterman's sign/Lauren Hutton sign is noted in(G)

a.scapho-lunate dissociation

b.perilunate dislocation

c.ulnar styloid fracture

d.radial styloid fracture

164.All are correctly matched except(G)

a.Boxer fracture---fracture of the fourth and fifth metacarpals

b.Bennet's fracture---fracture at the base of first metacarpal

c.Rolando fracture---- comminution of first metacarpal

d.Gamekeeper 's thumb/Skier's thumb--- disruption of radial collateral ligament of MCP of index finger

165.Boehler's angle is useful for assessment of (G)

a.fracture of talus

b.fracture of calcaneous

c.fracture of lower end of tibia

d.fracture of lower end of fibula

166.Lisfranc joint refers to(G)

a.tarsometatarsal joint

b.subtalar joint

d.tibio-fibular joint

d.matatarso-phalangeal joint

167.V anishing bone disease is also known as(G)

a.Gorham's disease

b.Maffusi's syndrome

c.candle wax disease

d.Cleidocranial dysplasia

168.Fibrous dysplasia is characetrised by except(G)

a.ground glass matrix

b.thick sclerotic margin(rind sign)

c.shepherd's crook deformity

d.delayed puberty

169.The best technique for identifying polysostotic variety of fibrous dysplasia(G)

a.CT

b.MRI

c.scintigraphy

d.PET

170.Singh index is related to(G)
a.index of osteopoross
b.index of osteopetrosis
c.index of fluorosis
d.all

171.Concertina deformity of lower limb and and beaded ribs may be found in(G)
a.osteogenesis imperfect
b.hyperparathyroidism
c.drug induced congenital abnormality
d.osteopetrosis.

172.Radiogrammetry refers to(G)
a.study of trabecular pattern of bone
b.measurement of cortical thickness
c.cerebral morphometry
d.all

173.Metacarpal shortening is noted in(G)
a.pseudo-pseudohypoparathyroidism
b.hyperparathyroidism
c.rickets
d.scurvy

174.Pseudofracture/Milkman's fracture is pathognomonic of(G)
a.osteomalacia
b.paget's disease
c.osteoporosis
d.osteopetrosis

175.Harrison's sulcus is seen in(G)
a.pseudo-pseudohypoparathyroidism
b.hyperparathyroidism
c.rickets
d.scurvy

176.The earliest radiographic changes in hands in case of rheumatoid arthritis is (G)
a.juxta-articular osteopenia
b.soft tissue swelling
c.both
d.none

177.Gull- wing deformity is noted in(G)
a.rheumatoid arthritis
b.erosive arthritis
c.juvenile osteoarthritis
d.primary osteo-arthritis

178.All are correctly matched except(G)
a.syndesmophyte-----ankylosing spondylitis
b.hook osteophytes----haemophilia
c.pencil-in-cup deformity----ankylosing spondylitis
d.tophi-----gout

179.Brodie abscess refers to(G)
a.intraosseous abscess with intense sclerosis
b.brain abscess with osteomyelitis
c. pharyngeal abscess
d.hepatic abscess

180.Mitten/Shock deformities of hands and feet noted in(G)
a.Apert syndrome
b.Treacher-Collin syndrome
c.Osteopetrosis
d.achodroplasia

181.Madelung deformity is noted in(G)
a.Down 's syndrome
b.Turner's syndrome
c.Apert 'ssyndrome
d.Sipple sndrome

182.The earliest radiographic sign of Perthes disease(G)
a.radiolucent subchondral fissure—crescent sign
b.loss of height
c.fragmentation
d.sclerosis of femoral head

183.The slip angle is relevant for(G)
a.slipped capital femoral epiphysis
b.fracture neck of femor
c.trochanteric fracture
d.fracture shaft of femur

184.Riser grade is important for(G)
a.scoliosis
b.slipped capital femoral epiphysis
c.kyphosis
d.hypothyroidism

185.'Hair-on-end appearance' and 'rodent facies' are seen in(G)
a.sickle cell anemia
b.thallessemia
c.iron deficiency anemia
d.megaloblastic anemia

186.The Salter-Harris classification is for(G)
a.epiphyseal injury
b.head injury
c.liver injury
d.splenic injury

187.Toddler fracture refers to(G)
a.displced ,oblique fracture of distal tibia
b. a.undisplced ,oblique fracture of distal tibia
c.undisplced ,transverse fracture of distal tibia
d.displced, transverse fracture of distal tibia

188.All fracture have high specificity of abuse except(G)

a.metaphyseal,rib and scapular fractures

b.fractures of outer third of clavicle

c.sternal fractures and spinous process fractures

d.greensick fractures

189.Rib-within-rib appearance on x ray of chest in found in(G)

a.sickle cell anemia

b.thalassaemia

c.haemochromatosis

d.osteopetrosis

190.The classical spinal lesion in eosinophilic granuloma (G)

a.vertebra plana

b.anterior wedging

c.anterior scalloping

d.scoliosis

191.Bony changes in haemophilia is all except(G)

a.enlargement of distal femoral and proximal tibial epiphyses

b.squaring of patella

c.widening of intercondylar notch

d.retarded bone age

192.Retarded skeletal maturation is seen in(C)

a.hypothyroidism

b.idiopathic sexual precocity

c.McCune Albright syndrome

d.Soto syndrome

193.Enchondrma and heamangioma is found in(C)

a.Ollier's disease

b.Maffuci'syndrome

c.Beckwith- Widerman's syndrome

d.Klippel-trenaunay –Weber syndrome

194.Hemihypertophy,macrglossia and umbilical hernia in seen in(C)

a.Ollier's disease

b.Maffuci'syndrome

c.Beckwith- Widerman's syndrome

d.Klippel-trenaunay –Weber syndrome

195.Hypertrophy of the skeleton and soft tissue of one limb or one side of body in association of an angiomatous malformation is found(C)

a.Ollier's disease

b.Maffuci'syndrome

c.Beckwith- Widerman's syndrome

d.Klippel-trenaunay –Weber syndrome

196.Multiple exostoses and enchodromatosis is found in (C)

a.Ollier's disease

b.Maffuci'syndrome

c.Beckwith- Widerman's syndrome

d.Klippel-trenaunay –Weber syndrome

197. Proximal limb shortening (rhizomelic) is noted in(C)

a.achondroplasia

b.Leri-Weil disease

c.Ellis-von Creveld syndrome

d.Jeune syndrome

198. Ellis-von Creveld syndrome is characterized by all except(C)

a.hexadactly

b.congenital heart disease

c.hypoplastic lateral tibial pateau characteristic in childhood

d.proximal limb shortening

199.Hitch-hiker thumb is noted in(C)

a.diastrophic dysplasia

b.Kneist syndrome

c.achondroplasia

d.cleidocranial dysplasia

200.H-shaped or inverted U-shaped vertebral bodies is noted in(C)

a.diastrophic dwarfism

b.thanatophoric dwarfism

c.achondroplasia

d.cleidocranial dysplasia

201.Telephone handle- shaped long bones is seen in(C)

a.thanatophoric dwarfism

b.diastrophic dwarfism

c.achondroplasia

d.cleidocranial dysplasia

202.X –linked mucoplysaccharidoses is(C)

a.Hurler

b.Hunter

c.Morquio

d.Moroteaux-Lamy

203.No cornaeal clouding is seen in(C)

a.Hurler

b.Hunter

c.Morquio

d.Moroteaux-Lamy

204.Generalised increased bone density is seen in all except(C)

a.osteopetrosis

b.fluorosis

c.Caffey'disease

d.scurvy

205.Solitary sclerotic bone lesion with a lucent centre is noted in (C)

a.osteoid osteoma

b.lymphoma

c.osteosarcoma

d.Ewing's sarcoma

206.Sclerotic bone metastases is noted in(C)
a.prostate
b.carcinoid
c.both
d.none

207.Expansile lytic metastases are noted in all except(C)
a.renal cell carcinoma
b.thyroid tumour
c.phaeochromocytoma
d.prostate

208.correct matching of location of bone lesions are all except(C)
a.chondrblastoma—epiphysis
b.osteosarcoma—metaphyses
c.Ewing's sarcoma—diaphyses
d.osteoblastoma—epiphyses

209.Fluid fluid level in CT and MRI is found in all except(C)
a.giant cell tumour
b.aneurysmal bone cyst
c Simle bone cyst
d.osteoid osteoma

210.Hair-on- end appearance is seen in all except(C)
a.Ewing's sarcoma
b.syphilis
c.Caffey's disease
d.osteosarcoma

211.Sunray periosteal reaction is seen in(C)
a.Ewing's sarcoma
b.syphilis
c.Caffey's disease
d.osteosarcoma

212.Multiple fractures with reducd bone density is seen in (C)
a.Cleidocranial dysplasia
b.osteogenesis imperfect
c.osteopetrosis
d.syphilis

213.Pseudoarthrosis is seen in all except(C)
a.nonunion of fracture
b.neurofibromatosis
c.Osteogenesis imperfecta
d.Paget's disease

214.Bone within bone appearance is noted in all except(C)
a.sickle-cell anemia
b.osteopetrosis
c.Gaucher's disease
d.fibrous dysplasia

215.Stippled epiphyses is noted in
a.congenital hypothyroidism
b.acromegaly
c.sickle cellanemia
d.none

216.Park's lines in bone noted in (C)
a.rickets

b.scurvy
c.growth arrest
d.lead poisoning
217.Celery stalk appearance is seen in(C)
a.osteopathia striata
b.congenital rubella
c.ricket
d.scurvy
218.Fraying and cupping of mataphyses is seen in(C)
a.scurvy
b.rubella
c.ricket
d.hypothyroidism
219.Erlemeyer Flask deformity is seen in all except(C)
a.Pyle'disease
b.Craniometaphyseal dysplasia
c.Gaucher 's disease
d.syphilis
220.Inferior rib notching is seen in all except(C)
a.coarctation of aorta
b.Blalock's operation
c.SVC obstruction
d.rheumatoid arthritis
221.Inferior rib notching is seen in all except(C)
a.aortic thrombosis
b.subclavian obstruction
c.pulmonary oligemia
d.hyperprarathyroidism

222.Superior rib nitching is seen in all except(C)
a.connective tissue disease
b.hyperparathyroidism
c.Marfan syndrome
d.coarctation of aorta
223.Madelung deformity is seen in all except(C)
a.Turner 's syndrome
b.Leri-Weil's disease
c.diaphyseal aclasis
d.thalessemia
224.Madelung deformity is noted in (C)
a.wrist
b.hip
c.ankle
d.facial region
225.Short metacarpals are seen in all except(C)
a.Turner's syndrome
b.pseudohypoparathyroidism
c. pseudopseudohypoparathyroidism
d.Down syndrome
226.Arachnodactly is noted in(C)
a.Marfan's syndrome
b.homocystinuria
c.both
d.none

227.Normal metacarpal index is (C)
a.2-4
b.5.4-7.9
c.8-10
d.11-12

228.Complete syndactly of digits II-V (mitten hand) and 'sock foot' noted in(C)
a.Apert syndrome
b.Holt-Oram syndrome
c.Poland's syndrome
d.diastrophic dysplasia

229.Intervertebral disc space is preserved in(C)
a.metastasis
b.infection
c.both
d.none

230.The most common cause of a solitary vertebra plana in childhood(C)
a.metastasis
b.Paget's disease
c.Langerhans cell histiocytosis
d.haemangioma

231.Fish shaped vertebra is noted in(C)
a.osteoporosis
b.neoplasm
c.infection
d.trauma

232.Enlarged vertebra may be found in all except(C)
a.acromegaly
b.Paget's disease
c.haemangioma
d.eosinophilic granuloma

233.Squaring of vertebral body may be seen in (C)
a.acromegaly
b.haemangioma
c.ankylosing spondylitis
d.osteoporosis

234.Ivory vertebral body may be seen in(C)
a.sclerotic metastases
b.Paget's disease
c.lymphoma
d.all

235.Central anterior vertebral body beaks is found in(C)
a.Hurler's syndrome
b.achonroplasia
c.Morqui's syndrome
d.Hunter syndrome

236.posterior scalloping of posterior vertebral bodies are found in all except(C)
a.tumours in spinal canal
b.neurofibromatosis
c.acromegaly
d.aortic aneurysm

237. Anterior scalloping of

posterior vertebral bodies are found in all except(C)

a.neurofibromatosis

b.lymphadenopathy

c.tuberculosis

d.aortic aneurysm

238.Gilula's arc is related to(SW)

a.wrist

b.elbow

c.foot

d.knee

239.Chondrocalcinosis is noted in(C)

a.hyperparathyroidism

b.alkaptonuria

c.Wilson'disease

d.all

240.Widening of symphysis pubis is noted in(C)

a.Exstrophy of bladder

b.ankylosing spondylitis

c.hypoparathyroidism

d.hyperthyroidism

241.All are correctly matched except(C)

a.coxa magna—wider and fatter femoral head

b.coxa plana—flattened femoral head

c.coxa valga—decreased femoral angle leading to more vertical femoral neck

d.cexa vara ----decreased femoral angle leading to more vertical femoral neck

242.Cobb 's method refers to(SW)

a.method of measurement of scoliosis

b.method of measurement of lordosis

c.method of measurement of kyphosis

d.method of measurement of iliac index

243.Osgood-Schlatter's disease refers to(SW)

a.ossification in the distal patellar tendon its insertion at tibial apophysis

b.ossification in distal femoral tendon at its insertion

c.ossification in distal triceps muscle tendon at its insertion

d.ossification in distal bicept tendon at its insertion

244.'Bare' orbit is seen in all except(C)

a.neurofibromatosis

b.orbit metastases

c.meningioma

d.congenital glaucoma

245.Concentric enlargement of optic foramen is seen in all except(C)

a.optic nerve glioma
b.neurofibroma
c.extension of retinoblastoma
d.raised intracranial pressure
246.Small or absent frontal sinuses are noted in all except(C)
a.congenital absence
b.hyperthyroidism
c.Down's syndrome
d.kartagener's syndrome
247.Gorlin syndrome is characterized by all except(C)
a.multiple radicular cyst
b.rib anomalies
c.lamellar falx calcification
d.multiple basal cell naevi
248.Causes of 'floating' teeth is noted in all except(C)
a.Langerhans cell histiocytosis
b.hyperparathyroidism
c.multiple myeloma
d.ameloblastoma
249.All are causes of J-shaped sella except(C)
a.neurofibromatosis
b.achondroplasla
c.mucoplysaccharidoses
d.pituitary adenoma
250.W-or omega-shaped sella is found in(C)
a.optic chiasm glioma
b.neurofibromatosls

b.achondroplasia
c.mucoplysaccharidoses
251.Diffuse involvement of the vault and skull base by multiple small 'punched out 'lesions is noted in(C)
a.multiple myeloma
b.Langerhans cell histiocytosis
c.hyperparathyroidism
d.haemangioma
252.Solitary round/ovoid punched out lesion with serrated and beveled edges in skull is seen in(C)
a.multiple myeloma
b.Langerhans cell histiocytosis
c.hyperparathyroidism
d.haemangioma
253.Geographical skull (multiple ovoid/serpiginous lucencies that cover large area of the calvarium) is noted in(C)
a.multiple myeloma
b.Hand-schuller-Christian disease
c.hyperparathyroidism
d.haemangioma
254.Pepper pot skull is seen in(C)
a.multiple myeloma
b.Hand-schuller-Christian disease
c.hyperparathyroidism

d.haemangioma

255.'Sunburst 'pattern of radiating spicules without discreet margin in skull is seen in(C)

a.multiple myeloma

b.Hand-schuller-Christian disease

c.hyperparathyroidism

d.haemangioma

256.Leontiasis ossea is noted in

a.Paget's disease

b.fluorosis

c.fibrous dysplasia

d.osteopetrosis

257.Soap bubble appearance of skull is seen in(C)

a. a.multiple myeloma

b.Hand-schuller-Christian disease

c.lacunar skull(luckenschadel)

d.haemangioma

258.Wormian bones is found in all except(C)

a.rickets

b.pyknodysostosis

c.Menkes syndrome

d.scurvy

259.Wormian bones is found in all except(C)

a.osteogenesis imperfect

b.hyperthyroidism

c.hypophosphatasia

d.down's syndrome

260.'Boat- shaped' skull is seen in(C)

a.sagittal synostosis

b.metopic synostosis

c.coronal synostosis

d.lambdoid synostosis

261.Triangular-shaped skull is seen in(C)

a.sagittal synostosis

b.metopic synostosis

c.coronal synostosis

d.lambdoid synostosis

262.Synostosis of multiple paired sutures produce (C)

a.Cloverleaf skull(kleeblattscheidel)/trilobular skull

b.Boat-shaped skull

c.triangular-shaped skull

d.cigar –shaped skull

263.Scaphocephaly /dolichocephaly is due to(C)

a.sagittal synostosis

b.metopic synostosis

c.coronal synostosis

d.lambdoid synostosis

264.Hair-on –end skull is noted in all except(C)

a.sickle cell anemia

b.thalassemia

c.hereditaty spherocytosis

d.fibrous dysplasia

265.All are skull features of achodroplasia except(C)

a.large skull

b.small base

c.large sella

d.small funnel shaped foramen magnum

266.Vertebral changes in achodroplasia are all except(C)

a.increasing interpedicular distance in lumbar vertebrae caudally

b.lumbar canal stenosis

c.posterior scalloping

d.short pedicles

267.Skeletal finding in achondrplasia are all except(C)

a.distal segment limb shortening

b.Champagne –glass pelvic cavity

c.Tident-shaped hands

d.Square iliac wings

268.Tufting of the terminal phalanges (arrow head appearance) and increased heel pad thicknes is seen in (C)

a.alkaptonuria

b.hyperthyroisism

c.acromegaly

d.coshing syndrome

269.Which joint show earliest change in ankylosing spondylitis(C)

a.hip joint

b.spine

c.sacroiliac joint

d.shoulder

270.Pattern of calcification seen in chondrosarcoma are all except(C)

a.popcorn

b.ring and arc

c.dot and comma

d.cloudy

271. Blount 's disease is associated with all except

a.internal tibial torsion

b.genu varum

c.genu recurvatum

d.external tibial torsion

272.Down's syndrome is characterized by all except(C)

a.brachycephaly and micrcephaly

b.hypopalasia of facial bones and sinuses

c.wide suture and delayed closures

d.hypertelorism

273.Down's syndrome is characterized by all except(C)

a.atlantoaxial subluxation

b.hypoplasia os posterior arch of C1

c.increased height and decreased AP diameter of lumbar vertebra

d.large acetabular index

274.Down's syndrome is characterized by all except(C)

a.narrow iliac wings

b.eleven pairs of ribs

c.clinodactly

d.multiple wormian bones

275.Onion skin periosteal reaction is noted in(C)

a.osteosarcoma

b.chodrosarcoma

c.Ewing's sarcoma

d.osteoblastoma

276.Fibrous dysplasia is characterized by all except(C)

a.ground glass opacity

b.endosteal scalloping

c.rind sign

d.exuberant periosteal reaction

277.Shepherd's crook deformity of the proximal femur is noted in(C)

a.Paget's disease

b.fibrous dysplasia

c.ankylosing spondylitis

d.Perthe's disease

278.Hurler's syndrome is characterized by all except(C)

a.J-shaped sella

b.anterior beaking of vertebra

c.Trident hands

d.anterior scalloping of vertebra

279.Pimary hyperthyroidism is characterized by all except(C)

a.subperiosteal bone resorption

b cortical tunneling

c.brown tumour

d.very common osteopenia

280.Rotting fence –post appearance of the proximal femur, basketwork appearance of cortex and pepper-pot skull are features of (C)

a.acromegaly

b.Cushing's syndrome

c.hyperprarathyroidism

d.hyperthyroidism

281. features of hyperparathyroidism are all except(C)

a.rotting fence-post appearance of proximal femur

b.basketwork appearance of cortex

c.triradiate pelvis

d.buffalo's hump

282Subpriosteal resorption seen in hyperparathyroidism particularly affect(C)
a. the radial side of distal phalanx of the middle finger
b. the ulnar side of diatalphalanx of the middle finger
c.the radial side of middle phalanx of the middle finger
d.the ulnar side of middle phalanx of the middle finger

283.Twisted ribbon's rib is found in(C)
a.neurofibromatosis
b.fibrous dysplasia
c.Paget's disease
d.eosinophilic granuloma

284.Rugger jersey spine noted in(C)
a.osteomalacia
b.pyknodysostosis
c.osteopetrosis
d.Paget's disease

285.All are features of osteopetrosis except(C)
a.decreasing bone sclerosis during childhood
b.bone- within- bone appearance
c.Rugger jersey spine
d.Erlenmeyer flask deformity

286.All are true of Paget's disease except(C)
a.'cotton wool' appearance of skull
b.'picture frame' vertebral body
c.Ivory vertebra
d.thinned out vault

287.Cup and pencil deformity is noted in(C)
a.rheumatoid arthritis
b.juvenile rheumatoid arthritis
c.psoriatic arthropathy
d.osteoarthritis

288.Rugger jersey spine ia noted in(C)
a.renal osteodytrophy
b.osteopetrosis
c.both
d.none

289.Rickets is characterized by all except(C)
a.widened growth plate
b.fraying ,splaying and cupping of the metaphysis
c.indistinct cortex
d.osteoporosis very common

290.Features of ricket is/are (C)
a.bowing of long bones
b.Triradiate pelvis
c.craniotabes
d.all

291.features of ricket ,all except(C)
a.cupping of anterior ends of ribs
b.Harrison's sulcus
c.scoliosis
d.looser zones common

292.Scurvy is characterized by all except(C)
a.Wimberger's sign
b.Trummerfeld zone
c.Pelkan spurs
d.no periosteal reaction

293.Loss of epiphyseal density with a pencil thin cortex in scurvy is known as(C)
a.Wimberger's sign
b.Trummerfeld zone
c.Pelkan spurs
d.none

294.All are features of scurvy except(C)
a.dense zone of provisional calcification
b.metaphyseal lucency(Trummerfeild zone)
c.metaphyseal corner fractures(Pelkan spur)
d.earliest signs seen at wrist joints

295.Hand-foot syndrome is seen in(C)
a.thalessemia
b.sickle cell anemia
c.lymphoma
d.psoriatic arthropathy

296.Simple bone cyst is characterized by all except(C)
a.metaphyseal lesion
b.most common in proximal humerous and femar
c.'fallen fragmant' sign
d.expansion always greater than width of epiphyseal plate

297.Marked ballooning of metaphyseal lesion of long bone with fluid-fluid level on CT/MRI is seen in(C)
a.simple bone cyst
b.aneurysmal bone cyst
c.giant cell tumour
d.none

298.Metaphyseal blanch sign is seen in(C)
a.scurvy
b.slipped capital femoral epiphysis
c.Perthe's disease
d.fibrous dysplasia

299.All are features of Turner's syndrome except(C)
a.short fourth metacarpal and/or metatarsal
b.Madelung deformity
c.enlargement of medial tibial plateau

d.cubitus varus in 70% cases
300.Whitish hyperdense foci
with areas of grey sinus
opacification on CT scan of
PNS is radiological hallmark
of(SW)
a.fungal sinusitis
b.bacterial sinusitis
c.allergic sinusitis
d.none
301.Facial bone fracture most
commonly involves(SW)
a.mandible
b.maxilla
c.zygomatic bone
d.none
302.Pilon fractures refers to
(SW)
a.fracture of distal end of tibia
b.fracture of distal end of
fibula
c.fracture of distal end of shaft
of both tibia and fibula
d.fracture of calcaneus
303.Fracture of the proximal
ulna with radial head
dislocation is known as(SW)
a.Monteggia fracture
dislocation
b.Galeazzi fracture
c.Piedmont fracture
c.Jefferson' fracture

304. Fracture of the shaft of
radius and radial ulnar
dislocation is known as(SW)
a.Monteggia fracture
dislocation
b.Galeazzi fracture /Piedmont
fracture
c.Pott's fracture
c.Jefferson' fracture
305.Clay Shoveler's injury
refers to(SW)
a.avulsion fracture of the
spinous process of C6 to T2
b.Trumatic spodylolisthesis of
C2
c.fracture of C2
d.fracture of C1 ring
306.The most common benign
bone tumour in
children(GRAINGER)
a.non-ossifying fibroma
b.ossifying bone fibroma
c.osteoblastoma
d.osteoid osteoma
307.A plain radiograph of
osteosarcoma shows all except
a.predilection for diaphyses of
long bones
b.destuctive lesions with
moth-eaten appearance
c.spiculated periosteal
reaction(sunburst appearance)

d.a cuff of periosteal new bone formation at the margin of soft tissue mass(Codman's triangle)

308.All are true regarding radiology of chondrosarcoma except

a.predilection for flat bones

b.lobular appearance

c.mottled ,annular,punctuate calcification

d.Codman's triangle

309.Radiologically,Ewing's sarcoma is characterized by all except

a.involve the metaphyseal region of long bones

b.onion peel periosteal reaction

c.soft tissue mass

d.affinity for flat bones

310.All are true regarding metasatic tumour of bone except

a.metastatic tumour more common than primary

b.prostate,breast and lung account for 80% of bone metastases

c.most frequently involved bone is femur

d.purely osteolytic lesions are best detected on radionuclide bone scan

312.Punched out lesions in skull radiography is characteristically seen in

a.thallessemia

b.multiple myeloma

c.leukemia

d.sickle cell anemia

313.Among the most common causes of bone infections

a.pneumococcus

b.staphylococcus

c.pseudomonas

d.E.coli

314. True regarding hematogenous osteomyelitis

a.x ray may be normal for up to 14 days after onset of symptoms

b.^{99m}Tc-phosphonate scanning often detects evidence of infection very late

c.least sensitive investigation is MRI

d. none

315.The most common cause of septic arthritis in native joint

a.pneumococcus

b.staphylococcus

c.pseudomonas

d.E.coli

316.The most common site of skeletal TB
a.hip joint
b.spine
c.knee
d.elbow

317.The most common site of Spinal TB in children
a.upper thoracic spine
b.lower thoracic and upper lumbar spine
c.lower lumbar spine
d.cervical spine

318.The most common site of Spinal TB in adult
a.upper thoracic spine
b.lower thoracic and upper lumbar spine
c.lower lumbar spine
d.cervical spine

319.The spinal tuberculosis is charcterised by all except
a.invlvement of two or more adjacent vertabra
b. no involvement of the intervertebral disk
c.kyphosis/gibbus formation due to collapse of vertebra
d.psoas abscess

320.Pott's disease refers to
a.spinal TB
b.TB of hip joint
c.pulmonary tuberculosis
d.none

321.Bilateral knee effusion in congenital syphilis is known as
a.Cluttion's joint
b.charcot's joint
c.neuropathic joint
d.none

322.Classic stigmata of congenital syphilis are all except
a.Hutchinson'teeth(centrally notched,widely spaced,peg-shaped lower central incisors)
b.mullberry's molar(sixth year molars with multiple poorly-developed cusps)
c.saddle nose
d.saber shins

323.cigar –shaped soft tissue calcification is noted in
a.csysticercosis
b.loa-loa
c.filaria
d.none

324.The most pathognomonic radiological finding of hydatid cyst
a.rounded mass of uniform density
b.cyst wall calcification

c.fluid layer of different opacity

d.daughter cyst within larger cyst

325.Snowflake sign in USG is seen in

a.echinococcus

b.teania solium

c.schistosomiasis

d.none

326.Fanconi anemia are characetrised by all except(N)

a.normal strature

b.microcephaly

c.thumb attached by thread

d.micrognathia

327.All are causes of osteoporosis except

a.hypogonadism

b.hyperthyroidism

c.hyperparathyroidism

d.fluorosis

328.The pulsating tumour of bone is

a.osteosarcoma

b.Ewing 's sarcoma

c.chondrosarcoma

d.Eosinophilic granuloma

329.Flaring of anterior end of ribs is characteristically seen in

a.NF

b.scurvy

c.ricket

d.hypothyroidism

330.The best view for fracture of C1 and C2

a.AP view

b.odontoid view

c.lateral view

d.oblique view

331.cyst associated with vertebral defect is

a.Bronchogenic cyst

b.neuroenteric cyst

c.myelocele

d.neuroblastoma

332.Milkman's fracture is a type of

a.clavicular fracture

b.humeral fracture

c.metacarpal fracture

d.pseudofracture

333.Blount 's disease refers to

a.genu valgum

b.genu varum

c.genu recurvatum

d.meniscal injury

334.Which fat pad is relatd to knee joint

a.Hoffa 's fat pad

b.Krager fat pad

c.Susan fat pad

d.Cart fat pad

d

BONE AND JOINT RADIOLOGY

ANSWERS

1.a---The most common form of chronic inflammatory polyarthritis is rheumatoid arthritis

2.a---The symmetric polyarthritis is seen in rheumatoid arthritis

3.a---Cartilge hair hypolasia involve metaphyseal ends

4.d---Cartilge hair hypoplasia is characterized by(H) short –limb dwarfism,metaphyseal dysostosis,sparse hair

5.b---Musculoskeletal manifestations of SLE are intermittent polyarthritis,none-erosive polyarthritis
may be ischemic necrosis of bone, hands, wrists and joints most commonly affected

6.d---The frequently involved joints in rheumatoid arthritis are (H) wrist joint,metecarpophalangeal joint(MCP),proximal interphalangeal joint(PCP)

7.d---The deformities seen in rheumatoid arthritis are(H),Swan neck deformity,Boutonniere deformity and Z-line deformity

8.a----The deformity showing hyperextension of the PIP joint with flexion of DIP joint is known as(H) Swan neck deformity

9.b----The deformity showing flexion of the PIP joint with hyperextension of DIP joint is known as(H) Boutonniere deformity

10.d----The rheumatoid arthritis involves(H)atlantoaxial joint,metatarsophalangeal joint(MTP) and temporomandibular joint

11.a---The initial radiographic finding in rheumatoid arthritis is(H) juxta articular osteopenia

12.a----Fifth MTP joint of foot is targeted first in rheumatoid arthritis(H)

13.d--- Features of joint involvement in acute rheumatic fever are(H) polyarthritis,migratory,almost always large joint and symmetric

14.a--Acro-osteolysis in noted in(H) systemic sclerosis

15.b---HRCT feature of systemic sclerosis ,(H)ground glass opacification doesnot predict rapid progression of disease.

16.a--- Symmetric sacroilitiis is often the earliest manifestations of ankylosing spondylitis(H)

17.c---Syndesmophyte is found in(H) ankylosing spodylitis

18.c---Bamboo spine is found in(H) ankylosing spodylitis

19.b--- ankylosing spondylitis shows ascending progression of disease

20.a----The earliest change in sacroiliac joint ankylosing spondylitis in x ray is(H) blurring of the subcotical margin of the subchondral bone

21.b----MRI is being increasingly used for diagnosis of ankylosing spondylitis(H)

22.a---Spondyloarthropathy shows periostitis with reactive bone formation is characteristic of(H)

23.d--Characteristic of peripheral psoriatic arthritis are a(H)DIP involvement,whiskering and small joint ankylosis

 24.d---Characteristic of peripheral psoriatic arthritis are a(H)pencil- in- cup deformity,osteolysis of phalangeal and metacarpal bones,telescoping of digits

25.d--Characteristic of peripheral psoriatic arthritis are a(H)pencil- in- cup deformity,osteolysis of phalangeal and metacarpal bones,periostitis and proliferative new bone formation at sites of enthesitis

26. d---The re is relative sparing of thoracolumbar spine in axial psoriatic arthritis

27. d---There is asymmetric sacroiliitis in axial psoriatic arthritis

28.a--pencil in cup deformity is seen in(H)psoriatic arthritis

29.a--Telescoping of digit is seen in(H) psoriatic arthritis

30.a---The most commonly used method to diagnose pulmonary involovement in sarcoidosis(H) is chest x ray

31.b---Stage 2 of pulmonary involvement in sarcoidosis refers to(H) hilar adenopathy +pulmonary infiltrates

32.d---Upper lobe chest non infectious disease are all except(H).sarcoidosis and silicosis,hypersensitivity pneumonitis,Langerhans cell histiocytosis

33.d---- upper lobe chest disease are all except(H)sarcoidosis,tuberculosis,pneumocystitis pneumonia

34.d---Sarcoidosis involve upper lobe (H)

35.d--- involvement of optic nerve favors multiple sclerosis (H)

36.a----Heberdon's node is noted in(H) osteoarthritis

37.a----Bouchard's node is noted in(H) osteoarthritis

38.b--.Location of Heberdon'S node is(H) DIP

39.a----Location of Bouchard'S node is(H) PIP

40.a---The preferred method for evaluation of Baker's cyst,rotator cuff tears,tendinitis and tendon injury and suspected early synovitis(H) is USG

41.a---^{99m}Tc is used for metastatic bone survey and evaluation of Paget's disease(H)

42.b---^{111}In-WBC radionuclide is used for prosthetic infection(H)

43.a---The most common type of arthritis is(H) osteoarthritis

44.b----Joints usually affected in osteoarthritis are (H) cervical and lumbosacral spine,knee joint and first metatarsophalangeal joint

45.d---Joints often spared in osteoarthritis are a(H)wrist joint,ankle joint,elbow joint

46.c---Joints of hand often involved in osteoarthritis are (H) PIP,DIP, the base of thumb

47.d---Characteristic features of advanced chronic tophaceous gout are(H) cystic changes,well-defined,erosion with sclerotic margins and overhanging bony edges

48a.Chondrocalcinosis is noted in(H) CPPD deposition disease

49.d--- (H) N.neisseria causes acute polyarticular arthritis

50.d---Episodic inflammation of joint is seen in (H) syphilis,lyme diseases,reactive arthritis following chlymdial urethritis

51.b----A reactive symmetric form of polyarthritis that affect a person with visceral or disseminated tuberculosis is known as(H) Poncet's disease

52.d--- (H)Tuberculous osteomyelitis typically involves thoracic and lumbar spine , The hip,knee and ankle joint are commonly involved joint.Reactiv arthritis may follow HIV urethritis

53.a---Acromegaly (H) shows increased intervertabral disc,hypertrophic anterior osteophyte,ligamental calcification and may simulate DISH

54.c--- Features of acromegaly(H) are barrell shaped chest,spadelike distal tuft increased heel pad and chondrocalcinosis

55.c---Second MCP and third MCP joints are often the first and prominent joints affected in arthropathy of hemochromatosis(H)

56.a---Knee joint is first joint affected in hemophilic arthropathy(H)

57.a---In sickle cell disease (H)Hand foot syndrome is rarely seen after five yers of age,osteomyelitis commonly involves long bones,there may be infarction of bone and bone marrow and avascular necrosis in humeral head.

58.d----osteomyelitis in sickle cell disease is particularly caused by(H) salmonella

59.b----there is no vascular necrosis in thallassemia(H)

60.a---The most frequent cause of neuropathic joint disease is(H) is diabetes mellitus

61.d-----Disorders associated with neuropathic joint disease are (H)diabetes mellitus,leprosy,syringomelia

62.d----Disorders associated with neuropathic joint disease are (H)tabes dorsalis ,meningomyelocele,peroneal muscular atrophy

63.d----The most commonly affected joints in tabes dorsalis are (H) knees,hips,ankles

64.a----The most commonly affected joints in syringomyelia are (H) glenohumeral joint.wrist joint,elbow

65.a-----The most commonly affected joints in diabetes mellitus are(H) tarsal joints and tarsometatarsal joints

???66.a---The Rocker foot is noted in(H)diabetes mellitus

67.a----The resorption and tapering of distal metatarsal bones is noted in(H) diabetes mellitus

8.a--The destructive changes at tarsometatarsal joints is known as(H) Lisfranc fracture dislocation

69.a----The most common rheumatic disease in children(N) juvenile rheumatic disease

70.d--Criteria for classification of JRA are (N) age of onset <16yrs,.arthritis=>1 joints,duration of disease =>6 weeks,polyarthritis variety =>5joints in first six month after onset

71.a---An 'exoskeleton' of calcium deposition may be seen in(N) juvenile dermatoyositis

72d---.Acro-osteolysis may be seen in systemic scleroderma

73.a---The most common chest finding in sarcoidosis(N) is isolated bilateral hilar lymphadenopathy

74a---.Coronary artery aneurysm may be seen in(N) Kawasaki's disease

75.b--- Takayasu arteritis is predominantly a large vessel vasculitis(N)

76.a---Classic beads on string appearance may be noted in(N) PAN

77.d---Late manifestation of congenital syphilis are (N)Olympian brow,saber shins and mulberry molars

78.d-----Late manifestation of congenital syphilis (N) Hutchinson teeth,saddle nose ,clutton joint and hutchinson's triad

79.a---Highoum Naki's sign(unilateral/bilateral thickening of sternoclavicular third of the clavicle) is feature (N)congenital syphilis

80.b---Olympian brow is seen in(N) congenital syphilis

81.d---- Congenital syphilis :(N) Wimberger's line,osteochondritis,periostitis of long bones and lucent metaphyseal line

82.a--Wimberger's line is noted in(N) congenital syphilis

83.b----Metaphyseal demineralistion of medial aspect of the proximal tibia in congenital syphilis is known as(N) Wimbeger 's line

84.a----Presence of Scoliosis is defined by(N) Cobb's angle > 10degrees

85.b---The most common primary malignant bone tumour in children and adolescent(N) osteosarcoma

86.b--- Osteochondroma grows away from the joint (N)

87.d---CT is better then MRI to detect the osteoid osteoma (N)

88.b----Ant eater sign on lateral view of foot is noted in calcaneonavicular coalition

90.c--Harish view of the heel refers to(N) axial view

91. c----Continuous C-sign lateral view of foot is noted in(N) talocalcaneal coalition

92.a---Blount's disease is characterized by (N) metaphyseal – diaphyseal angle >11 degrees,medial sloping of the epiphyses,widening of epiphyses,fragmentation of the mataphyses

93.a--Notch view of knee refers to(N) tunnel view

94.b---The diagnostic modality of choice for development dysplasia of hip(DDH) before 4-6months(N) is USG

95.a---(N)a normal alpha angle is >60 degrees ,a normal beta angle is <55degrees,alpha angle represents depth of acetabulum,beta angle represents the cartilaginous roof of acetabulun

96.a---Graf technique of USG is used for (N) hip joint

97.c---Regarding DDH(N),alpha angle < 60 degree imply acetabular dysplasia,beta angle increases as femoral head subluxates

98.d----Lines used for assessment of DDH are (N) Hilgrenreiner's line,Perkin's line and Shenton's line

99.a----Ossific nucleus of femoral head is normally located in(N) medial lower quadrant of intersection of Hilgrenreiner's and Perkin's line

100.d---(N)The Higrenreiner's line is drawn through the triradiate cartilage.The perkin's line is drawn perpendicular to the Hilgrenreiner's line at the lateral edge of acetabulum.The Shenton's line curves along the femoral metaphyses to lower border of superior pubic ramus.The acetabular index is angle between line drawn along the margin of the acetabulum and the Hilgrenreiner's line

101.b---(N)Ossific nucleus of femoral head is outside of medial lower quadrant inDDH.Shenton's line is broken in DDH.Normal acetabular angle should be no more than 30 degrees.The center-edge angle is a useful measure of femoal head coverage

102.d---X ray is the primary diagnostic tool for Legg-Calve-Perthes disease is(N)

103.c---Lauenstein(frog –leg) view of hip is used to diagnose(N) Legg-Calve-Perthes disease and Slipped capital femora epiphysis

104.b---Cage 's sign (a radiolucent horizontal V in the lateral aspect of the femoral physis) is feature of(N) Legg-Calve-Perthes disease

105.a--Lateral pillar classification of Legg-Calve-Perthes disease has been given by(N)Herring

106.c----'Blanch sign of Steel'on x ray of hip is noted in (N) slipped capital femoral epiphysis

107.d----Klein 's line is used to diagnose Sliped capital femoral epiphysis(N)

108.c--The pars on spine is best visualized on view(N)b oblique

109.c---Pars defect on oblique view of spine is known as(N) Scotty dog sign

110.a--For the diagnosis of atlantoaxial instability,atlantodens interval(ADI) should be(N)<5mm

111.b---A normal atlantodens interval in patients with Down 's syndrome is(N)<4.5mm

112.a--Sprengel's deformity refers to(N)congenital elevation of scapula

113.c---Madelung deformity is related to(N) wrist

114.a---Wassal classification is related to (N) thumb duplication

115.d---Torus(buckle fracture) fracture (N)is stable fecture

116.b--A fracture where bone is bent and fracture line does not propagate to concave side of bone is called(N) greenstick fracture

117.The most sensitive and specific test for osteomyelitis(N) is MRI

118.d--- In osteomyelitis(N)lytic changes in flat bone appear latter than long bones

119.c—CT is ideal for detecting gas in soft tissue(N)

120.d--- MRI in osteomyelitis(N) is more sensitive than CT or nuclear scan,is best imaging technique for identifying abscesses,is best imaging technique for differentiating bone and soft tissue infection,purulent pus appear hypointense on T1W and hyperintense on T2W

121.d--- Radionuclide study in a case of osteomyelitis(N) has ability to image entire skeleton to detect multiple foci,occurs uptake of radionuclide in third phase(4-6hrs),can detect infetion within 24-48 hrs of onset ,sensitivity in neonates is lower than adult

122.a-----^{99m}Tc metylene diphosphonate is used for imaging in osteomyelitis(N)

123.b---Obturator sign (medial displacement of obturator muscle in pelvis) is noted in(N) septic arthritis of hip

124.d----Telephone handle like femour is noted in thanotrophic dysplasia

125.a--Femur curved –like telephone receiver is noted in(N) thanotrophic dysplasia

126.c---Hitchhiker appearance (proximal displacement of thumb)is noted in(N) diastrophic dysplasia

127.d---Absent clavicle with multiple wormian bone is noted in(N) cleidocranial dysplasia

128.a----Iliac horn is seen in(N) nail-patella syndrome

129.c---Bone –in –bone appearance is seen in(N) osteopetrosis

130.d--Metatropic dysplasia is charecterised by (N)severe platyspondyly,dumbbell-shaped long bones,halbred appearance of pelvis

131.d---Dumbbell-shaped long bones and halbred appearance of pelvis is noted in(N) metatropic dysplasia

132.d---Caffey disease does not (N)involve phalanges and vertebral bodies

133.a----The most common genetic cause of osteoporosis(N) osteogenesis impefecta

134.c----The popcorn appearance of metaphyses is seen in(N) osteogenesis imperfecta

135.c---Silence classification is related to(N) osteogenesis imperfecta

136.c---Walker-Murdoch or wrist sign is noted in(N) Marfan syndrome

137.a---The Steinberg or thumb sign is noted in(N) Marfan syndrome

138.d--- Features of Marfan syndrome are(N)pectus excavatum/pectus carnatum,arachnodactly,camptodactyly
139.b---Hypophosphatasia radiologically resemble(N) ricket
140. d---Hyperphosphatasia is characterized by (N)bowing and thickening of diaphyses,large and thickened cranium,bony texture mix of teased cotton –wool appearance,lucent areas and pseudocysts
141.a---Pellegrini-Steida lesion lesion is noted in(G) knee
142.c---Magic angle phenomenon in MRI imaging (G) refers to artefactual increased signal from tendons on short TE imaging sequence,angle of alignment of tendon to static magnetic field is apprex.55 degree,magic angle effect is seen in ligament ,cartilage or menisci`,magic angle effect is not persistent on long TE sequence
143d---.Black synovium on MRI is noted in (G)pigmented villonodular synovitis,amyloid deposition,hemophiliac arthropathy
144.c---Water/edema in mri imaging(G) appears dark on T1W and bright on T2W images
145.d--The most common underlying process for pathological fracture is(G)metastatic disease
146.a---Orientation of pathological fracture in long bones(G) is transeverse
147.a----Transverse fracture noted in pathological fracture in long bones is known as(G) banana fracture
148.d----In stress fracture (G)fracture line is not easily identified
149.d----Radiographic 'five Ds'of diabetic neuropathic foot (G) are destruction and dislocation, disorganisation and debris ,density(heterotopic new bone and sclerosis)
150.b---Judet view is done to assesss(G) acetabula
151.a---In 'Open book' appearance of x ray of pelvis (G), there is disruption of both SI joint and pubic symphysis

152.d---Malgaigne complex ,a pattern of injury is noted in(G) pelvis

153.a---Straddle injury of pelvis is commonly seen in a bicycle accident(G)

154.c----Honda sign on scintigraphy of pelvis is noted in(G) sacral insufficiency fracture

155.a---Grashey view of x ray is done for(G) glenohumeral joint

156a---.Hill-Sachs deformity refers to(G) notch in the posterolateral head of humerous

157.a---Bankart's lesion refers to(G) fracture the antero-inferior glenoid rim

158.b---Light bulb sign on x ray of shoulder joint is seen in(G.posterior dislocation

159.a---X ray showing humeral head located inferomedial to the glenoid beneath the coracoids process suggest of (G) anterior dislocation

160.c--Positive fat pad sign and sail sign are indirect sign of(G) elbow joint effusion

161.d--Colles's fracture –impacted fracture of distal radius with dorsal displacement of distal fragment fracture.Smith's fracture--- fracture of distal radius with volarly displaced distal fragment fracture.Barton's fracture----displaced fracture of the volar lip of the distal radius without involvement of dorsal lip.Hutchinson's(Chauffeur's crank handle fracture)--- an isolated fracture of the radial styloid process

162.c--For suspected scaphoid fracture ,X ray may be taken to show fracture line(G) 7-10 days after original trauma

163.a---Terry Thomas sign/David Letterman's sign/Lauren Hutton sign is noted in(G) scapho-lunate dissociation

164.d--(G)Boxer fracture---fracture of the fourth and fifth metacarpals,Bennet's fracture---fracture at the base of first metacarpal involving matacarpophalangeal joint space,Rolando fracture----comminution of first metacarpal,Gamekeeper 's thumb/Skier's thumb---disruption of ulnar collateral ligament of MCP of index finger

165.b---Boehler's angle is useful for assessment of (G) fracture of calcaneous

166.a---Lisfranc joint refers to(G) tarsometatarsal joint

167.a---V anishing bone disease is also known as(G)Gorham's disease

168.d---Fibrous dysplasia is characetrised by(G)ground glass matrix,thick sclerotic margin(rind sign),shepherd's crook deformity

169.c--The best technique for identifying polysostotic variety of fibrous dysplasia(G) is scintigraphy

170.a---Singh index is related to(G) osteopoross

171.a ---Concertina deformity of lower limb and and beaded ribs may be found in(G) osteogenesis imperfect

172.b---Radiogrammetry refrs to(G) measurement of cortical thickness

173.a---Metacarpal shortening is noted in(G) pseudo-pseudohypoparathyroidism

174.a---Pseudofracture/Milkman's fracture is pathognomonic of(G) osteomalacia

175.c---Harrison's sulcus is seen in(G) rickets

176.c---The earliest radiographic changes in hands in case of rheumatoid arthritis is (G) juxta-articular osteopenia,soft tissue swelling

177.b---Gull wing deformity is noted in(G)erosive arthritis

178.c---Correctly matched (G) are syndesmophyte-----ankylosing spondylitis,hook osteophytes----haemophilia,tophi-----gout

179.a--Brodie abscess refrs to(G)intraosseous abscess with intense sclerosis

180.a --Mitten/Shock deformities of hands and feet noted in(G Apert syndrome

181.b---Madelung deformity is noted in(G) Turner's syndrome

182.a.The erliest radiographic sign of Perthes disease(G) is radiolucent subchondral fissure—crescent sign

183.a---The slip angle is relevant for(G) slipped capital femoral epiphysis

184.a---Riser grade is important for(G) scoliosis

185.b--'Hair-on-end appearance' and 'rodent facies' are seen in(G)thallessemia

186.a---The Salter-Harris classification is for(G) epiphyseal injury

187.b--Toddler fracture refers to(G) undisplced ,oblique fracture of distal tibia

188.d----Fracture having high specificity of abuse (G)are metaphyseal fracture ,rib and scapular fractures,fractures of outer third of clavicle ,sternal fractures and spinous process fractures

189.b---Rib-within-rib appearance on x ray of chest in found in(G) thalassaemia

190.a----The classical spinal lesion in eosinophilic granuloma (G) vertebra plan

191.d---Bony changes in haemophilia is (G) enlargement of distal femoral and proximal tibial epiphyses,squaring of patella ,widening of intercondylar notch

192.a----.Retarded skeletal maturation is seen in(C)hypothyroidism

193.a----Enchondrma and heamangioma is found in(C) Maffuci'syndrome

194.c---Hemihypertophy,macrglossia and umbilical hernia in seen in(C) Beckwith- Widerman's syndrome

195.d---Hypertrophy of the skeleton and soft tissue of one limb or one side of body in association of an angiomatous malformation is found(C) Klippel-trenaunay –Weber syndrome

196.a---Multiple exostoses and enchodromatosis is found in (C) Ollier's disease

197. a---Proximal limb shortening (rhizomelic) is noted in(C) achondroplasia

198.d--- Ellis-von Creveld syndrome is characterized by (C)hexadactly,congenital heart disease,hypoplastic lateral tibial pateau characteristic in childhood,middle and distal segment limb shortening

199.a---Hitch-hiker thumb is noted in(C)diastrophic dysplasia

200.b---H-shaped or inverted U-shaped vertebral bodies is noted in(C) thanatophoric dwarfism

201.c---Telephone handle- shaped long bones is seen in(C) thanatophoric dwarfism

202b---.X –linked mucoplysaccharidoses is(C) Hunter disease

203.b---No cornaeal clouding is seen in(C) Hunter

204.d---Generalised increased bone density is seen in(C)osteopetrosis,fluorosis,Caffey'disease

205.a---Solitary sclerotic bone lesion with a lucent centre is noted in (C) osteoid osteom

206.b---Sclerotic bone metastases is noted in(C) prostate,carcinoid

207.d---Expansile lytic metastases are noted in (C)renal cell carcinoma,thyroid tumour,phaeochromocytoma

208.d-- (C)chondrblastoma—epiphysis,osteosarcoma—metaphyses,Ewing's sarcoma—diaphyses,osteoblastoma—metaphyses

209.d---Fluid fluid level in CT and MRI is found in(C)giant cell tumour,aneurysmal bone cyst,Simle bone cyst

210.d---Hair-on- end appearance is seen in all except(C)Ewing's sarcoma,syphilis,Caffey's disease

211.d---Sunray periosteal reaction is seen in(C) osteosarcoma

212.b---Multiple fractures with reducd bone density is seen in (C) osteogenesis imperfect

213d---.Pseudoarthrosis is seen in (C)nonunion of fracture,neurofibromatosis,Osteogenesis imperfect

214.d---Bone within bone appearance is noted in (C) sickle-cell anemia,osteopetrosis,Gaucher's disease

215.a---Stippled epiphyses is noted in congenital hypothyroidism

216.c---Park's lines in bone noted in (C)growth arrest

217.b----Celery stalk appearance is seen in(C)congenital rubella

218.c----Fraying and cupping of mataphyses is seen in(C) ricket

219.d---Erlemeyer Flask deformity is seen in (C) Pyle'disease,Craniometaphyseal dysplasia,Gaucher 's disease

220.d---Inferior rib notching is seen in(C)coarctation of aorta,Blalock's operation,SVC ob struction

221.d---Inferior rib notching is seen in (C)aortic thrombosis,subclavian obstruction,pulmonary oligemia

222.d---Superior rib nitching is seen in (C)connective tissue disease,hyperparathyroidism,Marfan syndrome

223.d----Madelung deformity is seen in all(C)Turner 's syndrome,Leri-Weil's disease,diaphyseal aclasis

224.a---Madelung deformity is noted in (C)wrist

225.d---Short metacarpals are seen in (C)Turner's syndrome,pseudohypoparathyroidism,pseudopseudohypoparat hyroidism

226.c---Arachnodactly is noted in(C) Marfan's syndrome,homocystinuria

227.b---Normal metacarpal index is (C) 5.4-7.9

228.a---Complete syndactly of digits II-V (mitten hand) and 'sock foot' noted in(C) Apert syndrome

229.a---Intervertebral disc space is preserved in(C) metastasis

230.c---The most common cause of a solitary vertebra plana in childhood(C)Langerhans cell histiocytosis

231.a---Fish shaped vertebra is noted in(C) osteoporosis

232.d---Enlarged vertebra may be found in(C) acromegaly,Paget's disease,haemangioma

233.c---Squaring of vertebral body may be seen in (C) ankylosing spondylitis

234.d---Ivory vertebral body may be seen in(C) slcerotic metastases,Paget's disease,lymphoma

235.c---.Central anterior vertebral body beaks is found in(C) Morqui's syndrome

236.d---posterior scalloping of posterior vertebral bodies are found in(C) tumours in spinal canal,neurofibromatosis,acromegaly

237. a---Anterior scalloping of posterior vertebral bodies are found (C) lymphadenopathy, tuberculosis, aortic aneurysm,Down syndrome

238.a---Gilula's arc is related to(SW) wrist

239.d---Chondrocalcinosis is noted in(C) hyperparathyroidism,alkaptonuria,Wilson'disease

240.a----Widening of symphysis pubis is noted in(C) exstrophy of bladder

241.d---(C)coxa magna—wider and fatter femoral head,coxa plana—flattened femoral head,coxa valga—decreased femoral angle leading to more vertical femoral neck.coxa vara ---- decreased femoral angle leading to more horizontal femoral neck

242.a---Cobb 's method refers to(SW) method of measurement of scoliosis

243.a---Osgood-Schlatter's disease refers to(SW) ossification in the distal patellar tendon its insertion at tibial apophysis

244.d----'Bare' orbit is seen in all except(C)neurofibromatosis,orbit metastases,meningioma

245.d--Concentric enlargement of optic foramen is seen (C)optic nerve glioma,neurofibroma,extension of retinoblastoma

246.b--Small or absent frontal sinuses are noted in (C) congenital absence,Down's syndrome,kartagener's syndrome

247.a---Gorlin syndrome is characterized by (C) multiple dentigerous cyst,rib anomalies,.lamellar falx calcification,multiple basal cell naevi

248.d---Causes of 'floating' teeth is noted in (C)Langerhans cell histiocytosis.hyperparathyroidism,multiple myeloma

249.d--- Causes of J-shaped sella except(C) neurofibromatosis,achondroplasia,mucoplysaccharidoses

250.a---W-or omega-shaped sella is found in(C)optic chiasm glioma

251.a---Diffuse involvement of the vault and skull base by multiple small 'punched out 'lesions is noted in(C)multiple myeloma

252.b---Solitary round/ovoid punched out lesion with serrated and beveled edges in skull is seen in(C) Langerhans cell histiocytosis

253.b---Geographical skull (multiple ovoid/serpiginous lucencies that cover large area of the calvarium) is noted in(C)Hand-schuller-Christian disease

254.c---Pepper pot skull is seen in(C)hyperparathyroidism

255.d---'Sunburst 'pattern of radiating spicules without discreet margin in skull is seen in(C) haemangioma

256.c---Leontiasis ossea is noted(C) in fibrous dysplasia

257.c---Soap bubble appearance of skull is seen in(C) lacunar skull(luckenschadel)

258.d---Wormian bones is found in (C)rickets,pyknodysostosis,Menkes syndrome

259.b---Wormian bones is found in all (C)osteogenesis imperfect,hypophosphatasia,down's syndrome

260.a---'Boat- shaped' skull is seen in(C)sagittal synostosis

261.b---Triangular-shaped skull is seen in(C) metopic synostosis

262.a---Synostosis of multiple paired sutures produce (C) Cloverleaf skull(kleeblattscheidel)/trilobular skull

263.a---Scaphocephaly /dolichocephaly is due to(C) sagittal synostosis

264.d---Hair-on –end skull is noted in(C) sickle cell anemia,thalassemia,hereditaty spherocytosis

265.c---Skull features of achodroplasia are (C)large skull,small base,small sella,small funnel shaped foramen magnum

266.a---Vertebral changes in achodroplasia are (C)dereasing interpedicular distance in lumbar vertebrae caudally,lumbar canal stenosis,pesterior scalloping ,short pedicles

267.a---Skeletal finding in achondrplasia are (C)proximal segment limb shortening,Champagne –glass pelvic cavity,Tident-shaped hands,Square iliac wings

268.c---Tufting of the terminal phalanges (arrow head appearance) and increased heel pad thicknes is seen in (C) acromegaly

269.c---SI joint shows earliest change in ankylosing spondylitis(C)

270.d---Pattern of calcification seen in chondrosarcoma are (C) popcorn,ring and arc,dot and comma

271.d--- Blount 's disease is associated with internal tibial torsion,genu varum,genu recurvatum

272.d---Down's syndrome is characterized by (C) brachycephaly and micrcephaly,hypopalasia of facial bones and sinuses,wide suture and delayed closures,hypotelorism

273.d---Down's syndrome is characterized by (C) atlantoaxial subluxation,hypoplasia os posterior arch of C1,increased height and decreased AP diameter of lumbar vertebra and small acetabular index

274.a---Down's syndrome is characterized by (C) wide iliac wings,eleven pairs of ribs,clinodactly and multiple wormian bones

275.c---Onion skin periosteal reaction is noted in(C) Ewing's sarcoma

276.d---Fibrous dysplasia is characterized by (C) ground glass opacity,endosteal scalloping,rind sign

277.b---Shepherd's crook deformity of the proximal femur is noted in(C)fibrous dysplasia

278.d---Hurler's syndrome is characterized by all except(C)J-shaped sella,anterior beaking of vertebra,Trident hands,posterior scalloping of vertebra

279.d---Pimary hyperthyroidism is characterized by all except(C) subperiosteal bone resorption, cortical tunneling,brown tumour

280.c---Rotting fence –post appearance of the proximal femur, basketwork appearance of cortex and pepper-pot skull are features of (C) hyperprarathyroidism

281.d--- Features of hyperparathyroidism are(C)rotting fence-post appearance of proximal femur,basketwork appearance of cortex,triradiate pelvis

282.c---Subpriosteal resorption seen in hyperparathyroidism particularly affect(C)the radial side of middle phalanx of the middle finger

283.a---Twisted ribbon's rib is found in(C) neurofibromatosis

284.c---Rugger jersey spine noted in(C)osteopetrosis

285.a-- Features of osteopetrosis (C)increasing bone sclerosis during childhood,bone- within- bone appearance,Rugger jersey spine,Erlenmeyer flask deformity

286.d---Feature of Paget's disease are (C).'cotton wool' appearance of skull,'picture frame' vertebral body,Ivory vertebra,thick vertebra

287.c---Cup and pencil deformity is noted in(C) psoriatic arthropathy

288.c---Rugger jersey spine ia noted in(C)renal osteodytrophy,osteopetrosis

289.d----Rickets is characterized by (C)widened growth plate,fraying ,splaying and cupping of the metaphysic,indistinct cortex

290.d---Features of ricket are (C) bowing of long bones,Triradiate pelvis,craniotabes

291.d---features of ricket ,all except(C) cupping of anterior ends of ribs,Harrison's sulcus,scoliosis

292.d---Scurvy is characterized by (C)Wimberger's sign,Trummerfeld zone,Pelkan spurs andperiosteal reaction

293.a---Loss of epiphyseal density with a pencil thin cortex in scurvy is known as(C) Wimberger's sign

294.d---features of scurvy (C)dense zone of provisional calcification,metaphyseal lucency(Trummerfeild zone),metaphyseal corner fractures(Pelkan spur),earliest signs seen at knees

295.b---Hand-foot syndrome is seen in(C) sickle cell anemia

296.d---Simple bone cyst is characterized by (C) metaphyseal location,most common in proximal humerous and femar,'fallen fragmant' sign.expansion never more than width of epiphyseal plate

297.b---Marked ballooning of metaphyseal lesion of long bone with fluid-fluid level on CT/MRI is seen in(C)aneurysmal bone cyst

298.b---Metaphyseal blanch sign is seen in(C) slipped capital femoral epiphysis

299.d-- Features of Turner's syndrome are (C)short fourth metacarpal and/or metatarsal,Madelung deformity,enlargement of medial tibial plateau,cubitus valgus in 70% cases

300.a---Whitish hyperdense foci with areas of grey sinus opacification on CT scan of PNS is radiological hallmark of(SW)fungal sinusitis

301.a---facial bone fracture most commonly involves(SW)mandible

302.c---Pilon fractures refers to (SW)fracture of distal end of shaft of both tibia and fibula

303.a--Fracture of the proximal ulna with radial head dislocation is known as(SW) Monteggia fracture dislocation

304.b--- Fracture of the shaft of radius radial ulnar dislocation is known as(SW)Galeazzi fracture /Piedmont fracture

305.a---Clay Shoveler's injury refers to(SW) avulsion fracture of the spinous process of C6 to T2

306.a---The most common benign bone tumour in children(GRAINGER)non-ossifying fibroma

307.a---A plain radiograph of osteosarcoma shows predilection for metaphyses of long bones,destuctive lesions with moth-eaten appearance,spiculated periosteal reaction(sunburst appearance),a cuff of periosteal new bone formation at the margin of soft tissue mass(Codman's triangle)

308.d—Radiological feature of chondrosarcoma are predilection for flat bones,lobular appearance ,mottled ,annular,punctuate calcification

309.a---Radiologically,Ewing's sarcoma is characterized involvement of the diaphyseal region of long bones,onion peel periosteal reaction,.soft tissue mass,affinity for flat bones

310.c—Featruers of metasatic tumour of bone are metastatic tumour more common than primary,prostate,breast and lung account for 80% of bone metastases,most frequently involved bone is spine,purely osteolytic lesions are best detected on radionuclide bone scan

312.b---Punched out lesions in skull radiography is characteristically seen in multiple myeloma

313.b---Among the most common causes of bone infections is staphylococcus

314.a--- Xray may be normal for up to 14 days after onset of symptoms in osteomyelitis

315.b---The most common cause of septic arthritis in native joint is staphylococcus

316.b---The most common site of skeletal TB spine

317.a--The most common site of Spinal TB in children upper thoracic spine

318.c---The most common site of Spinal TB in adult is lower thoracic and upper lumbar spine

319.b---The spinal tuberculosis is charcterised by invlvement of two or more adjacent vertabra, involvement of the intervertebral disk,kyphosis/gibbus formation due to collapse of vertebra,psoas abscess

320.a---Pott's disease refers to spinal TB

321.a---Bilateral knee effusion in congenital syphilis is known as Cluttion's joint

322.a---Classic stigmata of congenital syphilis are Hutchinson'teeth(centrally notched,widely spaced,peg-shaped upper central incisors),mullberry's molar(sixth year molars with multiple poorly-developed cusps),saddle nose ,saber shins

323.a---cigar –shaped soft tissue calcification is noted in cysticercosis

324.d---The most pathognomonic radiological finding of hydatid cyst daughter cyst within larger cyst

325.a---Snowflake sign in usg is seen in echinococcus

326.a---Fanconi anemia are characetrised by all except(N) short strature,microcephaly,thumb attached by thread,micrognathia

327.d---Causes of osteoporosis are hypogonadism,hyperthyroidism,hyperparathyroidism

328.a---The pulsating tumour of bone is osteosarcoma

329.c---Flaring of anterior end of ribs is characteristically seen in ricket

330.b---The best view for fracture of C1 and C2 is odontoid view

331.b---cyst associated with vertebral defect is neuroenteric cyst

332.d---Milkman's fracture is a type of pseudofracture

333.b---Blount 's disease refers to genu varum

334.a—Hoffa fat pad is relatd to knee joint ,Krager fat pad is related to ankle joint

REFERENCE BOOKS

1. Harrison's principles of internal medicine, 18th edition,
2. Swartz's principle of surgery, 9th edition,
3. Nelson's textbook of paediatrics, 19th edition,
4. D.C.Dutta 's Textbook of Obstetrics, 7th edition
5. Diseases of Ear, Nose and Throat(PL Dinghra)
6. Grainger and Allison's Diagnostic Radiology, 5th edition,
7. Textbook of Radiology and imaging, 8th edition
8. Christensen's Physics of diagnostic radiology, 3rd edition
9. Farr's Physics for medical imaging, 2nd edition
10. Diagnostic Ultrasound(Rumack, Wilson), 4rd edition
11. Aids to Radiological Differential Diagnosis (Chapman and Nakielny), 5th edition

www.ingramcontent.com/pod-product-compliance
Lightning Source LLC
Chambersburg PA
CBHW051439170526
45166CB00001B/39